Self-Assessment Questions for the MRCP Part 2

Volume 1

Self-Assessment Questions for the MRCP Part 2

Volume 1

Dr Bilal Iqbal

Consultant Interventional Cardiologist, Royal Jubilee Hospital, Victoria, British Columbia, Canada
Professor of Medicine, University of Victoria Faculty of Medicine, University of British Columbia, Canada
Honorary Consultant Interventional Cardiologist, Royal Brompton and Harefield Hospitals, Middlesex, UK

Dr Amin Oomatia

Specialist Registrar in Nephrology, Royal Free Hospital, London, UK

Dr John Waters

Consultant in Acute Medicine and Nephrology, Addenbrooke's Hospital, Cambridge, UK

Dr Gautam Mehta

Associate Professor of Hepatology, University College London, London, UK

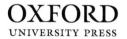

OXFORD
UNIVERSITY PRESS

Great Clarendon Street, Oxford, OX2 6DP,
United Kingdom

Oxford University Press is a department of the University of Oxford.
It furthers the University's objective of excellence in research, scholarship,
and education by publishing worldwide. Oxford is a registered trade mark of
Oxford University Press in the UK and in certain other countries

Published in the United States of America by Oxford University Press
198 Madison Avenue, New York, NY 10016, United States of America

British Library Cataloguing in Publication Data
Data available

Library of Congress Control Number: 2020946615

Set ISBN 978–0–19–879178–2
Volume 1 978–0–19–879179–9
Volume 2 978–0–19–879180–5

Printed and bound by
CPI Group (UK) Ltd, Croydon, CR0 4YY

DEDICATION AND ACKNOWLEDGEMENTS

I would like to thank my co-authors Gautam, John, and Amin for all their hard work, time, and patience without which this work would have never been completed. I am also grateful to all the contributors and reviewers for their knowledge, expertise, and valuable input. I cannot thank Fiona, from Oxford University Press, enough for her patience from outset with the idea and conception of the books to the completion of what once felt like a never-ending project.

These books have come together with years of hard work involving busy schedules, jobs, and not to mention the move and relocation from UK to Canada. I cannot be grateful enough to my wife, Nabila, and children, Adam, Anna, and Amelia, for their everlasting love, support, resilience, and patience at home, without which I would never had been able to complete this work.

Finally, I would like to dedicate these books to my wife and children, Nabila, Adam, Anna, and Amelia.

Bilal Iqbal

I would like to thank Gautam for involving me in this project, which has been a real privilege. Not only have I learnt a great deal of medicine from writing, editing, and re-drafting the countless versions of the manuscript, but it has reminded me how fascinating medicine actually is. We are truly lucky to be physicians in a day and age when not only do we know more than we ever have before about diseases, but we are also able to provide cutting edge treatment to our patients. I hope that after reading this book, our readers feel the same. A big thank you to Fiona Sutherland from Oxford University Press for being patient with us authors (especially when it came to missed deadlines) and being meticulous and thorough during the synthesis of this book.

Lastly, I'd like to dedicate my contribution in this book to my parents. To my mother, Masuma: thank you for always being patient and supportive, especially when I've been stressed and irritable. To my dad, Asgarali: without your hard work—which included studying for medical school under streetlights in 1960s' India—I would not have been granted so many amazing opportunities in my life and I certainly wouldn't have been inspired to go to medical school. Thank you both.

Amin Oomatia

I dedicate these books to my wife for her patience, my mother for her love, and to my late father for his lifelong dedication to his family.

John Waters

This book is dedicated to my parents, for their love and unfailing support in everything I do.

Gautam Mehta

CONTENTS

ABBREVIATIONS

AAIR	Asthma, Allergy, and Inflammation Research
ACC	American College of Cardiology
ACE	angiotensin converting enzyme
ADIP	acute inflammatory demyelinating polyradiculopathy
AEA	anti-endomysial antibodies
AHA	acquired haemophilia A/acquired factor VIII inhibition
AHA	American Heart Association
AHO	Albright's hereditary osteodystrophy
AIHA	autoimmune haemolytic anaemia
AIP	autoimmune pancreatitis
ALP	alkaline phosphatase
AML	acute myeloid leukaemia
ANA	anti-nuclear antibodies
ANA	anti-neutrophil antibody
ANCA	anti-neutrophil cytoplasmic antibody
Anti-HBc	hepatitis B core antigen
APCC	activated prothrombin complex concentrate
APP	activated protein C
ARDS	acute respiratory distress syndrome
ART	antiretroviral therapy
ASD	atrial septal defect
AVNRT	atrioventricular nodal re-entrant tachycardia
AVRT	atrioventricular re-entrant tachycardia
BCNE	blood culture-negative endocarditis
BMD	bone mineral density
BP	blood pressure
BPEG	British Pacing and Electrophysiology Group
CA	corticotroph adenomas
CAH	congenital adrenal hyperplasia
CAP	cellulose acetate precipitin
CASPAR	ClASsification of Psoriatic ARthritis

CDI	*Clostridium difficile* infection
CH	coeliac disease
CLL	chronic lymphocytic leukaemia
CMV	cytomegalovirus
CRH	corticotrophin releasing hormone
CRT	cardiac resynchronization therapy
CRT-D	cardiac resynchronization therapy combined with defibrillator therapy
CS	Cushing's syndrome
CSD	cat-scratch disease
DAT	direct antiglobulin test
DDDR	dual-chamber, rate-modulated pacing
DDP4	dipeptidylpeptidase-4
DEXA	dual energy X-ray absorptiometry
DH	dermatitis herpetiformis
DI	diabetes insipidus
DVT	deep vein thrombosis
ENaC	epithelial sodium channel
EVL	endoscopic variceal ligation
FDA	Food and Drug Administration
FEIBA	factor VIII inhibitor bypassing activity
FMTC	familial medullary thyroid carcinoma
FNAC	fine needle aspiration cytology
FNC	fine needle aspiration
FNHTR	febrile non-haemolytic transfusion reaction
GBS	Guillain-Barré syndrome
G-CSF	granulocyte-colony stimulating factor
GD	Graves' disease
GDH	glutamate dehydrogenase
GH	growth hormone
GO	Graves' ophthalmopathy
G6PD	glucose-6-phosphate dehydrogenase
GPI	glycosyl phosphatidylinositol anchor
HAART	highly active antiretroviral therapy
HBeAg	hepatitis B envelope antigen
HBIG	hepatitis B immunoglobulin
HBV	hepatitis B virus
hCG	human chorionic gonadotrophin
HRT	hormone replacement therapy
HSP	Henoch-Schönlein purpura

HSV	herpes simplex virus
HTLV-1	human T-lymphotropic virus type 1
ICD	implantable cardioverter defibrillator
IE	infective endocarditis
IFAT	immunofluorescent antibody test
IGRA	interferon-gamma release assay
IMWG	International Myeloma Working Group
IPSS	inferior petrosal sinus sampling
IPSS	International Prognostic Scoring System
IRIS	immune reconstitution inflammatory syndrome
ITP	idiopathic thrombocytopaenia purpura
JAK2	Janus kinase 2
LCHAD	long-chain 3-hydroxyacyl-CoA dehydrogenase
LEMS	Lambert Eaton syndrome
LH	luteinizing hormone
LLLB	left bundle branch block
LMWH	low-molecular-weight heparin
LP	lichen planus
MAT	microscopic agglutination test
MDR	multi-drug resistant
MDS	myelodysplastic syndrome
MEN2	multiple endocrine neoplasia type 2
MG	myasthenia gravis
MGUS	monoclonal gammopathy of uncertain significance
MNG	multinodular goitre
NASH	non-alcoholic steatohepatitis
NASPE	North American Society of Pacing and Electrophysiology
NCCT	Na-Cl co-transporter
NF1	neurofibromatosis type 1
NICE	National Institute for Health and Clinical Excellence
NOAC	new oral anticoagulant
NSBB	non-selective beta-blockers
NSTEMI	non-ST segment elevation MI
OGD	oesophago-gastroduodenoscopy
PAIR	percutaneous aspiration, injection, and re-aspiration
PAS	periodic acid Schiff
PCNSL	primary central nervous system lymphoma
PCR	polymerase chain reaction
PDA	persistent ductus arteriosus

PE	pulmonary embolus
PEP	post-exposure prophylaxis
PET	positron emission tomography
PHP	pseudohypoparathyroidism
Pi	protease inhibitor
PID	pelvic inflammatory disease
PIG-A	phosphatidylinositol glycan A
PLA	pyogenic liver abscesses
PML	progressive multifocal leukoencephalopathy
PNL	paroxysmal nocturnal haemoglobinuria
PPCI	primary percutaneous coronary intervention
PSC	primary sclerosing cholangitis
RBBB	right bundle branch block
rFVIIa	recombinant factor VIIa
rpoB	RNA polymerase B subunit
SeHCAT	selenium homocholic acid taurine
SHBG	sex hormone binding globulin
SJS	Stevens-Johnson syndrome
SLE	systemic lupus erythematosus
SPECT	single-photon emission CT
STEMI	ST segment elevation MI
SVT	supraventricular tachycardia
TB	*Mycobacterium tuberculosis*
TBM	TB meningitis
TEN	toxic epidermal necrolysis
TIPSS	trans-jugular intrahepatic porto-systemic shunt
TOE	transoesophageal echocardiography
TRALI	transfusion-related acute lung injury
TSH	thyroid function tests
TTE	transthoracic echocardiography
TTGA	tissue transglutaminase
USA	unstable angina
VDDR type I	vitamin D dependent rickets type 1
V-HeFT	Vasodilator-Heart Failure Trial
VHL	Von Hippel-Lindau disease
VSD	ventricular septal defect
VTE	venous thromboembolism
VZIG	varicella immunoglobulin
VZV	varicella zoster virus

CONTRIBUTORS

Dr Michelle E Allan
Specialist Registrar in Renal and General Internal Medicine
Royal London Hospital, Barts NHS Trust, London, UK

Dr Nicola Ambrose
Consultant Medical Oncologist and Consultant in Oncogenetics
The Royal Marsden Hospital, London, UK

Dr Abhishek Das
Senior Registrar in Microbiology
University College London Hospital, London, UK

Dr Angela George
Consultant Medical Oncologist and Consultant in Oncogenetics
The Royal Marsden Hospital, London, UK

Dr Theodore Gouliouris
Consultant in Microbiology and Infectious Diseases
Cambridge University Hospitals NHS Foundation Trust, Cambridge, UK

Dr Maria Ibrahim
Renal Registrar
Guy's and St Thomas' NHS Trust, London, UK

Dr Bilal Iqbal
Consultant Interventional Cardiologist
Royal Jubilee Hospital, Victoria, British Columbia, Canada
Professor of Medicine
University of Victoria Faculty of Medicine, University of British Columbia, Canada
Honorary Consultant Interventional Cardiologist
Royal Brompton and Harefield Hospitals, Middlesex, UK

Dr Emon Khan
Consultant Rheumatologist
University College London Hospital, London, UK

Dr Daniel Marks
Consultant Physician
University College London Hospital, London, UK

Dr Gautam Mehta
Associate Professor of Hepatology
University College London, London, UK

Professor Philip I Murray
Professor of Ophthalmology
University of Birmingham, Birmingham, UK

Dr Akshay Nair
Speciality Trainee in General and Older Adult Psychiatry
South London and Maudsley NHS Trust, London, UK

Dr Amin Oomatia
Specialist Registrar in Nephrology
Royal Free Hospital, London, UK

Dr Thomas Stoker
Specialty Registrar in Neurology
Addenbrooke's Hospital, Cambridge, UK

Dr John Waters
Consultant in Acute Medicine and Nephrology
Addenbrooke's Hospital, Cambridge, UK

Dr Mike Zandi

Consultant Neurologist, National Hospital for Neurology and Neurosurgery, and Honorary
Associate Professor, UCL Queen Square Institute of Neurology, London, UK

NORMAL VALUES

Category	Test	Unit	Range (All/Male)	Range Female
Haematology	Hb	g/L	130–180	115–160
	MCV	fL	80–98	
	WCC	× 10^9/L	4.0–11.0	
	Plt	× 10^9/L	150–400	
	Neut	× 10^9/L	1.5–7.0	
	Lymph	× 10^9/L	1.5–4.0	
	HCT	%	38.8–50	34.9–44.5
	MCV	fl/Red cell	79–98	
	MCH	pg/cell	27–33	
Urea and electrolytes	Sodium	mmol/L	135–145	
	Potassium	mmol/L	3.5–5.5	
	Creatinine	µmol/L	60–120	
	Urea	mmol/L	2.5–7.0	
	eGFR (MDRD)	mL/min/1.73m^2	>60	
	Bicarbonate	mmol/L	20–28	
	Chloride	mmol/L	95–107	
	Magnesium	mmol/L	0.6–1.0	
Bone	Corrected Ca2+	mmol/L	2.2–2.6	
	Phosphate	mmol/L	0.8–1.4	
	PTH	pmmol/L	0.9–5.4	
Liver	ALT	iU/L	1–31	
	AST	iU/L	1–31	
	GGT	iU/L	<50	
	ALP	iU/L	45–105	
	Bilirubin	µmol/L	1–22	
	Albumin	g/L	37–49	
	Amylase	iU/L	60–180	

Category	Test	Unit	Range (All/Male)	Range Female
Clotting	PT	s	11.5–15.5	
	APTT	s	30–40	
	INR		0.9–1.1	
	Fibrinogen	g/L	1.8–5.4	
Special haem	Reticulocyte	%	<2	
	HbA2	%	<2.5	
	HbF	%	0.3–4.4	
Misc	CRP	mg/L	<10	
	ESR	mm/1st Hr	<15	<20
	CK	iU/L	24–195	
	LDH	iU/L	10–250	
	Troponin T	ng/L	<14	
	Urate	μmol/L	200–420	
Endo	TSH	mU/L	0.4–5.0	
	T4 Serum free	pmol/L	10.0–22.0	
	T3 Serum free	pmol/L	3.0–70	
	HbA1c	mmol/mol	20–42	
	ACTH (9 am)	pmol/L	<18.0	
	Cortisol	nmol/L	138–635	
Lipids	Fasting glucose	mmol/L	4.0–7.0	
	Normal glucose	mmol/L	4.0–11.0	
	LDL	mmol/L	<3.36	
	HDL	mmol/L	>1.55	
	Total cholesterol	mmol/L	<5.2	
	Triglycerides	mmol/L	0.45–1.69	
CSF	Opening pressure	mmH20	12–250	
	Total protein	g/L	0.15–0.45	
	Glucose	mmol/L	2.5–4.4 (60–70% of serum glucose)	
Haematinics	Serum iron	μmol/L	12–30	
	TIBC (serum total iron binding capacity)	μmol/L	45–75	
	Transferrin saturation	%	15–50	
	Ferritin	μg/L	15–300	
	Transferrin	g/L	2.0–4.0	

Category	Test	Unit	Range (All/Male)	Range Female	
	Serum B12	ng/L	16–760		
	Serum folate	µg/L	2.0–11.0		
	Serum haptoglobin	g/L	0.13–1.63		
Autoimmune serology	Rheumatoid factor	iU/mL	<14		
ABG	pO2	kPa	11.3–12.6		
	pCO2	kPa	4.7–6.0		
	pH		7.35–7.45		
	HCO3−	mmol/L	21–29		
	H+	nmmol/L	35–45		
	BE	mmol/L	+/−2		
Antibodies	Total IgA	g/L	0.8–3		
	Total IgG	g/L	6.0–13.0		
	Total IgM	g/L	0.4–2.5		
Anti-cardio lipin	IgG	iU/L	<10		
	IgM	iU/L	<10		
	C3	g/L	0.8–1.6		
	C4	g/L	0.16–0.48		
Anti-TTG	<7 U/mL	Negative	>10 U/mL	Positive	In between Equivocal
Testosterone	Male	11–36	nmol/L		
	Female	0.8–3.1	nmol/L		
LH	Male	1.8–12	iU/L		
	Pregnant female	<1.5	iU/L		
	Post-menopausal	15–62	iU/L		
	Menstruating female, varies	Varies	iU/L		
FSH	Male	1.5–12.4	iU/L		
	Pregnant female		iU/L		
	Post-menopausal	25–135	iU/L		
	Menstruating female, varies	Varies	iU/L		
Oestradiol	Male	20–100	pmol/L		
Prolactin	Male	<450	miU/L		
	Non-pregnant women	100–550	miU/L		
	Pregnant women	1700–8500	miU/L		

CARDIOLOGY

QUESTIONS

1. **A 43-year-old man presented to the A&E department with a two-hour history of central crushing chest pain, nausea, and shortness of breath. He was a heavy smoker. On examination, the pulse rate was 104 beats per minute and regular, respiratory rate was 22 breaths per minute, and blood pressure (BP) was 95/50 mmHg. There was no radio-radial delay. Auscultation of the heart sounds revealed no murmurs. There were no other added heart sounds. The venous pressure was not elevated. The chest was clear to auscultation.**

```
Investigations:
  ECG: sinus rhythm, ST elevation V1-V4, ST depression in III
    and aVF
  CXR: borderline cardiomegaly, clear lung fields
```

He was treated with high-flow oxygen, morphine 10 mg IV, metoclopramide 10 mg IV, aspirin 300 mg PO, clopidogrel 300 mg PO, and metoprolol 50 mg PO.

What is the next most effective management step?

A. Anticoagulate with low molecular weight heparin and transfer to CCU.

B. Glycoprotein IIB/IIIA inhibitor.

C. Intravenous diuretics.

D. Primary percutaneous coronary intervention.

E. Thrombolysis.

2. **A 48-year-old man presented with a two-week history of persistent palpitations. There was no history of chest pain or breathlessness. He denied any systemic symptoms such as fever, weight loss, or diarrhoea. He had no significant past medical or family history. He consumed minimal alcohol but admitted occasional binges, including a binge about four weeks previously at a wedding reception. He did not smoke and worked as fitness instructor. On examination his pulse rate was 130 beats per minute, irregular, his respiratory rate was 18 breaths per minute, and his BP was 130/80 mmHg. Auscultation revealed a clear chest and normal heart sounds. There was no peripheral oedema.**

    ```
    Investigations:
      Hb                        140 g/L
      WCC                       8 × 10⁹/L
      Platelets                 180 × 10⁹/L
      Sodium                    136 mmol/L
      Potassium                 4.1 mmol/L
      Urea                      5 mmol/L
      Creatinine                118 μmol/L
      Magnesium                 1.1 mmol/L
      ECG: atrial fibrillation, ventricular rate 128/min
      CXR: normal heart size, clear lung fields
    ```

    ### What is the next best management step?

    A. An urgent echocardiogram
    B. Intravenous amiodarone
    C. Intravenous digoxin
    D. Oral beta blocker
    E. Synchronized DC cardioversion

3. **A 35-year-old Pakistani lady who migrated to the UK with her family four years previously, presented with worsening breathlessness and lower limb oedema. Her symptoms had begun two years previously and she had recently been prescribed diuretics for her lower limb oedema.**

On examination she was cyanosed, with no evidence of finger clubbing. The oxygen saturations were 81% on room air. The pulse rate was 100 beats per minute and BP was 90/60 mmHg. The jugular venous pressure was elevated. Auscultation of the heart sounds revealed a soft systolic murmur at the left lower sternal edge with a loud second heart sound. The chest was clear to auscultation. There was marked peripheral oedema to the thighs. She was admitted into hospital for further investigation. The following cardiac catheterization data was available (Table 1.1).

Table 1.1 Cardiac catheterization data

Chamber	Pressure (mmHg)	Oxygen saturation (%)
RA (high)	15	65
RA (low)	15	64
RV	108/42	64
PA	105/51	67
LV	95/40	95
Ascending Ao	95/60	95
Descending Ao	95/60	80

What is the most likely cause of this presentation?

A. Eisenmenger's syndrome
B. Patent foramen ovale
C. Persistent ductus arteriosus (PDA)
D. Pulmonary hypertension
E. Ventricular septal defect

4. **A 32-year-old Afro-Caribbean male was referred to the outpatient clinic. He had initially presented to the A&E department after sustaining an ankle injury during a game of football. Subsequent X-rays had not shown any evidence of fracture. Incidentally, his pulse rate was noted to be 40 beats per minute. His BP was 117/75 mmHg. A twelve-lead ECG showed complete heart block with a broad complex escape rhythm (ventricular rate of 40). On retrospective questioning, there was no history of dizziness, syncope, or unexplained collapse. He had been fit and well, with no previous medical complaints.**

    What is the management?

    A. Asthma, Allergy, and Inflammation Research (AAIR) permanent pacemaker insertion
    B. Arrange a 24-hour Holter monitor to look for evidence of significant pauses
    C. Dual-chamber, rate-modulated pacing (DDDR) permanent pacemaker insertion
    D. Reassure and discharge as currently asymptomatic
    E. Temporary pacing wire insertion

5. **A 45-year-old man was brought to the emergency department by the paramedic crew complaining of progressive shortness of breath and severe central chest pain. The pain varied with intensity and was initially alleviated by sitting forward and taking ibuprofen, but had worsened significantly over the preceding week. He reported generalized aches and pains and had felt increasingly nauseated and lethargic over the preceding few days, not eating and drinking much and passing little urine. He also reported becoming very short of breath on lying flat. There was no history of exertional chest pain. Aside from being prescribed a recent course of amoxicillin by his GP for a sore throat he was generally fit and well, and was taking no regular medications. He was a smoker and his father had died of ischaemic heart disease aged 48.**

    On examination he appeared pale, sweaty, and breathless, the respiratory rate was 28 beats per minute, pulse was 110 beats per minute, and BP was 220/115 mmHg. His JVP was raised at 7 cm. Auscultation of the heart revealed a quiet rub and of the lungs revealed bibasal crepitations. He also had bilateral ankle oedema. He had been treated by paramedics with high-flow oxygen, aspirin 300 mg PO, clopidogrel 300 mg PO, morphine 10 mg IV, and metoclopramide 10 mg IV.

    His ECG is shown in Figure 1.1.

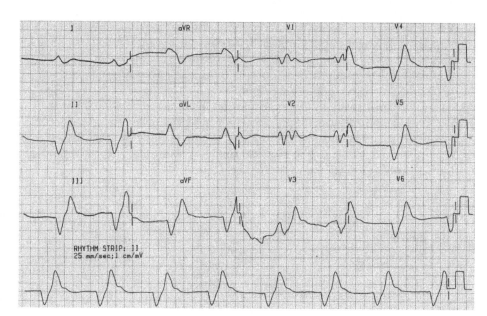

Figure 1.1 Patient's ECG.

Reproduced with permission from *Oxford Textbook of Medicine*, Fifth Edition. Edited by David A Warrell, Timothy M Cox, and John D Firth, Fig. 21.5.3, p. 3891. Oxford University Press, Oxford, UK, Copyright © 2010.

What is your immediate management?

A. Immediate thrombolysis

B. Request an urgent CT aorta

C. Request an urgent CXR

D. Request an urgent echocardiogram

E. Request urgent urea and electrolytes

6. **A 66-year-old man presented to hospital with a three-day history of exertional chest pain culminating in pain on minimal exertion. His past medical history included hypertension treated with bendroflumethiazide, asthma, for which he used a salbutamol inhaler PRN, and gastro-oesophageal reflux, for which he used gaviscon PRN. He was a heavy smoker. On examination his pulse rate was 90 beats per minute and BP was 135/80 mmHg. Physical examination was unremarkable. He was initially treated with high-flow oxygen, aspirin 300 mg PO, clopidogrel 300 mg PO, and low molecular weight heparin, and was subsequently pain free.**

```
Investigations:
  Hb                        140 g/L
  WCC                       8 × 10⁹/L
  Platelets                 180 × 10⁹/L
  Sodium                    136 mmol/L
  Potassium                 4.1 mmol/L
  Urea                      5 mmol/L
  Creatinine                118 µmol/L
  Total cholesterol         3.2 mmol/L
  LDL                       1.6 mmol/L
  Troponin T                1256 ng/L        (<14 ng/L)
  ECG: T wave inversion in leads II, III, and aVF
  CXR: normal heart size and clear lung fields
```

(a) What would your immediate management be?

  A. ACE inhibitor
  B. Beta blocker
  C. Morphine
  D. Nitrates
  E. Statin

(b) What is the best further management plan?

  A. Early inpatient coronary angiography.
  B. Inpatient dobutamine stress echocardiogram.
  C. Inpatient myocardial perfusion scan.
  D. Modified BRUCE protocol exercise treadmill test at day 4. If normal, allow home at day 5. If abnormal, then inpatient coronary angiography.
  E. To allow home after five days, but for inpatient coronary angiography only if he develops further chest pain.

7. A 61-year-old woman presented to a district general hospital with an eight-hour history of severe central crushing chest pain and nausea. Her cardiovascular risk factors included hypertension, hypercholesterolaemia, and she was a smoker. ECG on arrival showed 9 mm ST elevation in the anterior leads. There was no primary PCI service available on site, with the closest primary PCI centre two hours away via ambulance transport. The duty A&E doctors treated her with aspirin 300 mg PO, clopidogrel 300 mg PO, morphine 10 mg IV, metoclopramide 10 mg IV, metoprolol 50 mg PO, and IV reteplase. After 90 minutes, she still complained of chest pain. On examination, the pulse rate was 84 beats per minute and BP was 115/80 mmHg. Auscultation of the heart sounds revealed no murmurs. There were no other added heart sounds. The venous pressure was not elevated. The chest was clear. ECG showed minimal resolution of ST segment elevation with 7 mm ST elevation in the anterior leads. There were no Q waves.

Which treatment should this patient receive?

A. Further dose of beta blocker

B. GP IIB/IIIA inhibitor

C. Immediate transfer for rescue PCI

D. Intravenous nitrate infusion

E. Repeat thrombolysis

8. **A 43-year-old man was seen in the cardiology outpatient clinic for breathlessness on exertion. He had been very active up until six months previously, when he suffered a severe flu-like illness following which his symptoms began. Although he could manage 2–3 miles walking on the flat, he became breathless on climbing stairs quickly. There was no history of orthopnoea or paroxysmal nocturnal dyspnoea. On examination the pulse rate was 88 beats per minute and BP was 106/70 mmHg. The venous pressure was not elevated. Auscultation of the heart sounds was unremarkable with no added heart sounds. The chest was clear to auscultate. There was no pedal oedema.**

```
Investigations:
  Hb                        140 g/L
  WCC                       8 × 10⁹/L
  Platelets                 180 × 10⁹/L
  Sodium                    136 mmol/L
  Potassium                 4.1 mmol/L
  Urea                      4 mmol/L
  Creatinine                118 µmol/L
  ECG: sinus rhythm with left bundle branch block (LBBB)
  CXR: cardiomegaly with clear lung fields
  Echocardiogram: dilated LV cavity with severe global
    hypokinesis and severe impairment of LV systolic function
    (EF = 35%). Mild functional mitral regurgitation.
```

How would you treat this patient?

A. ACE inhibitor

B. ACE inhibitor and beta blocker

C. ACE inhibitor and diuretics

D. ACE inhibitor, beta blocker, and diuretics

E. ACE-inhibitor, beta blocker, and spironolactone

9. **A 56-year-old man was reviewed in the cardiology outpatient clinic for breathlessness on minimal exertion. He had a previous history of ischaemic heart disease, having suffered an anterior myocardial infarction followed by coronary artery bypass graft surgery seven years previously. He had been doing well up until the previous year, when he noticed progressive breathlessness on exertion. His exercise tolerance had reduced from being unrestricted to, after 50 yards on the flat, having to stop primarily due to breathlessness. There was no history of chest pain. He had been regularly followed up in the heart failure clinic and his medications had been regularly optimized. His medications included aspirin 75 mg od, simvastatin 40 mg od, ramipril 10 mg od, spironolactone 25 mg od, carvedilol 3.125 mg bd, digoxin 62.5 μg od, and furosemide 80 mg od.**

On examination his heart rate was 65 beats per minute and BP was 95/50 mmHg. Auscultation of the heart and chest was unremarkable. The venous pressure was not elevated. There was no peripheral oedema.

```
Investigations:
  Sodium                  132 mmol/L
  Potassium               4.3 mmol/L
  Urea                    8.5 mmol/L      (previously 7.3 mmol/L)
  Creatinine              158 μmol/L      (previously 145 μmol/L)
  ECG: sinus rhythm; anterior Q waves; first-degree heart block
  CXR: cardiomegaly with clear lung fields
  Echocardiogram: severe impairment of LV systolic function
    (EF = 25%); dilated LV cavity with global hypokinesis and
    extensive anteroseptal akinesis; mild functional mitral
    regurgitation
  Coronary angiography: patent grafts with no targets for
    revascularization
```

What alteration in pharmacotherapy would be appropriate?

A. Add candesartan 2 mg od
B. Increase furosemide to 80 mg bd
C. Reduce ramipril to 7.5 mg od
D. Stop carvedilol
E. Stop ramipril

10. **A 56-year-old man presented with breathlessness on minimal exertion. He had a significant past medical history of ischaemic heart disease. Six years previously, he suffered an inferior myocardial infarction subsequently requiring coronary artery bypass graft surgery. Two years previously, he suffered an anterior myocardial infarction with subsequent angioplasty to the distal left anterior descending artery. His progressive breathlessness had begun six months previously and his exercise tolerance was now reduced to 30 yards on the flat. There was no history of chest pain. He had been regularly followed up in the heart failure clinic and his medications had been appropriately optimized. His medication included aspirin 75 mg od, simvastatin 40 mg od, candesartan 8 mg od, spironolactone 50 mg od, bisoprolol 7.5 mg od, and bumetanide 2 mg bd.**

On examination his heart rate was 65 beats per minute and BP was 90/60 mmHg. Auscultation of the heart sounds revealed a soft pansystolic murmur at the apex. The venous pressure was not elevated. The chest was clear to auscultation. There was no peripheral oedema.

```
Investigations:
  ECG: sinus rhythm; first-degree heart block; left LBBB
  CXR: cardiomegaly with clear lung fields
  Echocardiogram: severe impairment of LV systolic function
    (EF = 20%); dilated LV cavity with anteroseptal and
    inferior akinesis; moderate functional mitral regurgitation
  Coronary angiography: patent grafts with no targets for
    revascularization
```

What therapy would improve symptoms and prognosis?

A. Cardiac resynchronization therapy

B. Dual chamber permanent pacemaker

C. Implantable cardioverter defibrillator

D. Mitral valve annuloplasty

E. Mitral valve replacement

11. **A 34-year-old man presented to A&E with a four-day history of fevers, night sweats, and breathlessness. This had been preceded by a three-week history of malaise, lethargy, and poor appetite. He had lost 6 kg in weight. There were no other systemic symptoms. He had been previously fit and well, and four weeks previously had a dental tooth extraction. On examination his temperature was 37.3°C, pulse rate was 105 beats per minute, BP was 115/50 mmHg, and oxygen saturations were 98% on air. There were no peripheral stigmata of endocarditis. The venous pressure was not elevated. Auscultation of the heart sounds revealed a loud pansystolic murmur at the apex. There were no added sounds. The chest was clear to auscultation. Abdominal examination was unremarkable.**

```
Investigations:
  Hb                      160 g/L
  WCC                     15 × 10⁹/L
  Platelets               490 × 10⁹/L
  Sodium                  136 mmol/L
  Potassium               4.1 mmol/L
  Urea                    11 mmol/L
  Creatinine              188 µmol/L
  CRP                     101 mg/L
  AST                     25 iU/L
  ALT                     35 iU/L
  ALP                     52 iU/L
  Bilirubin               10 µmol/L
  Albumin                 29 g/L
  CXR: normal heart size; clear lung fields
  ECG: sinus rhythm (rate 107); RBBB; normal PR interval
```

What is the next most important initial investigation?

A. Blood cultures

B. Renal ultrasound

C. Transoesophageal echocardiogram

D. Transthoracic echocardiogram

E. Urinalysis

12. **A 64-year-old man presented with a three-hour history of central crushing chest pain. An ECG confirmed an inferior ST segment elevation MI. He was treated with aspirin, clopidogrel, reteplase, and unfractionated heparin. After one hour, he was pain-free with good resolution of ST segments. On examination the heart rate was 35 beats per minute and BP was 135/70 mmHg. Auscultation of the heart sounds was unremarkable and the chest was clear to auscultation. The following ECG was obtained (Figure 1.2).**

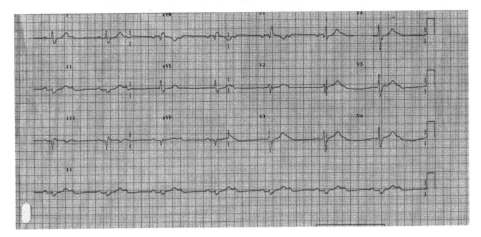

Figure 1.2 Twelve-lead ECG.

Reproduced with permission from *Oxford Textbook of Critical Care*, Second Edition. Edited by A Webb et al., Fig. 157.6. Oxford University Press, Oxford, UK, Copyright © 2016.

(a) **What does the rhythm strip demonstrate?**

   A. Atrial flutter
   B. Complete heart block
   C. First-degree heart block
   D. Second-degree heart block (Wenckebach)
   E. Second-degree heart block (Mobitz II)

(b) **What would your immediate management be?**

   A. Continue observation for deterioration
   B. External pacing
   C. Intravenous atropine
   D. Temporary pacing wire
   E. Urgent permanent pacemaker insertion

13. **A 43-year-old man was found to have an abnormal ECG during a routine medical check-up. His pulse was 50 beats per minute and irregular. His BP was 105/70 mmHg. Physical examination was unremarkable. The following rhythm strip was obtained (Figure 1.3).**

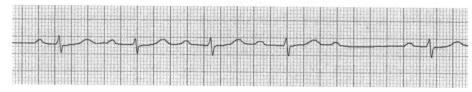

Figure 1.3 ECG rhythm strip.

Reproduced with permission from *Oxford Textbook of Critical Care*, Second Edition. Edited by A Webb et al., Fig. 157.5. Oxford University Press, Oxford, UK, Copyright © 2016.

(a) What does the rhythm strip demonstrate?

A. Complete heart block

B. First-degree heart block

C. Sino-atrial disease

D. Second-degree heart block (Mobitz I/Wenckebach)

E. Second-degree heart block (Mobitz II)

(b) What is the immediate management?

A. External pacing

B. Intravenous atropine

C. Permanent pacemaker insertion

D. Reassure and discharge

E. Temporary pacing wire

14. **A 73-year-old man presented with a four-day history of intermittent dizzy spells. He had experienced similar episodes over the preceding year but at the time of presentation they were more frequent. There was no history of chest pain. He complained of general lethargy and tiredness and over the preceding few months he had also experienced weight gain and cold intolerance. His past medical history included hypertension and hypercholesterolaemia. His medication included aspirin 75 mg od, ramipril 5 mg od, atenolol 25 mg od, and atorvastatin 20 mg od. On examination his pulse rate was 30 beats per minute and BP was 135/80 mmHg (lying) and 110/75 mmHg (standing). There was no neck swelling. Auscultation of the heart sounds revealed a soft pansystolic murmur at the apex. The venous pressure was not elevated. The chest was clear to auscultation. There was mild non-pitting lower limb oedema. His ECG rhythm showed complete heart block (not shown).**

(a) **What is the most likely cause of the intermittent dizzy spells?**

- A. Bradycardia
- B. Episodes of asystole
- C. Hypothyroidism
- D. Postural hypotension
- E. Ventricular tachycardia

(b) **What is the immediate management?**

- A. Intravenous atropine
- B. Intravenous glucagon
- C. Stop atenolol
- D. Temporary pacing wire
- E. Urgent thyroid function tests and thyroxine replacement

15. **A 63-year-old man presented with intermittent rapid palpitations and dizzy spells. He denied any chest pains. He had a previous history of hypertension and paroxysmal atrial flutter diagnosed five years previously which occurred only very occasionally in short paroxysms which he recognized well. His medications included warfarin, amiodarone 200 mg od, and candesartan 4 mg od. On examination his pulse rate was 80 beats per minute and BP was 150/95 mmHg. Physical examination was unremarkable.**

```
Investigations:
  Hb                    120 g/L
  WCC                   5 × 10⁹/L
  Platelets             210 × 10⁹/L
  Sodium                136 mmol/L
  Potassium             4.8 mmol/L
  Urea                  6 mmol/L
  Creatinine            96 µmol/L
  Magnesium             0.8 mmol/L
  Corrected calcium     2.2 mmol/L
  TSH                   <0.1 mU/L     (0.4-5.0 mU/L)
  Serum free T4         20 pmol/L     (10-22 pmol/L)
  ECG                   Figure 1.4
```

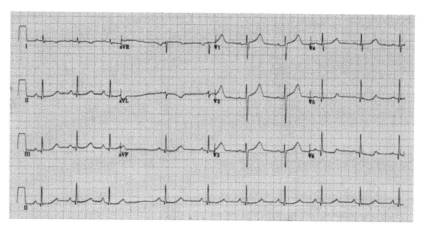

Figure 1.4 Twelve-lead ECG.

Reproduced with permission from *Training in Medicine*. Edited by E Jolly, A Fry, and A Chaudhry, Fig. 3.5, p. 67. Oxford University Press, Oxford, UK, Copyright © 2016.

What is the most likely cause of the presenting symptoms?

A. Atrial flutter

B. Bradycardia

C. Hypomagnesaemia

D. Polymorphic ventricular tachycardia

E. Thyrotoxicosis

16. **A 74-year-old lady presented with syncopal episode. She had a previous history of paroxysmal atrial fibrillation and hypertension. Her medications included sotalol 80 mg bd, bendroflumethiazide 2.5 mg od, and warfarin 3 mg od. On examination her pulse was 70 beats per minute and BP was 130/80 mmHg. Physical examination was unremarkable.**

```
Investigations:
  Hb                      140 g/L
  WCC                     7 × 10⁹/L
  Platelets               295 × 10⁹/L
  Sodium                  136 mmol/L
  Potassium               3.8 mmol/L
  Urea                    6 mmol/L
  Creatinine              96 µmol/L
  Magnesium               1.2 mmol/L
  Corrected calcium       2.4 mmol/L
  TSH                     2.5 mU/L        (0.4–5.0 mU/L)
  Serum free T4           17 pmol/L       (10–22 pmol/L)
  Her ECG rhythm strip is shown in Figure 1.5.
```

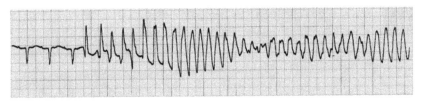

Figure 1.5 ECG rhythm strip.

Reproduced from *ESC CardioMed* (Third Edition) (online only product). Edited by Camm, Luscher, Maurer, and Serruys (2019) Fig. 48.11.10, www.oup.com. By permission of Oxford University Press and European Society of Cardiology.

What is the most effective immediate management step?

A. Intravenous amiodarone

B. Intravenous magnesium

C. Intravenous potassium

D. Stop sotalol

E. Synchronized DC shock

17. A 77-year-old man presented with a two-day history of dull central chest pain radiating up to the jaw and left arm which began initially on minimal exertion, but at time of presentation was also occurring at rest. Over the preceding two weeks he complained of a productive cough for which he completed a course of antibiotics. He had a past medical history of diabetes, hypertension, and hypercholesterolaemia. He had never smoked. His medications included aspirin 75 mg od, simvastatin 40 mg od, and ramipril 5 mg od. On examination, he was pain-free, his temperature was 37.5°C, oxygen saturations were 98% on room air, pulse rate was 80 beats per minute, and BP was 165/90 mmHg. Auscultation of the heart sounds revealed a soft fourth heart sound and no murmurs. The chest was clear to auscultation.

```
Investigations:
   Hb                        140 g/L
   WCC                       12 × 10⁹/L
   Platelets                 180 × 10⁹/L
   Sodium                    132 mmol/L
   Potassium                 4.1 mmol/L
   Urea                      5 mmol/L
   Creatinine                118 µmol/L
   CRP                       88
   Troponin T                <1 ng/L          (<14 ng/L)
   ECG: sinus rhythm; T wave inversion in II, III, aVF, V5,
      and V6
   CXR: normal heart size, clear lung fields
```

What is the most likely diagnosis?

A. Atypical pneumonia

B. Myopericarditis

C. Non-ST elevation myocardial infarction

D. Pulmonary embolism

E. Unstable angina

18. **A 25-year-old female was admitted with breathlessness on exertion, intermittent palpitations, and syncope. Table 1.2 shows the cardiac catheter data obtained.**

Table 1.2 Cardiac catheterization data

Chamber	Pressure (mmHg)	Oxygen saturation (%)
RA (high)	a = 15; v = 23	64
RA (mid)	a = 15; v = 23	66
RA (low)	a = 15; v = 23	84
RV	88/20	83
PA	92/40	84
PCWP	A = 15; v = 25	
LV	110/15	97
Ascending Ao	108/68	97
Descending Ao	109/69	96

What features are likely to be present on the twelve-lead ECG?
A. LBBB with left axis deviation
B. LBBB with prolonged PR interval
C. LBBB with right axis deviation
D. Right bundle branch block (RBBB) with left axis deviation
E. RBBB with right axis deviation

19. **Table 1.3 shows cardiac catheter data for a 42-year-old man complaining of breathlessness.**

Table 1.3 Cardiac catheterization data

Chamber	Pressure (mmHg)	Oxygen saturation (%)
RA (high)		64
RA (mid)		66
RA (low)		68
RV	30/9	83
PA	28/13	84
LV	128/8	97
Ascending Ao	125/68	97
Descending Ao	109/69	96

What would be the most likely auscultatory finding in this patient?
A. A continuous murmur at the upper right sternal edge
B. Ejection systolic murmur at the upper left sternal edge
C. Ejection systolic murmur at the upper right sternal edge
D. Loud pulmonary component to the second heart sound
E. Pansystolic murmur at the lower left sternal edge

20. **A 51-year-old man presented with a one-year history of exertional breathlessness and syncope. He had a previous history of atrial septal defect that was closed surgically as a child, as well as a long-standing history of asthma, hypertension, and hypercholesterolaemia. His current medication included aspirin 75 mg od, atenolol 25 mg od, ramipril 5 mg od, simvastatin 20 mg od, and salbutamol inhaler PRN.**

The following investigations including cardiac catheter data (Table 1.4) are available.

```
Left ventriculogram: preserved left ventricular systolic
    function
CXR: normal heart size; clear lung fields
```

Table 1.4 Cardiac catheterization data

Chamber	Pressure (mmHg)	Oxygen saturation (%)
RA		64
RV	50/18	67
PA	49/20	67
LV	168/14	97
Ascending Ao	100/68	97

What is the most appropriate management?

A. Add furosemide 40 mg od
B. Add ISMN 10 mg bd
C. Increase ramipril to 7.5 mg od
D. Stop beta blocker
E. Stop ramipril

21. **A 68-year-old man presented with progressive breathlessness over the preceding few weeks. He reported marked leg swelling and difficulty lying flat. There was no history of chest pain, cough, sputum, or haemoptysis but he reported some weight loss despite fluid retention. His past medical history included asthma, hypertension, diabetes, and lymphoma that was treated with chemotherapy four years previously. He took aspirin 75 mg od, atenolol 25 mg od, gliclazide 80 mg bd, becotide inhaler two puffs bd, and salbutamol inhaler PRN.**

On examination, he was pale and sweaty with cool peripheries. His temperature was 37.4°C, pulse was 110 beats per minute, respiratory rate was 30 per minute, and BP was 85/49 mmHg. Oxygen saturations were 96% on room air. The venous pressure was elevated. Auscultation of the heart revealed quiet heart sounds with no added sounds, and of the lung fields revealed reduced air entry at both bases. There was a smooth non-tender liver edge palpable 4 cm below the costal margin. There was sacral oedema with pitting leg oedema up to the mid-thighs.

```
Investigations:
  Hb                      100 g/L
  WCC                     11 × 10⁹/L
  Platelets               145 × 10⁹/L
  Sodium                  131 mmol/L
  Potassium               5.1 mmol/L
  Urea                    11 mmol/L
  Creatinine              196 µmol/L
  AST                     55 iU/L
  ALT                     75 iU/L
  ALP                     155 iU/L
  Bilirubin               23 µmol/L
  Albumin                 28 g/L
  CRP                     12 mg/L
  Urine dipstick:         blood + protein +
  ECG: sinus tachycardia; LBBB
  CXR: cardiomegaly; bilateral blunting of costophrenic angles
  ABG (air)               pH 7.30
  pO₂                     12 kPa
  pCO₂                    3.5 kPa
  HCO₃⁻                   14
  BE                      −6.1
```

What is the cause of this patient's breathlessness?

A. Acute pulmonary oedema

B. Liver failure

C. Nephrotic syndrome

D. Pericardial tamponade

E. Pulmonary embolism

22. **A 70-year-old lady complained of exertional breathlessness. She had undergone a percutaneous cardiac procedure 25 years previously, which significantly improved her breathlessness. Over the recent years, her breathlessness had once again returned and she had breathlessness on minimal exertion. On examination her pulse rate was 75 beats per minute and her BP was 125/80 mmHg. Table 1.5 shows the cardiac catheter data obtained.**

Table 1.5 Cardiac catheterization data

Chamber	Pressure (mmHg)	Oxygen saturation (%)
RA (high)	a = 10 v = 20	65
RA (mid)	a = 10 v = 20	83
RA (low)	a = 10 v = 20	82
RV	52/18	83
PA	50/21	83
PCWP	26	
LV	135/7	95
Ascending Ao	126/82	95

What procedure is this patient likely to have had in the past?

A. Aortic valve annuloplasty
B. Aortic valve replacement
C. Atrial septal defect closure
D. Mitral valve annuloplasty
E. Mitral valve replacement

23. **Table 1.6 shows cardiac catheter data for an 18-year-old female complaining of exertional breathlessness and dizziness.**

Table 1.6 Cardiac catheterization data

Chamber	Pressure (mmHg)	Oxygen saturation (%)
SVC		61
IVC		62
RA (high)	a = 3 v = 4	64
RA (mid)	a = 3 v = 4	84
RA (low)	a = 3 v = 4	84
RV	26/9	82
PA	21/11	81
PCWP	5	
LV	133/4	97
Ascending Ao	131/72	97

What two features would be present on the twelve-lead ECG?

A. LBBB with right axis deviation
B. LBBB block with right ventricular deviation
C. Normal axis with prolonged PR interval
D. RBBB with right axis deviation
E. RBBB with right ventricular hypertrophy

24. **A 12-year-old girl complained of deteriorating breathlessness. She struggled to participate in school sporting activities. On examination, her fingers were clubbed and there was peripheral and central cyanosis. The pulse rate was 90 beats per minute and BP was 125/70 mmHg. Table 1.7 shows the cardiac catheter data obtained.**

Table 1.7 Cardiac catheterization data

Chamber	Pressure (mmHg)	Oxygen saturation (%)
RA (high)	a = 11 v = 17	50
RA (mid)	a = 11 v = 17	51
RA (low)	a = 11 v = 17	51
RV	110/20	50
PA	110/28	50
PCWP	9	
LV	107/13	70
Ascending Ao	120/70	71
Descending Ao	120/70	69

Which diagnosis best fits the data in Table 1.7?

A. Atrial septal defect
B. Eisenmenger's complex
C. Eisenmenger's syndrome
D. Fallot's tetralogy
E. Ventricular septal defect

25. **Table 1.8 shows cardiac catheter data obtained from an 18-year-old female with central cyanosis. She had a long-standing history of anorexia and there was previous history of appetite suppressant use.**

Table 1.8 Cardiac catheterization data

Chamber	Pressure (mmHg)	Oxygen saturation (%)
SVC		68
IVC		67
RA	5	67
RV	95/11	66
PA	25/15	66
PCWP	5	
LV	117/5	96
Ascending Ao	110/70	81
Descending Ao	110/70	81

Which is the diagnosis?

A. Eisenmenger syndrome
B. Fallot's tetralogy
C. Persistent ductus arteriosus
D. Primary pulmonary hypertension
E. Pulmonary stenosis

26. **A 76-year-old man was found to have a murmur. There was no history of chest pain, but he complained of breathlessness on heavy exertion. He had no previous cardiovascular history other than hypertension for which he took bendroflumethiazide. On examination the pulse rate was 80 beats per minute and BP was 190/50 mmHg. Results of investigations are shown in Table 1.9.**

Table 1.9 Cardiac catheterization data

Chamber	Pressure (mmHg)	Oxygen saturation (%)
RA	5	67
RV	22/5	66
PA	23/15	66
PCWP	15	
LV	190/18	96
Ascending Ao	190/50	95
Descending Ao	190/50	95

```
Left ventriculogram: dilated and hyperdynamic left ventricle
  (EF = 70%)
Coronary angiogram: normal coronary arteries
CXR: cardiomegaly; clear lung fields
```

What is the most appropriate treatment?

A. Add amlodipine 5 mg od
B. Add bisoprolol 2.5 mg od
C. Add furosemide 40 mg od
D. Add ISMN 10 mg bd
E. Add ramipril 2.5 mg od

27. **A 68-year-old man presented with sudden onset of chest pain, breathlessness, and palpitations. He had a previous history of myocardial infarction seven years previously for which he had subsequent coronary artery bypass graft surgery. Over the preceding few years he had experienced exertional breathlessness and orthopnoea. A repeat coronary angiogram two years before had documented patent grafts with no targets for revascularization. An echocardiogram showed extensive anteroseptal akinesis with severe impairment of LV systolic function (EF = 30%). His medications included aspirin, ramipril, simvastatin, ezetimibe, furosemide, and bisoprolol. On examination, the patient was clammy, his pulse rate was 132 beats per minute and BP was 80/60 mmHg. Auscultation of the heart sounds revealed a third heart sound. The venous pressure was not elevated. Auscultation of the lung fields revealed bibasal crepitations. There was no pedal oedema. His twelve-lead ECG is shown in Figure 1.6.**

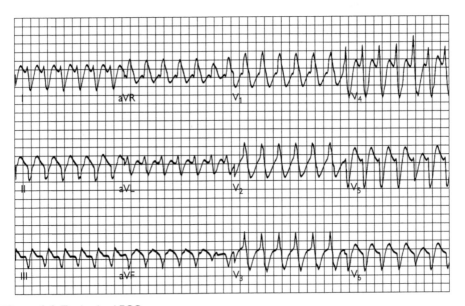

Figure 1.6 Twelve-lead ECG.

Reproduced with permission from *Mayo Clinic Internal Medicine Board Review*, Eleventh Edition. Edited by CM Wittich, Fig. 3.11. p. 39. Oxford University Press, Oxford, UK, Copyright © 2016.

What is the immediate management?

A. IV adenosine

B. IV amiodarone

C. IV magnesium

D. Synchronized DC cardioversion

E. Thrombolysis

28. A 56-year-old man presented with acute shortness of breath. There was no history of chest pain. He had a history of hypertension, hypercholesterolaemia, diet-controlled diabetes, and benign prostatic hyperplasia. His medications included aspirin 75 mg od, simvastatin 40 mg od, amlodipine 5 mg od, and tamsulosin 400 µg od. A twelve-lead ECG showed sinus tachycardia with ST depression in V4, V5, and V6. A chest X-ray showed pulmonary oedema and an echocardiogram demonstrated impaired systolic LV function with an ejection fraction of 35%. He was diagnosed with decompensated congestive cardiac failure. A urinary catheter was inserted, he was fluid restricted and treated with intravenous diuretics and nitrate infusion.

```
Admission electrolytes:
  Sodium                    136 mmol/L
  Potassium                 4.1 mmol/L
  Urea                      7 mmol/L
  Creatinine                141 µmol/L
```

The amlodipine was discontinued and he was started on ramipril 2.5 mg od. Forty-eight hours after admission, he had made good progress and was switched to oral diuretics. His urine output then fell to 15 mL/hour. On examination he was comfortable, his respiratory rate was 18 breaths per minute, pulse rate was 80 beats per minute, and BP was 135/88 mmHg. Auscultation of the chest revealed normal heart sounds but scattered bibasal crepitations. The venous pressure was not elevated. Abdominal examination was unremarkable and there was no palpable bladder. There was no peripheral oedema.

```
Repeat electrolytes and urinalysis:
  Sodium                    130 mmol/L
  Potassium                 5.1 mmol/L
  Urea                      24 mmol/L
  Creatinine                350 µmol/L
  Urinalysis                protein + blood ++
```

(a) What is the immediate management?

    A. Cautious 250 mL intravenous fluid challenge
    B. Stop ACE inhibitor
    C. Stop oral diuretics
    D. Switch back to intravenous diuretics
    E. Urgent haemofiltration

(b) What is the next best investigation to identify the cause of the acute deterioration in renal function?

    A. Captopril renogram
    B. Renal angiography
    C. Renal biopsy
    D. Renal ultrasound scan
    E. Transrectal ultrasound

29. **A 66-year-old man presented with gradual deterioration in breathlessness over the preceding week. He had a past medical history of hypertension and hypercholesterolaemia. Previously, angiography had confirmed renovascular disease unmasked after starting an ACEi, which was then discontinued. His medications included aspirin 75 mg od, atenolol 50 mg od, and rosuvastatin 10 mg od. On examination the pulse was 105 beats per minute, saturations on air were 89%, and BP was 120/60 mmHg. The venous pressure was elevated. Auscultation of the heart sounds revealed a third heart sound and a pansystolic murmur at the apex. There was pitting ankle oedema.**

```
Investigations:
  Hb                        110 g/L
  WCC                       6 × 10⁹/L
  Platelets                 180 × 10⁹/L
  Sodium                    132 mmol/L
  Potassium                 3.9 mmol/L
  Urea                      10.1 mmol/L
  Creatinine                172 μmol/L
  Troponin I                <1 ng/L          (<14 ng/L)
  ECG: sinus rhythm; LBBB
  CXR: cardiomegaly; pulmonary oedema
  Echocardiogram: dilated LV cavity with global hypokinesis;
    severe impairment of LV systolic function (EF = 30%);
    moderate functional mitral regurgitation
```

The atenolol was discontinued and the patient responded well to 48 hours of intravenous diuretics and a nitrate infusion, after which he was started on oral diuretics. His pulse was 80 beats per minute and BP was 107/60 mmHg. The chest was clear to auscultation.

What medications would you add?

A. Amlodipine 5 mg od and bisoprolol 1.25 mg od

B. Bisoprolol 1.25 mg od and digoxin 62.5 μg od

C. Bisoprolol 1.25 mg od and spironolactone 12.5 mg od

D. Candesartan 2 mg od and spironolactone 12.5 mg od

E. ISDN 10 mg bd and hydralazine 25 mg bd

30. **A 38-year-old man presented to the A&E department with a one-week history of intermittent palpitations. He described them as short-lived episodes of rapid regular palpitations which terminated spontaneously but were increasing in frequency. There were no obvious precipitating factors. Other than mild discomfort in the chest during these episodes he reported no other symptoms. He was a smoker and consumed 14 units of alcohol per week. He had a past medical history of childhood asthma but had been symptom free for many years. During examination, he developed symptoms once more. His pulse was 150 beats per minute and BP was 107/75 mmHg. Auscultation of the heart sound revealed normal heart sounds.**

```
Investigations:
   Hb                            160 g/L
   WCC                           5 × 10⁹/L
   Platelets                     170 × 10⁹/L
   Sodium                        136 mmol/L
   Potassium                     4.1 mmol/L
   Urea                          5 mmol/L
   Creatinine                    118 µmol/L
   Magnesium                     0.7 mmol/L
   Corrected calcium             2.1 mmol/L
   Troponin I                    <1 ng/L          (<14 ng/L)
   ECG Rhythm strip: Figure 1.7
```

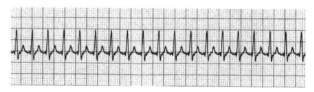

Figure 1.7 ECG Rhythm strip.

Reproduced from *Oxford Handbook of Cardiac Nursing*, Second Edition. Edited by K Olson, Fig 12.1, p. 246. Oxford University Press, Oxford, UK, Copyright © 2014.

What is the best initial management?

A. IV adenosine

B. IV amiodarone

C. IV digoxin

D. IV magnesium

E. IV verapamil

1. D) Primary percutaneous coronary intervention

This man has presented with an acute myocardial infarction. The ECG demonstrates an anterior ST elevation MI with reciprocal changes in the inferior leads. In the context of ST elevation MI early reperfusion therapy is the most crucial management step. This can be using the more traditional method of thrombolysis or more recently primary percutaneous coronary intervention (PPCI). PPCI is superior to thrombolysis and is therefore the most effective management step. Anticoagulation with low molecular weight heparin and the use of glycoprotein 2B/3A inhibitors would be appropriate in the setting of a non-ST elevation MI or unstable angina (USA). Diuretics would be appropriate if there was clinical or radiographic evidence of pulmonary congestion.

Tutorial

The most important immediate management steps for patients presenting with an acute coronary syndrome is to achieve respiratory and haemodynamic stabilization followed by prompt anti-platelet therapy. This is usually aspirin 300 mg and clopidogrel 300 mg PO. With the results of the PLATO trial, ticagrelor has become the more dominant second anti-platelet agent, as this novel $P2Y_{12}$ inhibitor has shown superior outcomes when compared to clopidogrel. The dosing for ticagrelor is 180 mg PO followed by 90 mg bd regimen. Additionally, it is worth noting that caution should be taken when giving oxygen to normoxic patients as a recent study (AVOID) showed that patients with saturations above 94% on room air randomized to receiving supplement oxygen therapy had higher serum titres of creatinine kinase and troponin, as well as larger infarction size on cardiac MRI six months post events. The mechanism of which is thought to be due to hyperoxia-mediated vasoconstriction. Analgesia can be given which can include intravenous opiates coupled with an anti-emetic agent. Sublingual GTN can be used to dilate coronary vasculature, but the BP needs to be monitored. Beta blockers should be started early if there are no contraindications (bradycardia, hypotension, heart block, or pulmonary oedema).

In ST elevation MI early reperfusion therapy is the most crucial management step. For over two decades, thrombolysis has been the cornerstone in the acute management of ST segment elevation MI (STEMI), with streptokinase achieving a significant 19% reduction in mortality and a greater reduction in those treated early. Thrombolysis has important limitations (see Box 1.1) and PPCI offers an alternative by mechanically disrupting the occlusive thrombus and opening the underlying stenosis, rapidly restoring blood flow and achieving recanalization rates greater than 90%. There is a large body of evidence that demonstrates superiority of PPCI over thrombolysis. Pooled data from 23 trials has shown PPCI is superior to in-hospital thrombolysis at reducing short- and long-term mortality, re-infarction, and stroke, independent of the thrombolytic agent used. PPCI is now widely available in addition to thrombolysis. If available, PPCI is regarded as the reperfusion strategy of choice for patients with ST-elevation MI with a four-fold increase in PPCI in England and Wales over the last two years. As only a minority of patients with STEMI present directly to PPCI centres, patients may either receive thrombolysis at the presenting centre or be transferred for PPCI. Even with transfer times up to three hours, PPCI remains superior to immediate in-hospital thrombolysis, with a 42% reduction in the combined end point of death, re-infarction, and stroke (95% CI: 29–53%, p<0.001).

The acute management of non-ST elevation MI or USA comprises aspirin, clopidogrel/ticagrelor, beta blockers, low-molecular weight heparin, and glycoprotein IIB/IIIA inhibitors.

Box 1.1 Advantages and disadvantages of PPCI compared to thrombolysis

Advantages

- Greater patency rates of infarct-related artery (streptokinase: 55%, rt-PA: 60%, and PPCI: >90% at 90 minutes)
- Reduced re-occlusion and re-infarction rates
- Reduced haemorrhagic stroke
- Avoids the risk associated with thrombolysis, such as bleeding
- Reduced mortality
- Better residual left ventricular function
- More rapid electrocardiographic normalization
- Haemodynamic and coronary anatomy data from angiography
- Improved risk stratification with identification of patients suitable for coronary artery bypass surgery
- Can be performed where thrombolysis is contraindicated (5–20% of patients)

Disadvantages

- High procedural costs
- Cardiac catheterization facilities not readily available
- Risks of cardiac catheterization and percutaneous intervention
- Reperfusion arrhythmias are more common

Further Reading

Dalby M, Bouzamondo A, Lechat P, Montalescot G (2003). Transfer for primary angioplasty versus immediate thrombolysis in acute myocardial infarction: a meta-analysis. *Circulation* 108: 1809–1814.

Iqbal M, Westwood M, Swanton R (2008). Recent developments in acute coronary syndromes. *Clinical Medicine* 8: 42–48.

Keeley E, Boura J, Grines C (2003). Primary angioplasty versus intravenous thrombolytic therapy for acute myocardial infarction: a quantitative review of 23 randomised trials. *Lancet* 361: 13–20.

2. D) Oral beta blocker

This man presents with acute persistent atrial fibrillation, greater than 48 hours onset. There is no evidence of haemodynamic compromise, thus no indication for emergency DC cardioversion. If the onset of atrial fibrillation is clear and within 48 hours of onset, then cardioversion, both electrically and chemically, would be appropriate. However, in cases where the duration of the arrhythmia is greater than 48 hours or uncertain, then cardioversion, both electrically and chemically, should be avoided, as there is a risk of atrial thrombus formation and subsequent risk of stroke. Thus, in this case, chemical cardioverting agents, for example amiodarone and flecainide, will not be appropriate. The most appropriate management will be ventricular rate control which can be achieved either by a beta blocker or calcium channel antagonist. Digoxin is no longer routinely recommended as a primary treatment unless the patient has concomitant pulmonary oedema or if used in conjunction with other rate controlling agents. Although an echocardiogram is important in the management of atrial fibrillation to assess heart structure and function, there is no urgency for this.

Tutorial

Atrial fibrillation can be classified as paroxysmal, persistent, or permanent based on the temporal pattern of the arrhythmia (Figure 1.8). When first presenting with atrial fibrillation, acute causes must be excluded (Table 1.10). Lone atrial fibrillation is defined as atrial fibrillation without an apparent cause. Patients presenting with atrial fibrillation within 48 hours of onset should be cardioverted (chemically or electrically). This patient presents with persistent atrial fibrillation (duration greater than 48 hours), without a clear cause (lone atrial fibrillation). Atrial fibrillation 'begets' atrial fibrillation. It induces both electrophysiological and structural atrial re-modelling which facilitate its persistence. Thus, the greater the duration of atrial fibrillation, the less successful the cardioversion is likely to be. Therefore, it would be reasonable to schedule this gentleman, at the earliest opportunity, for an elective DC cardioversion. In such cases, initially it is important to optimize ventricular rate control, as poor ventricular rate control is associated with a tachycardiomyopathy (reversible left ventricular dysfunction). The rate control agents which can be used have been discussed in the first part of the answer to this question, though it is worth noting that a combination of beta blockers and rate-slowing calcium antagonists is usually avoided due to a combined negative inotropic effect, but may be used in selected cases. It is also worth noting that a beta blocker, sotalol, is avoided because its class III anti-dysrhythmic effects mean it has cardioverting potential. Whilst this may initially seem ideal, there is actually a great risk to patients of thromboembolism, which is discussed further below, which must be addressed prior to cardioversion.

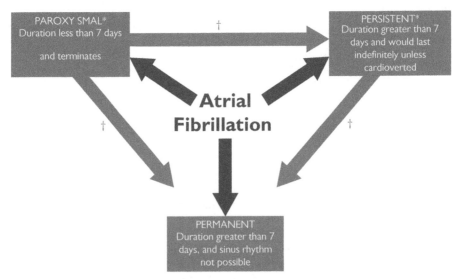

Figure 1.8 Classification of atrial fibrillation (based on the temporal pattern of arrhythmia).

* When a patient has had two or more episodes of atrial fibrillation, this is termed recurrent. Both paroxysmal and persistent atrial fibrillation are potentially recurrent arrhythmias.

† With time, paroxysmal atrial fibrillation may become persistent. Likewise, both paroxysmal and persistent atrial fibrillation may become permanent.

During or following a cardioversion, there is a risk of any left atrial thrombus becoming dislodged and embolizing. For this reason, patients are anticoagulated for at least four weeks, usually with warfarin, prior to DC cardioversion to allow for resolution of any potential atrial thrombus. An alternate approach is to proceed immediately to cardioversion once the patient is fully

Table 1.10 The causes of atrial fibrillation (* denotes the most common causes)

Cardiovascular causes	Non-cardiovascular causes
Ischaemic heart disease*	**Metabolic causes**
Hypertension*	Thyrotoxicosis*
Mitral valve disease	$\downarrow K^+$, $\downarrow Mg^{2+}$, $\downarrow Ca^{2+}$, Acidosis
• Mitral stenosis	Pheochromocytoma
• Mitral regurgitation	Drugs (sympathomimetics)
• Mitral valve prolapse	Alcohol ('holiday heart syndrome')
Mitral stenosis*	Post-operative (non-cardiac surgery)
Mitral regurgitation	Hypothermia
Mitral valve prolapse	**Respiratory causes**
Rheumatic heart disease	Pneumonia
Heart failure	Carcinoma of the lung
Cardiomyopathy	Pulmonary embolism
Pericarditis	Trauma
Endocarditis	Thoracic surgery
Myocarditis	**Other causes**
Congenital heart disease	Vagal atrial fibrillation
Sinus node dysfunction	Adrenergic atrial fibrillation
Cardiac tumours	Intracranial haemorrhage
Post-cardiac surgery	'Lone' atrial fibrillation
Supraventricular arrhythmia	
• Wolff-Parkinson-White Syndrome	
• AV nodal re-entrant tachycardia	

anticoagulated, providing it has been demonstrated on transoesophageal echocardiogram that there is no left atrial thrombus. Providing the patient has been cardioverted back into sinus rhythm, anticoagulation should then be continued for at least four weeks after DC cardioversion, to prevent any further clot formation, whilst allowing mechanical atrial activity to fully resume.

All patients with atrial fibrillation must have a routine echocardiogram to assess left ventricular function, exclude structural and valvular heart disease, and assess left atrial diameter. An enlarged left atrial diameter reduces the chance of successful cardioversion and increases the rate of recurrence of atrial fibrillation.

Further Reading

Iqbal M, Taneja A, Lip G, Flather M (2005). Recent developments in atrial fibrillation. *British Medical Journal* 330: 238–243.

National Institute for Clinical Excellence. The management of atrial fibrillation [CG180]. June 2014, updated August 2014. Available at: http://www.nice.org.uk/guidance/CG180

3. C) Persistent ductus arteriosus (PDA)

Given the patient's age and presentation, it is likely she has a congenital heart disease which has progressed to make her dyspnoeic. The patient has clinical features of both (a) Eisenmenger's syndrome (reversal of a left-to-right cardiac shunt): peripheral cyanosis and right ventricular pressure > left ventricular pressure; and (b) pulmonary hypertension: raised pulmonary artery and right ventricular pressures, a soft systolic murmur left lower sternal edge of functional tricuspid regurgitation, and subsequent peripheral oedema. Whilst pulmonary hypertension can be primary, it is usually secondary to another pathology. Eisenmenger's syndrome is always secondary to another cardiac abnormality which can be an atrial, ventricular, atrio-ventricular septal defect, or a PDA. The exact aetiology can be identified by analysing the cardiac catheterization data in a logical systematic approach. It is clear that right ventricular and pulmonary artery pressures are significantly elevated. This itself would constitute the diagnosis of pulmonary hypertension and given that the right ventricular pressure is greater than the left ventricular pressure, it implies a right-to-left (Eisenmenger's shunt). Next, when analysing the saturations, the obvious abnormality is a drop in saturations between the ascending and descending aorta. This would suggest a right-to-left shunt at the level of the aorta. The only possibility is a PDA.

It is worth noting the reasons for two important missing signs that are usually associated with a PDA and Eisenmenger's syndrome: clubbing and the 'machinery' murmur of a PDA. Clubbing is a cardinal feature of right-to-left shunts with the proposed mechanism being growth-factors such as prostaglandins, which are usually broken down by the lungs, being able to get into the systemic circulation and drive nailbed epidermal growth. However, with a PDA, because the shunt occurs into the descending aorta after the origin of the subclavian arteries, clubbing occurs in the toes but not the hands. With regards to the machinery murmur of a PDA which is normally loud in infancy, it usually becomes quiet as right ventricular pressures rise and can disappear completely when the shunt reverses.

Tutorial

A PDA is the persistence of a normal foetal structure between the main pulmonary artery and the proximal descending aorta, just after the origin of the left subclavian artery. From the sixth week of foetal life, the ductus is responsible for most of the right ventricular outflow. It contributes to 60% of the total cardiac output throughout the foetal life. Only about 5–10% of its outflow passes through the lungs. The ductus arteriosus is an important structure in foetal development as it contributes to the flow of blood to the rest of the foetal organs. Closure of the ductus before birth may lead to right heart failure. At birth, the ductus normally undergoes closure. Persistence beyond ten days of life is considered abnormal. In uncomplicated cases it is associated with left-to-right shunting, and in such cases, cardiac catheterization data will show a step up in oxygen saturation in the pulmonary artery. The increased pulmonary blood flow, with time, can result in pulmonary hypertension, but, whilst the aortic pressures exceed those of the pulmonary artery, the shunt continues in a left-to-right direction. With time, as pulmonary hypertension worsens, there is equalization of pressures in the pulmonary artery and aorta and resulting right-to-left shunting. This is Eisenmenger's syndrome.

Further Reading

Pandya B, Cullen S, Walker F (2016). Congenital heart disease in adults. *British Medical Journal* 28: 354: i3905.

4. C) DDDR permanent pacemaker insertion

This patient has complete heart block with a broad ventricular escape rhythm, so there is increased risk of asystole. Untreated, complete heart block can also predispose to ventricular arrhythmias. In the absence of a permanent pacemaker system, complete heart block is associated with an annual mortality exceeding 15%. In this case, the aim would be to pace both the atrium and the ventricle to maintain physiological rhythm, and therefore, the patient should receive a dual chamber permanent pacemaker system. A temporary pacing wire would only be indicated if this patient was to become hypotensive or develop significant pauses, and then it would serve as a bridge to a permanent pacemaker system. There is clear evidence of complete heart block and this patient undisputedly requires a permanent pacemaker system. Thus, there is no role for a Holter monitor in this setting.

Tutorial

It is important to be aware of the pacing nomenclature, and the different types of pacemaker systems that are available. A three-letter code describing the basic function of the various pacing systems was first proposed in 1974 by the American Heart Association (AHA) and the American College of Cardiology (ACC). Since then, the code has been updated by North American Society of Pacing and Electrophysiology (NASPE) and the British Pacing and Electrophysiology Group

(BPEG, now known as Heart Rhythm UK). The complete code is referred to as the NBG code for pacing and comprises five letters: 12345. This is explained in more detail in Box 1.2. Common pacemaker systems are explained in Box 1.3.

Box 1.2 Pacemaker coding explained

Letter 1: the chamber(s) being paced. **A** = atrium, **V** = ventricle, and **D** = both.

Letter 2: the chamber(s) being sensed. **A** = atrium, **V** = ventricle, and **D** = both.

Letter 3: refers to how the pacemaker responds to a sensed event.

- **I** = sensed event inhibits the output pulse
- **T** = sensed event triggers an output pulse
- **D** = dual modes of response (both inhibit and trigger). This designation is restricted to dual chamber systems. An event sensed in the atrium inhibits the atrial output but triggers a ventricular output. There is a programmable delay between the sensed atrial event and the triggered ventricular output to mimic the normal PR interval. If the ventricular lead senses a native ventricular signal during the programmed delay, it will inhibit the ventricular output.
- **O** = no response to sensed input.

Letter 4: rate response facility (if present) is denoted by the letter **R.** This indicates that the pacemaker has rate response facility and adjusts its programmed paced heart rate in response to patient activity. A number of mechanisms are used to detect patient's activity, that is, vibration, respiration, and pressure.

Letter 5: when present, specifies only the location or absence of multisite pacing, defined as stimulation sites in both atria, both ventricles, more than one stimulation site in any single chamber, or a combination of these. This feature is uncommon, and the fifth letter is usually omitted. The most common application of multisite pacing is biventricular pacing (CRT) for the management of heart failure.

- O = no multisite pacing
- A = multisite pacing in the atrium
- V = multisite pacing in the ventricle or ventricles
- D = dual multisite pacing in both atrium and ventricle

As most pacemakers don't multisite pace (i.e. are an O), the fifth number is usually just missed off.

Box 1.3 Common setups of pacemakers

DDD/DDDR pacemaker systems:

- One lead in the right atrium and one lead in the right ventricle
- Common indications include second- or third-degree AV block

VVI/VVIR pacemaker systems:

- One lead in the right ventricle only
- Common indications are slow flutter or fibrillation +/− pauses

AAIR pacemaker systems:

- One lead in the right atrium only
- Used in patients with pure sinus node dysfunction without evidence of atrial fibrillation and AV block at rapid heart rates
- Often patients with sick sinus syndrome have a DDDR system implanted, as many go on to develop AV block in later life

Further Reading

Madhaven M, Mulpuru S, McLeod C, et al. (2017). Cardiac pacemakers: function, troubleshooting, and management: part 2 of a 2-part series. *Journal of American College of Cardiology* 69(2): 211–235.

Mulpuru S, Madhaven M, McLeod C, et al. (2017). Cardiac pacemakers: function, troubleshooting, and management: part 1 of a 2-part series. *Journal of American College of Cardiology* 69(2): 189–210.

5. E) Request urgent urea and electrolytes

The patient's chest pain along with examination findings point to a likely diagnosis of pericarditis. Given the marked hypertension, evidence of pulmonary and pitting oedema, along with symptoms of non-specific aches and pains, nausea, and lethargy should raise a suspicion of uraemia and fluid overload secondary to acute renal failure. The preceding history of a flu-like illness may relate to the onset of a vasculitic glomerulonephritis as a possible aetiology.

On examining the ECG, the initial impression is that of LBBB, and given a strong cardiovascular risk profile coupled with chest pain and nausea and with signs of pulmonary congestion, one could diagnose acute myocardial infarction with new onset LBBB. The answer lies, however, in closer examination of ECG and retrospective analysis of the history. The ECG shows very broad complexes initially resembling LBBB morphology. However, closer examination shows considerable widening of the QRS complexes; as they do so, they appear 'sinusoidal'. The ECG features are suggestive of severe hyperkalaemia (with imminent cardiac arrest).

Therefore, the most important initial investigation is urea and electrolytes, and subsequent appropriate treatment of hyperkalaemia. As the ECG gives the impression of LBBB, given the history of chest pain, one may diagnose an acute myocardial infarction. Even if the ECG represented true LBBB, thrombolysis would be contraindicated with uncontrolled hypertension. A chest X-ray may help confirm a diagnosis of pulmonary congestion, and similarly a cardiac echocardiogram may demonstrate a pericardial effusion. However, neither of these will explain the ECG changes or the overlying diagnosis. The history of chest pain, oliguria, and severe hypertension in a young patient may also lead one to consider aortic dissection as a unifying diagnosis causing hypertension, chest pain, and renal failure. However, the pain described is not characteristic of aortic dissection and did not precede the symptoms of uraemia. Even if it was the underlying cause of the presentation, the patient's ECG still suggests hyperkalaemia and this would require confirmation and treatment prior to any other investigation.

Tutorial

Peaked T waves are the first ECG abnormality to be seen in hyperkalaemia. They are classically described as tall, narrow, and symmetrical. Other features are summarized in Box 1.4. Electrophysiologically, hyperkalaemia causes the resting membrane potential to become less negative, which leads to partial inactivation of the sodium channels. As a result, influx of sodium ions is impaired, phase 0 of depolarization is decreased, and conduction is slowed, accounting for QRS widening and AV dissociation. Hyperkalaemia also inhibits depolarization of the atria, and thus P waves become less visible and eventually absent. As hyperkalaemia worsens, conduction becomes so slow that QRS widening produces 'sinusoidal waves'. Ultimately, the myocyte membranes become totally unexcitable, resulting in asystole.

The immediate treatment for hyperkalaemia is to stabilize the membrane potential by administering intravenous calcium gluconate or calcium chloride. This acts in minutes and the effects last for up to one hour. During this time, treatment with insulin and dextrose is necessary, as insulin drives potassium into cells. In patients with renal failure, insulin and dextrose must be given with close monitoring, as insulin is primarily metabolized by the kidneys, and this may predispose to severe hypoglycaemia.

Box 1.4 ECG features of hyperkalaemia

- Tall peaked symmetrical T waves
- QRS widening
- Flattened P waves
- Absent P waves (atrial standstill)
- Shortening of PR interval
- Sinusoidal QRS complexes
- AV dissociation
- Asystole

Further Reading

Diercks D, Shumaik G, Harrigan R (2004). Electrocardiographic manifestations: electrolyte abnormalities. *Journal of Emergency Medicine* 27, 153–160.

6. B) Beta blocker

This question tests the knowledge of the initial management of unstable angina (USA) and non-ST segment elevation MI (NSTEMI). It is important to know which therapeutic agents have prognostic benefit. The initial management comprises aspirin, clopidogrel/ticagrelor, low molecular weight heparin, beta blocker (if no contraindications), and GP IIB/IIIA inhibitors (in high-risk cases). There is overwhelming evidence for their prognostic benefit. Nitrates and morphine only help symptoms, but do not improve prognosis. Furthermore, these agents would not be indicated as the patient is pain free. Verapamil and diltiazem lower the heart rate, thereby reducing myocardial oxygen consumption. Verapamil should not be used routinely in the acute management, due to its negatively inotropic effect. Diltiazem is often used in patients who are not able to tolerate beta blockers. However, both verapamil and diltiazem do not have the prognostic benefit that is associated with beta blockers. This patient has a history of asthma, and this is a *relative* contraindication to beta blockers, these agents should not be routinely withheld in patients with obstructive airways disease. More than often, these agents are often well tolerated, particularly the more cardio-selective beta$_1$ blockers. ACE inhibitors and statins should be started early in all patients with acute coronary syndromes but do not fall into the immediate management. Patients with a positive troponin are often classified as high risk, and there is strong evidence to support the use of GP IIB/IIIA inhibitors in the early management of NSTEMI, which if it had been listed as an option, would also have been correct.

A) Early inpatient coronary angiography

This gentleman presents with chest pain and T wave inversion in the inferior leads, associated with positive cardiac biomarkers (troponin). The diagnosis is NSTEMI. Currently, an early invasive approach with coronary angiography +/− revascularization is considered to be the optimum strategy and is associated with better outcomes. Myocardial perfusion imaging, dobutamine stress echocardiography, and exercise treadmill testing are useful for demonstrating inducible ischaemia.

Tutorial

Beta blockers should be started early in patients with acute coronary syndromes in the absence of contraindications (heart block, hypotension, and pulmonary oedema). Peripheral vascular disease and obstructive airways disease are relative contraindications and, if necessary, these patients may be given a beta blocker with a short half-life (e.g. metoprolol) or a greater beta$_1$-selective agent (e.g. bisoprolol) and observed closely for adverse effects. In patients who have survived a myocardial infarction and have obstructive airways disease beta blockers are associated with a 40% reduction in total mortality. Diltiazem is an alternative to beta blockers in reducing ventricular rate and thus myocardial oxygen consumption but is not as prognostic as beta blockers.

Intravenous GP IIb/IIIa inhibitors have been extensively evaluated and three agents have been developed to be administered with adjuvant UFH/LMWH: abciximab (Reopro), tirofiban (Aggrastat), and eptifibatide (Integrilin). Initially developed for use with coronary angioplasty to reduce procedure-related thrombotic complications, more recent studies have focused on GP IIb/IIIa inhibitors in the primary medical management of USA/NSTEMI. Patients at high-risk with elevated troponin or those undergoing early PCI derive greater benefit from GP IIb/IIIa inhibitors. Even in patients with USA/NSTEMI who are not scheduled for early coronary revascularization, the greatest benefit was seen in patients with elevated troponin. Current NICE guidelines state:

- GP IIb/IIIa inhibitors should be used with aspirin, clopidogrel, and heparin in the initial medical management of USA/NSTEMI in patients who are at high risk. Patients at high risk include those with ongoing chest pain, haemodynamic instability, dynamic ST/T wave changes on the electrocardiogram, and an elevated troponin. Another tool to identify high risk is a TIMI score ≥3 (see Further Reading).
- Though, early angiography is desirable for high-risk patients, in situations where PCI does not occur or is not immediately available, initial medical management with GP IIb/IIIa inhibitors is still recommended.

ACE inhibitors decrease morbidity and mortality in patients with established left ventricular dysfunction and in patients with left ventricular dysfunction post-MI. More recently, ACE inhibitors have shown benefit in patients with coronary artery disease and preserved left ventricular systolic function. ACE inhibitors should be started in all patients with acute coronary syndromes, provided there are no contraindications, even in those with preserved left ventricular function. In those who cannot tolerate ACE inhibitors, angiotensin II antagonists can be used. Numerous landmark trials have shown the benefits of statins in patients at high risk with or without clinical evidence of coronary artery disease in all sex and age groups, irrespective of initial cholesterol levels. Statins reduce recurrent ischaemic events in patients with acute coronary syndromes and should be started early. Although ACE inhibitors and statins should also be started early, their initiation would not fall into the immediate management of acute coronary syndrome.

Many studies have compared clinical outcomes associated with early invasive strategy versus an early conservative therapy in patients with USA or NSTEMI. An early conservative strategy involves aggressive medical therapy, with coronary angiography and revascularization reserved only for patients with recurrent or inducible ischaemia. In an early invasive strategy, all patients undergo early coronary angiography, within 12–48 hours of presentation, and revascularization if indicated. Current evidence suggests that a routine early invasive strategy in USA and NSTEMI is associated with better long-term outcomes, particularly in high-risk patients. In the TACTICS-TIMI 18 trial, the benefits of an early invasive strategy were only observed in patients with high risk, defined as troponin elevation, ST segment deviation, or TIMI risk score ≥3 (NB: candidates are not expected to memorize scoring systems for the MRCP part 2 exam, but for those interested a reference is included in the Further Reading section). Pooled data from seven trials has shown that although a routine invasive strategy is associated with higher early mortality during initial hospitalization, it is associated with better long-term outcomes following discharge with a significant reduction in death, myocardial infarction, recurrent angina, and re-hospitalization. These benefits were only observed in patients at high risk with elevated cardiac biomarkers. Based on recent robust evidence, an early invasive strategy should be routine in the management of NSTEMI.

Further Reading

Mehta S, Cannon C, Fox K, et al. (2005). Routine vs selective invasive strategies in patients with acute coronary syndromes: a collaborative meta-analysis of randomized trials. *Journal of American Medical Association* 293: 2908–2917.

National Institute for Clinical Excellence. Acute coronary syndromes in adults [QS68]. September 2014. Available at: www.nice.org.uk/guidance/qs68

7. C) Immediate transfer for rescue PCI

This lady has presented with acute anterior STEMI. She has had failed thrombolysis as evidenced by failure of ST segment resolution and ongoing chest pain. Current evidence supports rescue PCI as opposed to repeat thrombolysis as the treatment of choice for patients with failed thrombolysis. GP IIB/IIIA inhibitors have a role as adjunctive therapy in primary PCI, and thus no role in the current management of this patient. An intravenous nitrate infusion can be used for symptoms but has no prognostic benefit. The heart rate does permit up-titration of beta blocker, and this should be strongly considered as adjunctive therapy in this patient. However, the most important management step is to arrange immediate transfer for rescue PCI.

Tutorial

All patients should be re-assessed at 90 minutes following thrombolysis for evidence of ongoing ischaemia. The presence of ongoing ischaemic pain, or more importantly failure of ST elevation to resolve by greater than 50%, is generally classified as failed thrombolysis. Patients in whom thrombolysis fails may either have repeat thrombolysis or urgent angiography (rescue PCI). The MERLIN trial showed no difference in mortality between rescue PCI and repeat thrombolysis. However, rescue PCI was associated with significantly improved event-free survival, largely due to a reduction in subsequent revascularization. On the contrary, the REACT trial showed that rescue PCI was superior to repeat thrombolysis and significantly improved event-free survival, with a significant reduction in mortality, re-infarction, and revascularization. Although there were important differences between the two trials, the conflicting results have led to controversy concerning the optimal management of failed thrombolysis. A recent meta-analysis supports the use of rescue PCI following failed thrombolysis, with a significant reduction in mortality and re-infarction, when compared to repeat thrombolysis. Current evidence supports rescue PCI as opposed to repeat thrombolysis as the treatment of choice for patients with failed thrombolysis.

Further Reading

Collet J, Montalescot G, Le May M, et al. (2006). Percutaneous coronary intervention after fibrinolysis: a multiple meta-analyses approach according to the type of strategy. *Journal of American College of Cardiology* 48: 1326–1335.

Gershlick A, Stephens-Lloyd A, Hughes S, et al. (2005). REACT Trial Investigators. Rescue angioplasty after failed thrombolytic therapy for acute myocardial infarction. *New England Journal of Medicine* 353: 2758–2768.

Sutton A, Campbell P, Graham R, et al. (2004). A randomized trial of rescue angioplasty versus a conservative approach for failed fibrinolysis in ST-segment elevation myocardial infarction: the Middlesbrough Early Revascularization to Limit Infarction (MERLIN) trial. *Journal of American College of Cardiology* 44: 287–296.

8. B) ACE inhibitor and beta blocker

This man has severe impairment of LV systolic function, most likely secondary to a viral myocarditis six months ago. He currently has NYHA II cardiac status. This question tests the knowledge of the chronic management of stable heart failure. All patients with NYHA I–II cardiac status should receive an ACE-inhibitor followed by beta blocker therapy. It would be appropriate to initiate ACE inhibitor prior to beta blocker therapy. There are no signs of fluid overload and the CXR does not demonstrate pulmonary congestion; thus, diuretics are not indicated. Often in clinical practice, unnecessary diuretic use leads to hypotension and renal impairment, and this prevents the appropriate up-titration of prognostic therapy.

Tutorial

The medical management of heart failure has revolutionized with the emergence of trial evidence and data. A low cardiac output in the context of heart failure activates the renin-angiotensin system and the sympathetic system in an attempt to restore the circulation. This has an adverse effect on the compromised heart which leads to volume overload, fibrosis, and abnormal cardiac remodelling with progressive deterioration in cardiac function. The primary aims in the chronic management of heart failure are to improve symptoms and prognosis. The management is multidisciplinary, ranging from patient education, lifestyle modifications, pharmacotherapy, device therapy, and surgical intervention.

All patients with left ventricular systolic dysfunction should be started on ACE inhibitors, irrespective of functional status, provided there are no contraindications. If they are not tolerated, then angiotensin II receptor blockers can be used. These agents inhibit the renin-angiotensin system. The serum creatinine needs to be monitored, and a rise of >25% after starting an ACE inhibitor or angiotensin II receptor blocker suggests underlying renovascular disease, and in such cases, they must be discontinued until this is excluded. The presence of hypotension is not an absolute contraindication to starting ACE inhibitors. Patients often have low BP readings in the context of a low cardiac output, which is usually well tolerated and unaccompanied by symptoms. Therapy may be initiated in patients with systolic BPs as low as 90 mmHg, provided they do not become symptomatic as a result of hypotension. This applies to other pharmacotherapeutic agents in heart failure.

Beta blockers should not be commenced in the acute stages of heart failure. Once considered a contraindication, there is now overwhelming data to support the use of beta blockers in stable heart failure. They should be initiated with NYHA class I–II status but may also be used cautiously in patients with NYHA class III–IV status. Beta blockers that are licensed for use in heart failure include bisoprolol, carvedilol, metoprolol, and nebivolol. Beta blockers increase diastolic filling time and improve stroke volume, prevent arrhythmias, and prevent adverse cardiac remodelling by inhibiting the sympathetic and thus the renin-angiotensin system. Current guidelines suggest that all patients with stable heart failure should initially be started on an ACE inhibitor, followed by initiation of beta-blocker therapy.

Spironolactone should be used for patients in NYHA class III–IV status, or those with an ejection fraction of less than 30%. It is important to monitor the renal function and for hyperkalaemia (given that such patients are also on ACE inhibitors or angiotensin II receptor blockers). Digoxin should be used as first-line treatment with ACE inhibitors in all patients with heart failure and atrial fibrillation. For patients in NYHA class III–IV status in sinus rhythm, digoxin has been shown to improve symptoms and reduce hospitalization, but without a reduction in mortality. Patients with NYHA III–IV status who are on maximal medical therapy (ACE inhibitor, beta blocker, spironolactone, and digoxin) with evidence of interventricular conduction delay (LBBB; QRS>120 mm) may be considered for cardiac resynchronization therapy (CRT) (biventricular pacemaker).

Further Reading

National Institute for Clinical Excellence. Chronic heart failure in adults: diagnosis and management [NG106]. September 2018. Available at: http://www.nice.org.uk/guidance/ng106

Yancy C, Jessup M, Bozkurt B, et al. (2013). 2013 ACCF/AHA guideline for the management of heart failure: executive summary: a report of the American College of Cardiology Foundation/American Heart Association Task Force on practice guidelines. *Circulation* 128(16): 1810–1852.

9. A) Add candesartan 2 mg od

This patient has an ischaemic cardiomyopathy with severe impairment of LV systolic function. He currently has NYHA class III cardiac status. This question tests the knowledge of chronic management of heart failure and optimization of heart failure therapy. There has been a slight deterioration in renal function, but this should not be an indication for stopping or reducing the doses of ACE inhibitors. However, it would be important to monitor the renal function closely. This patient is currently not fluid overloaded, and thus there is no clear indication for increasing diuretics. However, in some cases, increasing diuretics may help symptoms, by reducing pulmonary venous congestion (but this would be supported by clinical and radiographic findings). This patient has stable heart failure symptoms, thus stopping beta blockers would not be appropriate. He is at present on maximal medical therapy for heart failure (ACE inhibitor, beta blocker, spironolactone, and digoxin). The use of angiotensin II receptor blockers, in addition to ACE inhibitor therapy, has also been shown to provide symptomatic and prognostic benefit. If this patient had LBBB on the ECG, then consideration for CRT would be appropriate.

Tutorial

Renal function should be monitored closely on initiation of ACE inhibitor therapy, and if there is an increase in creatinine >25% from baseline, then this suggests renovascular disease, and ACE inhibitors should only be used when this is excluded. It is also important to remember, that deterioration of renal function with ACE inhibitors in the context of renovascular disease is an idiosyncratic effect and reducing the dose of ACE inhibitors is futile in such cases. If renovascular disease is suspected, then ACE inhibitors should be stopped. The CHARM study has shown that additive therapy with an angiotensin II receptor blocker in patients already on an ACE inhibitor provides prognostic benefit. However, patients must be monitored closely for development of hyperkalaemia.

Further Reading

McMurray J, Ostergren J, Swedberg K, et al, for the CHARM Investigators and Committees (2003). Effects of candesartan in patients with chronic heart failure and reduced left-ventricular systolic function taking angiotensin-converting-enzyme inhibitors: the CHARM-Added trial. *Lancet* 362: 767–771.

10. A) Cardiac resynchronization therapy

This patient has ischaemic cardiomyopathy (NYHA class III) and appears to be on optimum medical therapy. There are no options for further coronary revascularization. He is euvolaemic. The mitral regurgitation is moderate in severity and is secondary to left ventricular dysfunction (annular dilatation). This is not an indication for mitral valve replacement. Whilst mitral valve annuloplasty is often an adjunctive therapy for severe functional mitral regurgitation during cardiac surgery, it is not usually a primary indication for surgery. This patient has first-degree heart block and LBBB. LBBB is due to left ventricular systolic dysfunction. Whilst a combination of first-degree heart block and LBBB may signify conduction disease, it would itself not constitute a primary indication for permanent pacemaker insertion, especially in a patient with no symptoms to suggest bradycardia. Furthermore, he has tolerated beta-blocker therapy. Thus, there is no indication for dual chamber pacemaker insertion. Whilst an implantable cardioverter defibrillator (ICD) has prognostic benefit for patients with left ventricular dysfunction (EF <30%) and LBBB, it does not have symptomatic benefit. For patients on optimum medical therapy with LBBB on the ECG the appropriate option would be CRT, which has been shown to provide symptomatic and prognostic benefit. The prognostic benefit is increased if this is combined with defibrillator therapy (CRT-D).

Tutorial

In systolic dysfunction, the loss of synchronized ventricular contraction is associated with intraventricular conduction delay, predominately due to LBBB. This can further impair cardiac function. It is estimated that 15% of all patients with heart failure and 30% of those with moderate to severe heart failure have LBBB. Furthermore, studies have shown that heart failure patients with LBBB and QRS time >200 ms have a mortality rate five times that of patients with normal QRS. The development of LBBB is associated with ventricular remodelling, leading to a number of physiological effects, including increased end diastolic stress, mitral regurgitation, and, most importantly, decreased left ventricular contractility. The electrical correction of ventricular desynchrony has become the basis for CRT. With the development of sophisticated electronic technology, devices have been developed that can now synchronize depolarization of the left and right ventricle. This resynchronization leads to reverse remodelling, an improvement in ventricular systolic function, and a decrease in functional mitral regurgitation. CRT has shown improvement in symptoms in both patients with ischaemic and non-ischaemic cardiomyopathy. The recent CARE-HF and COMPANION trials clearly established the benefit of both CRT alone, and in conjunction with CRT-D.

In CARE-HF, patients with NYHA Class III–IV cardiac status, an ejection fraction <35% and a QRS time >120 ms were randomized to either CRT or continuation of their standard medical therapy. CRT therapy was associated with a 36% decrease in mortality or hospitalization for cardiovascular symptoms and a 36% decrease in death from any cause. In addition, CRT therapy decreased mitral regurgitation, increased ejection fraction, and improved symptoms and quality of life. COMPANION was a randomized trial comparing CRT and CRT-D with standard medical therapy in patients with NYHA Class III–IV cardiac status, an ejection fraction <35%, normal sinus rhythm and QRS duration of >120 ms. All patients were treated with ACE inhibitors, beta blockers, and spironolactone. CRT therapy alone led to a 19% decrease in death and hospitalization for any cause compared with medical treatment. CRT-D decreased the same end point by 20%. Death from or hospitalization due to cardiovascular disease was decreased by 25% in the CRT alone group, and by 28% in the CRT-D treated patients. Furthermore, CRT alone reduced the risk of death from any cause by 24% and CRT-D resulted in a decrease in all-cause mortality by 36% compared with standard medical therapy. Both CARE-HF and COMPANION indicate that CRT alone improves symptoms and quality of life, and that it is an important adjunct to standard medical therapy for heart failure in patients with sinus rhythm and LBBB.

To summarize, patients who have intraventricular conduction delay other than LBBB do not achieve any benefit from CRT, while patients with ischaemic and non-ischaemic cardiomyopathy benefit equally. In patients with LBBB who continue to experience significant symptoms whilst on optimum medical therapy, CRT can provide an important therapeutic option with or without an ICD.

Further Reading

Bristow M, Saxon L, Boehmer J, et al. (2004). Comparison of Medical Therapy, Pacing, and Defibrillation in Heart Failure (COMPANION) Investigators. Cardiac-resynchronization therapy with or without an implantable defibrillator in advanced chronic heart failure. *New England Journal of Medicine* 350: 2140–2215.

Cleland J, Daubert J, Erdmann E, et al. (2005). The effect of cardiac resynchronization on morbidity and mortality in heart failure. *New England Journal of Medicine* 352: 1539–1549.

National Institute for Clinical Excellence (2014). Implantable cardioverter defibrillators and cardiac resynchronisation therapy for arrhythmias and heart failure [TA314]. June 2014. Available at: http://www.nice.org.uk/ta314

11. A) Blood cultures

This man gives a history of fever, malaise, and weight loss with a murmur of mitral regurgitation on examination and no other obvious focus of infection. There is a leucocytosis with raised inflammatory markers. All of these features, in an otherwise previously fit and well patient, make infective endocarditis the most likely diagnosis. Blood cultures are the single most important investigation in infective endocarditis. Whilst an echocardiogram is important in making the diagnosis, it would not be the most important initial investigation. There is evidence of renal impairment, indicating glomerulonephritis, and a urinalysis and renal ultrasound would be important investigations in due course.

Tutorial

Infective endocarditis (IE) is defined as an infection of the endocardial surface of the heart (valves, mural endocardium, or septal defect). The clinical presentation is traditionally classified as either acute or sub-acute. Acute IE frequently involves normal valves, with an aggressive clinical course, caused by virulent organisms, such as S. aureus. Subacute IE typically affects abnormal valves, that is, pre-existing valvular pathology, and usually has a more latent clinical course that may extend over many weeks to months, often caused by beta-haemolytic streptococci or enterococci. The most commonly affected valve is the mitral valve, followed in order of frequency by aortic valve, combined mitral and aortic valve, the tricuspid valve, and, rarely, the pulmonary valve. Bacteraemia can result from various invasive procedures, ranging from oral surgery, to sclerotherapy of oesophageal varices, to abdominal and urological surgery. Common procedures include endoscopy, colonoscopy, dental extractions, and transurethral resection of the prostate. The history should enquire about invasive procedures and recreational drug use that may be causing the bacteraemia. Intravenous drug users are at increased risk of tricuspid valve endocarditis. Most subacute disease caused by S. viridans infection is related to dental disease and transient bacteraemia secondary to gingivitis. Symptoms of endocarditis often appear within two weeks of dental or other bacteraemia-prone procedure. The clinical features of endocarditis are summarized in Table 1.11.

Blood cultures remain the key in making the diagnosis of IE. Never draw only one set of blood cultures—'one is worse than none'. Two sets of blood cultures have greater than 90% sensitivity when bacteraemia is present, and serial blood cultures should be taken, as a single set of blood cultures may not reveal the culprit organism. Blood cultures are positive in 90–95% of cases. In 5–10% of cases, the blood cultures will be negative, and the most common cause for culture negative endocarditis is prior treatment with antibiotics. For this reason, blood cultures should always be taken prior to commencing antibiotic therapy. Causes of culture positive and culture-negative endocarditis are given in Table 1.12. Echocardiography is considered the diagnostic investigation of choice, especially in patients who present with a clinical picture of IE but who have negative cultures. In most cases, transthoracic echocardiography (TTE) is sufficient. TTE may be normal, as vegetations less than 3 mm will not be seen. The sensitivity of TTE is approximately 60%. Transoesophageal echocardiography (TOE) has greater sensitivity (greater than 90%) in identifying vegetations. TOE is indicated in suspected IE when TTE is negative despite the presence of clinical features of IE; in patients with mechanical prosthetic valves, right-sided lesions; and for detection of myocardial abscesses. Note, it is important to remember that TOE has the potential to cause bacteraemia.

The diagnosis of IE can never be completely excluded based on negative echocardiogram findings alone, either from TTE or from TOE—approximately 15% of cases of IE do not demonstrate any detectable vegetations at the time of the echocardiogram. Proteinuria and microscopic haematuria are present in approximately 50% of cases. The ECG often shows nonspecific changes, but first-degree heart block and new interventricular conduction delays may signal septal involvement in aortic valve disease with the potential for abscess formation. The CXR may be normal but may show pulmonary congestion with haemodynamically significant aortic and mitral regurgitation. Pulmonary embolic phenomena strongly suggest tricuspid valve involvement (common in

Table 1.11 Clinical features of endocarditis

Clinical Feature	Notes
Fever	Almost always present (90%).
Petechiae	Conjunctivae, dorsum of hands and feet, oral mucosa, soft palate, chest, and abdominal wall.
Splinter haemorrhages	Subungual haemorrhages affecting hands and feet that may also result from trauma to nails or psoriasis; if present for entire length of nail, they are more likely to reflect trauma (a true splinter usually occurs 3–5 mm proximal to free edge of nail).
Clubbing	Previously this was almost a universal finding, but now present in less than 10% of cases; occurs in patients who have extended course of untreated endocarditis.
Osler nodes	Tender nodules; red-purple; present in pulp of finger and toes, soles of the feet; thenar and hypothenar eminences of hands; appearance often preceded by neuropathic pain; present for hours to days and remain tender for up to two days.
Janeway lesions	Erythematous non-tender macules (1–4 mm diameter); palms, soles, and around ankles.
Arthritis	Occurs in patients who have extended course of untreated endocarditis; asymmetrical and limited to 1–3 joints. An acute septic mono-arthritis is associated with S. aureus infection.
Murmur	Present in 85% of cases. However, in right-sided endocarditis only a third of patients have a detectable murmur. Valvular involvement (in descending order of frequency): mitral, aortic, mitral and aortic, tricuspid, and pulmonary valves.
Splenomegaly	Occurs in patients who have extended course of untreated endocarditis; may persist after treatment.
Roth spots	Retinal haemorrhages with pale centres, near the optic disc. Other causes include SLE, polyarteritis nodosa, anaemia, and leukaemia.

Table 1.12 Causes of culture positive and negative endocarditis

Culture positive endocarditis	Culture negative endocarditis
• Streptococcus viridans • Staphylococcus aureus • Coagulase-negative Staphylococcus aureus (prosthetic valve) • Streptococcus faecalis • Enterococcus • Group A, C, D, and G Streptococcus • Group B Streptococcus (in pregnancy)	• Prior antibiotic therapy • Nutritionally deficient variants of Streptococcus viridians* • Brucella spp • Neisseria spp • Legionella spp • Mycoplasma • HACEK group of oropharyngeal bacteria: (Haemophilus, Actinobacillus, Cardiobacterium, Eikenella, and Kingella) • Chlamydia spp • Fungi (Candida and Aspergillus spp) • Histoplasmosis • Coxiella spp • Bartonella spp • Tropherema whippeli (Whipple's disease)

intravenous drug users). Clinically, the modified Duke's criteria are used for a more definitive diagnosis for infective endocarditis and is fulfilled in the presence of two major criteria; one major criterion and three minor criteria; or five minor criteria. These are summarized in Table 1.13.

Table 1.13 Modified Duke's Criteria

Criterion	Notes
Major criteria	
Positive blood culture for infective endocarditis	This includes (a) typical microorganism consistent with IE from two separate blood cultures, with *either* S. viridans, S. bovis, or HACEK group, *or* community-acquired S. aureus or enterococci, in the absence of a primary focus); (b) Microorganisms consistent with IE from persistently positive blood cultures, defined two positive cultures of blood samples drawn >12 hours apart *or* all of three or a majority of four separate cultures of blood (with first and last sample drawn one hour apart); and (c) a single positive blood culture for C. burnetii; or antiphase I IgG antibody titre >1:800.
Evidence of endocardial involvement	Positive echocardiographic findings for IE *or* new valvular regurgitation (worsening or changing of pre-existing murmur not sufficient). Positive echocardiographic findings for IE include: oscillating intracardiac mass on valve or supporting structures, in the path of regurgitant jets, or on implanted material in the absence of an alternative anatomic explanation, abscess, and new partial dehiscence of prosthetic valve.
Minor criteria	
Predisposition	Predisposing heart condition or intravenous drug use.
Fever	Temperature >38.0°C (100.4°F).
Vascular phenomena	Major arterial emboli, septic pulmonary infarcts, mycotic aneurysm, intracranial haemorrhage, conjunctival haemorrhages, and Janeway lesions.
Immunological phenomena	Glomerulonephritis, Osler's nodes, Roth spots, and rheumatoid factor.
Microbiological phenomena	Positive blood culture but does not meet a major criterion as noted above[a] or serological evidence of active infection with organism consistent with IE.
PCR findings	Broad-range PCR of 16S.
Echocardiographic findings	Consistent with IE but do not meet a major criterion as noted above.

Reproduced from Li JS, Sexton DJ, Mick N, et al., Proposed modifications to the Duke criteria for the diagnosis of infective endocarditis. *Clinical Infectious Diseases* 2000;30:633–8, by permission of Oxford University Press and Infectious Diseases Society of America

Further Reading

Gould F, Denning D, Elliott T, et al. (2012). Guidelines for the antibiotic treatment of endocarditis in adults: report of the Working Party of the British Society for Antimicrobial Chemotherapy. *Journal of Antimicrobial Chemotherapy* 67: 269–289.

Li J, Sexton D, Mick N, et al. (2000). Proposed modifications to the Duke criteria for the diagnosis of infective endocarditis. *Clinical Infectious Disease* 30: 633–638.

12. E) Second-degree heart block (Mobitz II)

A) Continue observation for deterioration

The rhythm strip demonstrates two P waves followed by a narrow QRS complex (Figure 1.9). The PR interval is fixed, when a QRS complex follows a P wave. Therefore, this represents second-degree (Mobitz II) heart block with 2:1 conduction block. Some candidates may confuse this with atrial flutter. Remember, in atrial flutter, there is often a characteristic undulating

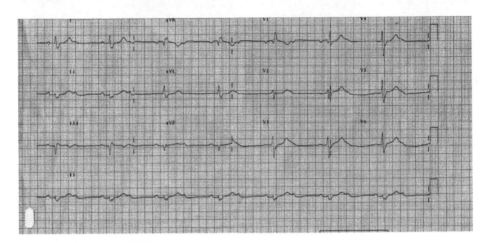

Figure 1.9 Twelve-lead ECG.

Reproduced with permission from *Oxford Textbook of Critical Care*, Second Edition. Edited by A Webb et al., Fig. 157.6. Oxford University Press, Oxford, UK, Copyright © 2016.

saw-toothed baseline, and atrial rate (P wave rate) is 300 per minute. There is no haemodynamic compromise. Heart block which occurs following an inferior or infero-posterior MI is often temporary and patients can simply be observed. In the presence of haemodynamic compromise, intravenous atropine may be administered acutely, as a bridge to urgent transvenous temporary pacing wire insertion.

Tutorial

Following an inferior or infero-posterior ST segment elevation MI, heart block can occur. Often, this is temporary and resolves after reperfusion therapy. If this is not associated with haemodynamic compromise, that is, hypotension, then simple observation of haemodynamic status and avoidance of rate-slowing drugs is all that is needed, and often the heart block will resolve within 48 hours. If there is haemodynamic compromise, then a temporary pacing wire is indicated. In such cases, if the heart block resolves, as is often the case, the temporary pacing wire can be removed after 24 hours with no need for a permanent pacemaker system. If heart block persists, then a permanent pacemaker system would be indicated.

Further Reading

Silverman M, Upshaw C, Lange H (2004). Woldemar Mobitz and His 1924 classification of second-degree atrioventricular block. *Circulation* 110(9): 1162–1167.

Strasberg B, Amat-Y-Leon F, Dhingra R, et al. (1981). Natural history of chronic second-degree atrioventricular nodal block. *Circulation* 63(5): 1043–1049.

13. D) Second-degree heart block (Mobitz I/Wenckebach)

D) Reassure and discharge

The rhythm strip demonstrates progressive prolongation of the PR interval followed by a P wave that is not followed by a QRS complex (Figure 1.10). This cycle then repeats itself. This is an example of Mobitz I second-degree heart block or Wenckebach phenomenon. The QRS complexes are narrow, indicating that the site of delay is likely to be in the AV node. Often the patients are asymptomatic, and this requires no further intervention. If patients are symptomatic, then a permanent pacemaker may become necessary.

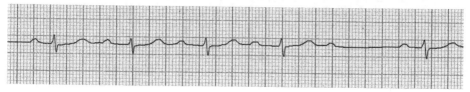

Figure 1.10 ECG rhythm strip.

Reproduced with permission from *Oxford Textbook of Critical Care*, Second Edition. Edited by A Webb et al., Fig. 157.5. Oxford University Press, Oxford, UK, Copyright © 2016.

Tutorial

The Mobitz I second-degree heart block (Wenckebach) is characterized by progressive prolongation of the PR interval, which results in a progressive shortening of the R-R interval. Ultimately, the atrial impulse fails to conduct. The PR interval is shortest in the first beat in the cycle, when the R-R interval is the longest. Mobitz type I block is caused by conduction delay in the AV node in 70% of patients and by conduction delay in the His-Purkinje system in the remaining 30%. The presence of a narrow QRS complex suggests the site of the delay is more likely to be in the AV node. However, a wide QRS complex may be observed with either AV nodal or infra-nodal conduction delay. Mobitz I block localized to the His-Purkinje system is associated with a risk of progression to complete heart block.

The most common cause of Wenckebach phenomenon is an incidental finding in young, and often, athletic individuals. Other causes include (a) rate-slowing drugs, that is, beta blockers, non-dihydropyridine calcium antagonists (verapamil and diltiazem), amiodarone and digoxin; (b) structural heart disease; (c) myocardial ischaemia; (d) aortic valve disease; and (e) Lyme disease.

Further Reading

Silverman M, Upshaw C, Lange H (2004). Woldemar Mobitz and His 1924 classification of second-degree atrioventricular block. *Circulation*110(9): 1162–1167.

Strasberg B, Amat-Y-Leon F, Dhingra RC, et al. (1981). Natural history of chronic second-degree atrioventricular nodal block. *Circulation* 63(5): 1043–1049.

14. B) Episodes of asystole

C) Stop atenolol

This patient has a pulse rate of 30 beats per minute and has an ECG which shows complete heart block as the underlying cause. They have clinical features consistent with hypothyroidism, which is associated with a bradycardic state. However, this is unlikely to be the cause of complete heart block, and the presence of complete heart block represents an underlying structural or conduction defect. As in this case, patients may remain stable with complete heart block prior to presentation. The intermittent dizzy spells are likely to represent short runs of asystole leading to decreased cerebral perfusion and thus dizziness. A rare complication of untreated complete heart block with a broad escape rhythm is ventricular tachycardia, but this far less common than brief periods of asystole. Hypothyroidism in itself does not cause dizziness. The patient's symptoms are not reported as orthostatic and thus postural hypotension is not the correct answer for this patient. Though it is worth noting that patients with heart block can present with such symptoms as they are unable to mount the usual compensatory reflex tachycardia in response to standing up. This is especially the case if they also have peripheral vascular disease or autonomic dysfunction which also results in a blunted physiological response to change in posture.

The treatment for this patient is cessation of rate-slowing medications. If the patient is haemodynamically compromised or symptomatic with the above rhythm, then intravenous atropine (up to 3 mg) may be administered. Intravenous glucagon may be used to reverse the effect of beta blockers and non-dihydropyridine calcium antagonists. If the patient remains haemodynamically compromised or symptomatic despite these measures, then insertion of a temporary pacing wire is necessary, as a bridge to a permanent pacemaker system. This patient is haemodynamically stable at present. The immediate treatment is cessation of rate-slowing medications, admission into hospital with cardiac monitoring, and ultimately insertion of a dual chamber permanent pacemaker system.

Tutorial

Third-degree heart block (complete heart block) occurs when where there is no conduction through the AV node, resulting in complete dissociation of atrial and ventricular activity. It is characterized by QRS complexes being conducted at their own rate and totally independently of the P waves. The ventricular escape mechanism can occur anywhere from the AV node to the bundle-branch Purkinje system. A high ventricular focus, that is, above the His bundle, produces a narrow QRS complex escape rhythm, while a lower ventricular focus, that is, at or below the His bundle, produces a wide QRS complex. A broad complex escape rhythm is associated with an increased risk of asystole. A rare complication of untreated complete heart block with a broad escape rhythm is ventricular tachycardia. When the block is at the level of the AV node, the escape rhythm is often junctional with a rate of 45–60 beats per minute. These patients are often haemodynamically stable and their heart rate increases in response to exercise and atropine. When the block is below the AV node, the escape rhythm arises from the His bundle or the bundle-branch Purkinje system at rates less than 45 beats per minute. These patients generally are haemodynamically unstable and their heart rate is unresponsive to exercise and atropine.

Causes of complete heart block include (a) rate-slowing drugs, that is, beta blockers, non-dihydropyridine calcium antagonists (verapamil and diltiazem), amiodarone and digoxin; (b) structural heart disease; (c) myocardial ischaemia; (d) severe hyperkalaemia; (e) aortic valve disease (especially following aortic valve surgery); (f) Lyme disease; (g) *Trypanosoma cruzi* infection; and (h) maternal anti-Ro and anti-La antibodies (congenital complete heart block).

Further Reading

Kojic E, Hardarson T, Sigfusson N, Sigvaldason H (1999). The prevalence and prognosis of third-degree atrioventricular conduction block: the Reykjavik study. *Journal of International Medicine* 246(1): 81–86.

15. D) Polymorphic ventricular tachycardia

The ECG demonstrates a prolonged QT interval, most likely secondary to amiodarone therapy. There are many causes of QT prolongation, but the most common cause is drug-induced (Box 1.5). This man has a history of paroxysmal atrial flutter, which he is able to recognize, and in his case is not associated with symptoms, thus making this unlikely as a cause for the presenting symptoms. A depressed TSH is suggestive of thyrotoxicosis, but unlikely with a normal serum free T4. Amiodarone therapy can alter thyroid function tests, and a complete assessment using both TSH and serum free T4 should be made. In the context of QT prolongation, the most likely cause for the intermittent palpitations and dizziness would be polymorphic ventricular tachycardia (torsade de pointes). Whilst hypomagnesaemia is a cause for QT prolongation, this is often seen with severe long-standing hypomagnesaemia—a slightly reduced serum magnesium, as in this case, is unlikely to be the primary cause. Furthermore, hypomagnesaemia is not the cause of the symptoms. The best answer is polymorphic ventricular tachycardia.

Tutorial

Torsade de pointes is defined as polymorphic ventricular tachycardia, in which the morphology and axis of the QRS complexes varies from beat to beat. This was originally described as regular variation of the QRS vector from positive to negative and was termed torsade de pointes or 'twisting of points' (Figure 1.11). This often occurs in the setting of a prolonged QT interval (often ≥600 ms). Torsade usually occurs in bursts and is often not sustained. The ventricular rate can be in the range of 150–250 beats per minute. The underlying basis for this rhythm disturbance is prolongation of phase III of the cardiac action potential. Torsade is inherently an unstable rhythm and can degenerate into ventricular fibrillation. Therapy should begin as soon as the diagnosis is made.

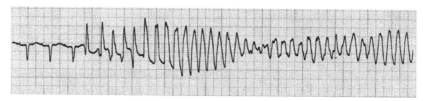

Figure 1.11 Polymorphic ventricular tachycardia (torsade de pointes).

Reproduced from *ESC CardioMed* (Third Edition) (online only product). Edited by Camm, Luscher, Maurer, and Serruys (2019) Fig. 48.11.10, www.oup.com. By permission of Oxford University Press and European Society of Cardiology.

If a patient is haemodynamically compromised, then synchronized DC cardioversion is indicated. The most effective initial treatment is the administration of intravenous magnesium (2–4 g). Magnesium is very effective, even in those with normal magnesium levels. If this fails, then a repeat dose of magnesium can be given, but beware of hypermagnesaemia (depression of neuromuscular

---

Box 1.5 Causes of QT prolongation

- Electrolyte disturbance
  - Hypokalaemia
  - Hypomagnesaemia
  - Hypocalcaemia
- Drugs
  - Class IA (procainamide, quinidine, disopyramide)
  - Class IC (flecainide)
  - Class III (sotalol, amiodarone)
  - Antihistamines (astemizole, terfenadine)
  - Macrolides (erythromycin, clarithromycin)
  - Fluoroquinolones (ciprofloxacin, nitrofurantoin)
  - Anti-psychotics (tricyclic anti-depressants, phenothiazines, lithium)
  - Anthracycline chemotherapeutics (doxorubicin, daumomycin)
  - Antifungals (ketoconazole)
  - High dose methadone
- Hypothermia
- Congenital
  - Jervell-Lange-Neilson syndrome (AR, deafness)
  - Romano-Ward syndrome (AD, not associated with deafness)
  - Channelopathies (LQT1-8; LQT1-3 account for most cases)

function). Hypokalaemia should be corrected if present. Approximately 80% of torsade rhythms are initiated by a pause. Thus, in cases of sustained torsades, other therapies include an isoprenaline infusion, atropine, or overdrive pacing (up to 140 beats per minute) to prevent such pauses and reduce the QT interval.

However, in cases of torsades secondary to congenital prolonged QT syndromes, the primary abnormality is with an abnormally high sympathetic tone, and isoprenaline infusions should be avoided. In such cases the treatment is with beta blockers. If the use of beta blockers results in symptomatic bradycardia, then a permanent pacemaker system is indicated in the long-term management of these patients, so that beta blockers can be given.

Further Reading

Wellens H (2001). Electrophysiology: ventricular tachycardia: diagnosis of broad QRS complex tachycardia. *Heart* 86(5): 579–585.

16. B) Intravenous magnesium

The rhythm strip demonstrates sinus rhythm, which is followed by a broad complex tachycardia, which twists about the isoelectric line. This is polymorphic ventricular tachycardia (torsade de pointes). The patient is not haemodynamically compromised. Hypokalaemia should be corrected, and the potassium in this case is low in the normal range. It will not be harmful to administer potassium. Sotalol should be stopped immediately. However, the most effective *initial* treatment is intravenous magnesium, as this will often terminate the arrhythmia. Magnesium should be administered even if magnesium levels are normal. Amiodarone should not be used in such cases, as this itself may prolong the QT interval. A synchronized DC shock would be indicated if the patient was haemodynamically compromised.

Tutorial

In torsade, if a patient is haemodynamically compromised, then synchronized DC cardioversion is indicated. Whilst this is often not sustained, it is inherently an unstable rhythm, and can degenerate into ventricular fibrillation, and thus therapy should begin as soon as the diagnosis is made. If the patient is haemodynamically stable, the most effective initial treatment is the administration of intravenous magnesium (2–4 g). Magnesium is very effective, even in those with normal magnesium levels. If this fails, then a repeat dose of magnesium can be given, but beware of hypermagnesaemia (depression of neuromuscular function). Hypokalaemia should be corrected if present. Approximately 80% of torsade rhythms are started by a pause. Thus, in cases of sustained or recurrent torsades, other therapies include an isoprenaline infusion, atropine, or overdrive pacing (up to 140 beats per minute) should be considered to prevent such pauses and shorten the QT interval.

Further Reading

Pellegrini C, Scheinman M (2010). Clinical management of ventricular tachycardia. *Current Problems in Cardiology* 35(9): 453–504.

17. E) Unstable angina

This gentleman has a strong cardiovascular risk profile. The recent history of chest pain is characteristic of cardiac ischaemia. His ECG shows regional changes with infero-lateral ischaemia. The troponin is negative. This would be best described as USA. The fact that this patient has recently been treated for respiratory tract infection, the presence of leucocytosis, and raised inflammatory markers suggest a diagnosis of myocarditis or myopericarditis. However, leucocytosis and raised inflammatory markers may be observed in acute coronary syndromes, representing myocardial necrosis. ECG changes in myocarditis or myopericarditis are often global, and often the pain is atypical, pleuritic, and positional. The characteristic nature of the pain in this case, in the presence of significant cardiovascular risk factors, with localized ECG changes indicates coronary ischaemia and points to a diagnosis of USA. If the troponin were positive, then the diagnosis would be non-ST elevation MI. A low sodium and mildly deranged LFTs may prompt the candidate to consider the diagnosis of atypical pneumonia. Atypical pneumonia is unlikely given the normal CXR. The deranged LFTs may be secondary to statins and/or antibiotics. Pulmonary embolism would be associated with hypoxia and pleuritic chest pain. Regional infero-lateral ischaemic ECG changes are not characteristically seen in pulmonary embolism.

Tutorial

Acute coronary syndromes include USA, NSTEMI, and STEMI. Those without persistent ST-elevation represent a continuum from USA to NSTEMI and can be further classified on the basis of troponin release, a biochemical marker of myocardial cell death (Figure 1.12).

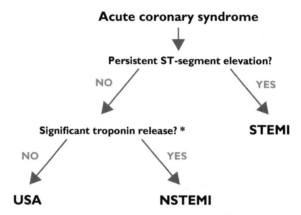

Figure 1.12 Classification of acute coronary syndromes.

* Non-ST segment elevation acute coronary syndrome represents a continuum from USA to NSTEMI. Differentiating NSTEMI from USA depends upon the troponin release being greater than the cut-off point. This varies between different laboratories and troponin assays used. Troponin levels should be measured after 12 hours from the onset of chest pain.

Further Reading

Basra S, Virani S, Paniagua D, et al. (2016). Acute coronary syndromes: unstable angina and non-ST elevation myocardial infarction. *Heart Failure Clinics* 12(1): 31–34.

18. D) RBBB with left axis deviation

Cardiac catheter data show a step up in oxygen saturation in the low RA, suggesting a left-to-right shunt at this level. There are elevated RV and PA pressures indicating pulmonary hypertension. The large 'V' waves in the RA and LA (PCWP) suggest tricuspid and mitral regurgitation. The diagnosis which best fits this is an ostium primum atrial septal defect with pulmonary hypertension. A step up in oxygen saturation in the high RA would suggest a sinus venosus atrial septal defect and in the mid RA would suggest an ostium secundum atrial septal defect. The ECG in ostium primum defects shows partial or complete RBBB with left axis deviation, whereas in ostium secundum defects there is partial or complete RBBB with right axis deviation. Right ventricular hypertrophy would also be seen on the ECG given the pulmonary hypertension, but this option is not available.

Tutorial

Atrial septal defect (ASD) is characterized by a defect in the inter-atrial septum allowing pulmonary venous return from the left atrium to pass directly to the right atrium. There are four types of ASDs: (a) ostium secundum—the most common type of ASD accounting for 75% of cases; (b) ostium primum—the second most common type of ASD accounting for 15–20% of cases; it is a form of atrioventricular septal defect and is commonly associated with mitral and tricuspid valve abnormalities; (c) sinus venosus ASD—seen in 5–10% of all ASDs; the defect is located along the superior aspect of the atrial septum and often associated with anomalous connection of the right-sided pulmonary veins; and (d) coronary sinus ASD—a rare defect characterized by an unroofed coronary sinus and a persistent left superior vena cava that drains into the left atrium.

The size of the left-to-right shunt depends on the defect size, the relative compliance of the ventricles, and the pulmonary and systemic vascular resistance. With small ASD, left atrial pressure may exceed right atrial pressure, whereas with large ASD, mean atrial pressures are nearly always identical. Shunting across the interatrial septum is usually left to right and occurs predominantly in late ventricular systole and early diastole. Left-to-right shunting may not be explained by pressure gradients alone, as the right and left atrial pressures may be similar. The right atrium is more compliant than the left atrium, and this encourages left-to-right shunting. However, transient and small right-to-left shunts may occur, especially during deep inspiration (decreasing intrathoracic pressure with increased venous return), even in the absence of pulmonary hypertension. A chronic left-to-right shunt results in increased pulmonary blood flow that can alter the pulmonary vascular resistance leading to pulmonary arterial hypertension, and even shunt reversal: Eisenmenger's syndrome. ASDs can remain undiagnosed for decades and even moderate-to-large ASDs may not cause symptoms in childhood. Common childhood symptoms include easy fatigability, exertional breathlessness, and recurrent respiratory infections. In childhood, the diagnosis is often considered after incidental detection of a heart murmur or after an abnormal CXR or ECG finding. If undetected in childhood, symptoms can develop gradually over decades and reflect changing ventricular compliance with age, pulmonary hypertension, atrial arrhythmias, and, sometimes, those associated with mitral valve disease in an ostium primum ASD. Most patients with ASD who survive beyond the sixth decade will be symptomatic. Clinical deterioration in older patients occurs due to: (a) age-related decrease in left ventricular compliance augmenting the left-to-right shunt; (b) atrial arrhythmias, which increase in frequency after the fourth decade and can precipitate right ventricular failure; (c) development of pulmonary hypertension in the presence of a persistent large left-to-right shunt; or (d) development of clinically significant mitral regurgitation associated with an ostium primum ASD.

Characteristic findings in patients with secundum ASD are (a) right-axis deviation; and (b) rSR' pattern in V_1 or RBBB (delayed postero-basal activation of the ventricular septum and enlargement of the right ventricular outflow tract). Characteristic findings in patients with primum ASD are (a) left-axis deviation; and (b) rSR' pattern in V_1 or RBBB (delayed postero-basal activation of the ventricular septum and enlargement of the right ventricular outflow tract). Left-axis deviation and a negative P wave in lead III suggest a sinus venosus defect. Increasing pulmonary hypertension can cause loss of the rSR' pattern in V_1 with the development of tall monophasic R waves. A prolonged P-R interval can be seen in familial ASD or ostium primum ASD secondary to left atrial enlargement with an increased distance between the SA and AV node produced by the defect itself. In the presence of a clinically significant left-to-right shunt, the CXR will show (a) cardiomegaly owing to dilatation of the right atrium and right ventricle; and (b) prominent pulmonary artery and pulmonary vascular markings. Diagnosis can be made using transthoracic or transoesophageal echocardiography. Transoesophageal echocardiography is required to image a sinus venosus ASD. Cardiac catheterization can help confirm the diagnosis, demonstrating a step up in oxygen saturations at the level of the shunt. If high oxygen saturation is present in the superior vena cava or if the catheter enters a pulmonary vein directly from the right atrium, a sinus venosus ASD is likely.

Patients with small defects and normal pulmonary artery pressures require reassurance. Those with larger defects with pulmonary hypertension and/or right ventricular failure require diuretics for congestive symptoms, treatment of pulmonary hypertension, and ASD closure (surgical or percutaneous) if no contraindications exist. The indication for ASD closure is increasing pulmonary: systemic blood flow (Q_p:Q_s >2:1). The development of severe pulmonary hypertension is associated with shunt reversal and development of Eisenmenger's syndrome. If the pulmonary hypertension is irreversible, then closure is contraindicated. However, if one can demonstrate reversible pulmonary hypertension, then closure may be undertaken, if there is evidence of: (a) pulmonary reactivity with a pulmonary vasodilator challenge or (b) lung biopsy findings consistent with reversible pulmonary arterial changes.

Further Reading

O'Connor M, McDaniel N, Brady W (2008). The paediatric electrocardiogram part III: congenital heart disease and other cardiac syndromes. *American Journal of Emergency Medicine* 26(4): 497–503.

19. E) Pansystolic murmur at the lower left sternal edge

There is a step up in oxygen saturation in the RV, thus suggesting a left-to-right shunt at this level, that is, a ventricular septal defect (VSD). There is no evidence of pulmonary hypertension. Atrial septal defects will classically show a step up in oxygen saturation in the RA. A patent ductus arteriosus will show a step up in oxygen saturation in the PA. A VSD is classically associated with a harsh pansystolic murmur at the sternal edge. An ejection systolic murmur at the upper left sternal edge (pulmonary area) would be heard with pulmonary stenosis or increased pulmonary flow (as in ASD, though this would be associated with fixed splitting of the second heart sound). A loud pulmonary component of the second heart sound is present in pulmonary hypertension. A continuous murmur (through systole and diastole) at the upper right sternal edge is heard in a patient with patent ductus arteriosus.

Tutorial

VSD is an embryologic malformation of the ventricular septum resulting in abnormal communication between the left and right ventricles. It can occur as an isolated lesion or in combination with other congenital cardiac anomalies. A left-to-right shunt occurs at the level of the ventricles, which increases pulmonary blood flow. Occasionally perimembranous defects can result in a left ventricle to right atrium shunt (Gerbode defect). Spontaneous closure of small defects occurs in approximately 50% of patients, often in early childhood (by two years of age). Closure is uncommon after four years of age. This is most frequently observed in muscular (80%) followed by perimembranous (35–40%) defects. Chronically increased pulmonary blood flow results in pulmonary hypertension and left ventricular volume and pressure overload. A small VSD with high resistance to flow permits only a small left-to-right shunt and has no significant haemodynamic consequences. A moderate-large defect allows a large left-to-right shunt, and with time can result in haemodynamic consequences. A small VSD usually causes no symptoms. Patients with moderately sized VSDs frequently have a history of one or more episodes of pneumonia and/or upper respiratory tract infection per year. Patients with VSDs complicated by pulmonary hypertension and shunt reversal (i.e. Eisenmenger's complex) may present with exertional breathlessness, syncope, haemoptysis, cyanosis, clubbing, and polycythaemia. Infective endocarditis is a recognized complication, irrespective of the size of the defect.

The most common physical finding is a harsh pansystolic murmur along the left sternal border, often loudest at the third and fourth intercostal spaces, and widely transmitted over the precordium. The murmur does not radiate to the left axilla, as with mitral regurgitation, and does not increase in intensity with inspiration, as with tricuspid regurgitation. Generally, the smaller the defect, the more turbulent the blood flow through it and the louder the murmur. A systolic thrill can commonly be palpated in the region of the murmur along the lower left sternal border. A systolic thrill is less common with large defects. When the left-to-right shunt is large, a mid-diastolic, low-pitched murmur can be heard over the left sternal border and apex, suggesting increased flow through the mitral valve. As pulmonary hypertension and Eisenmenger's complex develops, the murmur and thrill disappear, and signs of pulmonary hypertension are present. A pansystolic murmur in this setting is likely to represent tricuspid regurgitation.

The CXR is often normal with small defects. In larger defects, there may be cardiomegaly indicating left ventricular +/− right ventricular enlargement, left atrial enlargement, prominent pulmonary vascular markings, and pulmonary congestion. The ECG is often normal with small defects, though a deeper-than-normal S wave in the right precordial leads or a mildly increased R wave in lead V_5 or V_6 sometimes indicates mild left ventricular hypertrophy and volume overload. With larger defects there may be features of left +/− right ventricular hypertrophy. Biventricular hypertrophy is often present in large defects accompanied by equiphasic RS complexes in the mid-precordial leads (Katz-Wachtel phenomenon). The defect can be seen on transthoracic echocardiography. Cardiac catheterization shows a step in oxygen saturation at the level of the ventricles and provides precise information about the magnitude of the shunt as well as pulmonary artery pressures and pulmonary vascular resistance.

Patients with small defects and normal pulmonary artery pressure require re-assurance only. Those with larger defects with pulmonary hypertension and heart failure may require diuretics for congestive symptoms; treatment of left ventricular dysfunction; treatment of pulmonary hypertension; and VSD closure (surgical or percutaneous) if no contraindications exist. Indications for VSD closure include: (a) increasing pulmonary: systemic blood flow (Q_p:Q_s > 2:1); (b) left ventricular dilatation; (c) left ventricular dysfunction; (d) recurrent endocarditis; (e) development of (at least mild) aortic regurgitation through prolapse of the right coronary cusp of the aortic valve in supracristal defects; and (e) acute rupture of interventricular septum complicating acute myocardial infarction. A contraindication to VSD closure is the presence of irreversible severe pulmonary hypertension (defined as pulmonary vascular resistance $\geq$ ⅔ systemic vascular resistance). If one can demonstrate reversible pulmonary hypertension, then closure may be undertaken (evidence of pulmonary reactivity with a pulmonary vasodilator challenge, or lung biopsy findings consist with reversible pulmonary arterial changes).

Further Reading

Frank J, Jacobe K (2011). Evaluation and management of heart murmurs in children. *American Family Physician* 84(7): 793–800.

20. E) Stop ramipril

Cardiac catheter data show no intracardiac shunting but evidence of pulmonary hypertension. However, the most striking abnormality is a pressure drop from the LV into the ascending aorta, that is, a pressure gradient of 68 mmHg across the aortic valve. This is often termed 'aortic pull-back gradient', as the catheter tip is pulled back from the LV cavity across the aortic valve into the ascending aorta. An aortic pull-back gradient of 68 mmHg represents severe aortic stenosis. This patient has severe symptomatic aortic stenosis. The left ventriculogram indicates preserved left ventricular systolic function. Vasodilator therapy, that is, the use of nitrates, ACE inhibitors, and angiotensin II receptor blockers are contraindicated in severe aortic stenosis, and thus stopping ramipril is the most appropriate initial management step. The definitive management for this patient will be aortic valve replacement. This patient has a long-standing history of asthma, and with a recent history of progressive breathlessness, beta-blocker therapy is unlikely to be the cause of the deteriorating symptoms. Obstructive airways disease is a relative contraindication to beta blockers, though these are often well tolerated in these patients. If not tolerated, then more cardio-selective beta$_1$ blockers, for example bisoprolol, may be considered. There is no indication for diuretics as the CXR does not show pulmonary congestion.

Tutorial

Common causes of aortic stenosis include bicuspid aortic valve defect (most common cause in the young), degenerative calcification (most common cause in the elderly), and rheumatic valve disease (which has declined dramatically). Rare causes include congenital, infective endocarditis, hyperuricaemia, alkaptonuria, and Paget's disease of the bone. The severity of aortic stenosis can be classified using the valve area and/or transvalvular pressure gradient. The normal aortic valve orifice is 3–4 cm^2 in area, and current guidelines have graded aortic stenosis as mild (valve area >1.5 cm^2), moderate (valve area: 1.5–1.0 cm^2) and severe (valve area <1.0 cm^2). Transthoracic echocardiography is the most useful method for assessing severity of aortic stenosis and provides a physiological maximum instantaneous gradient across the aortic valve. The gradient is calculated using the modified Bernoulli equation ($\Delta P = 4v^2$, where v = peak velocity across the aortic valve). Echocardiography also allows calculation of aortic valve area. The mean gradient across the aortic valve is calculated using the Gorlin formula which incorporates the aortic valve area, cardiac output, and heart rate. Reduction in valve area to 1.5 cm^2 is associated with little haemodynamic disturbance. However, beyond this, any further decrement in aortic valve area produces a steep rise in left ventricular outflow obstruction. As a general rule, severe aortic stenosis is defined as a mean gradient >50 mmHg. A pull-back gradient, as obtained during cardiac catheterization, represents the difference between the peak systolic pressures in the left ventricular cavity and the ascending aorta, that is, peak-peak gradient. In fact, peak aortic and peak left ventricular systolic pressures do not occur simultaneously (left ventricular systolic pressure peaks before that of the ascending aorta). Thus, the peak-peak gradient is lower than the maximum instantaneous gradient across the aortic valve measured at echocardiography.

Complications of aortic stenosis include: left ventricular failure; sudden death (predominantly in symptomatic aortic stenosis); pulmonary hypertension; arrhythmias (atrial fibrillation and ventricular tachycardia); heart block (calcification of the conduction system); infective endocarditis; systemic embolic complications (disintegration of aortic valve apparatus); haemolytic anaemia; and iron deficient anaemia (Heyde's syndrome—association between aortic stenosis and occult gastrointestinal bleeding, usually from colonic angiodysplastic lesions). The primary indication for aortic valve replacement in aortic stenosis is symptomatic severe aortic stenosis (mean gradient >50 mmHg). For asymptomatic patients, indications for valve replacement include either moderate/severe aortic stenosis undergoing other cardiac surgery, that is, coronary artery bypass surgery, aortic surgery or other valve surgery; or severe aortic stenosis *and* any of the following: (a) left ventricular systolic dysfunction (mean gradient >40 mmHg); (b) an abnormal BP response to exercise (on *supervised* exercise treadmill testing); (c) ventricular tachycardia; or (d) valve area <0.6 cm^2.

In patients without left ventricular outflow obstruction, a decrease in systemic vascular resistance (as occurs during exercise) results in increased cardiac output so that BP is subsequently maintained. If severe aortic stenosis is present, cardiac output cannot increase in response to decreased systemic vascular resistance. As a result, BP falls, leading to hypotension and syncope. For this reason, vasodilator therapy, for example nitrates, ACE inhibitors, and angiotensin II receptor blockers are relatively contraindicated in severe aortic stenosis. However, ACE inhibitors may have an emerging role in the management of patients with aortic stenosis. Sclerotic aortic valve tissues demonstrably express angiotensin II and ACE, which may contribute to valve inflammation, calcification, and disease progression. ACE inhibitors may be beneficial for left ventricular hypertrophy, apoptosis, and fibrosis which are all consequences of aortic stenosis. Patients with mild-moderate aortic stenosis often tolerate ACE inhibitors well. However, the routine use of ACE inhibitors in severe aortic stenosis is not currently recommended.

Further Reading

Alame A, Karatasakis A, Karacsonyi J, et al. (2017). Comparison of the American College of Cardiology/American Heart Association and the European Society of Cardiology Guidelines for the management of patients with valvular heart disease. *Journal of Invasive Cardiology* 29(9): 320–326.

Newby D, Cowell S, Boon N (2006). Emerging medical treatments for aortic stenosis: statins, angiotensin converting enzyme inhibitors, or both? *Heart* 92: 729–734.

21. D) Pericardial tamponade

This patient presents with a one-week history of progressive breathlessness. He is currently in shock with a raised venous pressure, hypotension, and cool peripheries. The differential diagnosis of raised venous pressure and hypotension includes: (a) pericardial tamponade; (b) tension pneumothorax; (c) massive pulmonary embolism; and (d) congestive cardiac failure (cardiogenic shock). The presence of LBBB and cardiomegaly with blunting of the costophrenic angles support pulmonary oedema, but with acute cardiogenic shock due to new onset LBBB (classified as a STEMI) one would expect chest pain and also expect a greater degree of hypoxia. Furthermore, the presence of small bilateral pleural effusions may be seen with pericardial effusions and secondary to hypoalbuminaemia. Tension pneumothorax has been ruled out by the presence of breath sounds bilaterally and a normal chest X-ray. Pulmonary embolism is unlikely since any massive pulmonary embolism which could cause hypotension to this degree would undoubtedly be associated with hypoxia. The patient does have low albumin and mild derangement of liver function tests, but this is likely due to hepatic congestion rather than acute liver failure. Urine dipstick shows only +1 of protein which likely represents underlying diabetic kidney disease. A protein:creatinine ratio would be the definitive test to diagnose nephrotic range proteinuria but is unlikely to be significantly raised given there is only +1 protein on urinary dipstick (though it is worth noting the proteinuria due to myeloma kidney can often be negative or low on urinary dipstick testing). Furthermore, proteinuria would not result in such profound hypotension or cause cardiomegaly.

Thus, the most likely diagnosis that fits the history and examination findings is pericardial tamponade, probably secondary to a relapse of underlying lymphoproliferative disorder given his weight loss.

Tutorial

Pericardial tamponade is a medical emergency caused by the accumulation of fluid in the pericardial space that reduces ventricular filling with subsequent haemodynamic compromise. The pericardial space normally contains 20–50 mL of fluid. The amount of pericardial fluid needed to impair the diastolic filling of the heart depends on the rate of fluid accumulation and the compliance of the pericardium. The causes of pericardial effusions are listed in Box 1.6. As tamponade develops, there is marked reduction in diastolic filling because the transmural distending cardiac pressures are insufficient to overcome the increased pericardial pressures. Rapid accumulation of as little as 150 mL of fluid can result in a marked increase in pericardial pressure and severely restrict cardiac output, whereas chronic accumulation of 1000 mL of fluid may occur without any significant effect on diastolic filling of the heart. Chronic accumulation results in adaptive stretching of the pericardium, and a more compliant pericardium can allow considerable fluid accumulation without haemodynamic insult. Because the heart is compressed throughout the cardiac cycle due to increased pericardial pressures, the venous return is also impaired and right ventricular collapse occurs. This can be seen on echocardiography.

Box 1.6 Causes of pericardial effusion

- Idiopathic
- Infectious:
  - Viral: coxsackievirus A and B, hepatitis viruses, HIV
  - Bacterial: pneumococci, streptococci, staphylococci, *Mycoplasma*, *Legionella*, *Mycobacteria*
  - Fungal: histoplasmosis, coccidioidomycosis, *Candida*
- Malignancy:
  - Lung
  - Breast
  - Lymphoma
  - Leukaemia
  - Kaposi sarcoma
- Post-operative/post-procedural:
  - Post-cardiac surgery
  - Post percutaneous coronary intervention
  - Post myocardial biopsy
- Autoimmune disease:
  - Systemic lupus erythematosus
  - Rheumatoid arthritis
  - Ankylosing spondylitis
  - Scleroderma
  - Wegener granulomatosis
- Drugs:
  - Hydralazine
  - Isoniazid
  - Minoxidil
  - Anticoagulants
- Other:
  - Uraemia
  - Myxoedema
  - Radiation therapy
  - Acute myocardial infarction (free wall rupture)
  - Aortic dissection
  - Trauma

Pericardial tamponade is a clinical diagnosis. Beck's triad comprises a clinical complex of: (a) raised jugular venous pressure; (b) hypotension; and (c) diminished heart sounds. Pulsus paradoxus may be present. Other causes of pulsus paradoxus include constrictive pericarditis, severe asthma, restrictive cardiomyopathy, massive pulmonary embolism, and right ventricular infarction with shock. Pulsus paradoxus may be absent in patients with significantly elevated LV diastolic pressures, ASD, pulmonary hypertension, and aortic regurgitation. Kussmaul's sign, a paradoxical increase in venous pressure during inspiration, is usually observed in patients with constrictive pericarditis but is occasionally observed in patients with tamponade. Ewart's sign (also known as Pins sign) is dullness to percussion beneath the angle of the left scapula owing to compression of the left lung by pericardial fluid.

Echocardiography is the imaging modality of choice for the diagnosis of pericardial effusion, as the test can be performed rapidly and in unstable patients. Pericardial effusion appears as an echo-free space between the visceral and parietal pericardium. Early effusions tend to accumulate posteriorly owing to an expandable postero-lateral pericardium. Right ventricular diastolic collapse is a feature on echocardiography. Pericardiocentesis serves as both a diagnostic and therapeutic intervention.

Further Reading

Hoit B (2007). Pericardial disease and pericardial tamponade. *Critical Care Medicine* 35(8): 355–364.

Little W, Freeman G (2006). Pericardial disease. *Circulation*. 113(12): 1622–1632.

22. D) Mitral valve annuloplasty

The cardiac catheter data demonstrate a number of findings: (a) the large 'V' wave in the right atrial pressure suggests tricuspid regurgitation; (b) the presence of an 'a' wave in the right atrial pressure suggests underlying sinus rhythm; (c) there is a step up in oxygen saturation in the mid RA, suggesting left-to-right shunting at this level—this would otherwise be in keeping with an ostium secundum atrial septal defect; (d) the elevated PA pressures indicate pulmonary hypertension; and (e) there is a diastolic pressure gradient (19 mmHg) across the mitral valve (PCWP—LV diastolic pressure). This would be in keeping with severe mitral stenosis. Tricuspid regurgitation is often present in patients with mitral stenosis, even after mitral valve annuloplasty/surgery, and reflects underlying pulmonary hypertension.

The two main structural abnormalities are the presence of mitral stenosis and a left-to-right shunt at the level of the interatrial septum. These may represent two separate pathologies, that is, mitral stenosis or an ostium secundum atrial septal defect. Given that this patient has previously had a successful percutaneous cardiac procedure for breathlessness, and now presents with recurrent breathlessness and the presence of severe mitral stenosis, the above data would be consistent with previous percutaneous mitral valve annuloplasty (balloon valvotomy). This involves inflating a balloon across the stenosed mitral valve and is used in selected patients. The best results are seen with thin mobile leaflets that have commissural fusion, little calcification or subchordal thickening. The presence of significant mitral regurgitation is a contraindication, as balloon valvuloplasty may result in a significant increase in the degree of regurgitation.

The balloon is introduced via the venous circulation into the right side of the heart and passed into the left atrium via a transseptal puncture creating an iatrogenic ASD. This combination of mitral stenosis and ASD is termed the Lutembacher syndrome. Lutembacher syndrome is defined as a combination of mitral stenosis and a left-to-right shunt at atrial level, typically via an ostium secundum defect. Both these defects can be either congenital or acquired. Initially, Lutembacher described this syndrome in 1918 in a 61-year-old patient who was thought to have congenital mitral stenosis and ASD. In fact, the mitral stenosis was rheumatic in origin, and thus it was eventually defined as congenital ASD and acquired mitral stenosis. In many cases, mitral annuloplasty is often used to treat mitral stenosis, which results in an iatrogenic ASD secondary to transseptal puncture. This is more common that a congenital ASD.

Tutorial

The most common cause of mitral stenosis is rheumatic fever. Other causes include congenital mitral stenosis, rheumatoid arthritis, systemic lupus erythematosus, carcinoid syndrome, mucopolysaccharidoses, Fabry's disease, methysergide therapy, and Whipple's disease. The normal area of the mitral valve orifice is 4–6 cm². Narrowing of the valve area to less than 2.5 cm² impedes the free flow of blood between the left atrium and left ventricle and increases left atrial pressure. This is required to maintain transmitral flow and patients start to develop symptoms. Severe mitral stenosis occurs when the opening is reduced to 1 cm². At this stage, a left atrial pressure of 25 mmHg is required to maintain a normal cardiac output. With progressive stenosis, flow restriction reduces cardiac output. The left atrium enlarges and pulmonary venous and capillary pressures increase. The resulting pulmonary congestion and reduced cardiac output can mimic primary left ventricular failure, but left ventricular contractility is normal in most cases. Chronic elevation of left atrial pressure leads to pulmonary hypertension; tricuspid and pulmonary regurgitation; and secondary right heart failure. The severity of mitral stenosis can be assessed using echocardiography that can measure both mitral valve orifice area and mean pressure gradient.

The most common symptom of mitral stenosis is exertional breathlessness. Haemoptysis may occur if the bronchial veins rupture, due to elevation in pulmonary venous pressure. Hoarseness can develop from compression of the left recurrent laryngeal nerve against the pulmonary artery by the enlarged left atrium (Ortner's syndrome). Compression of bronchi by the enlarged left atrium can cause persistent cough. Pregnant women with mild mitral stenosis may become symptomatic during their second trimester because of the increase in blood volume and cardiac output. Atrial fibrillation is common, although some patients may be in sinus rhythm. Other ECG findings include left atrial hypertrophy (bifid P waves in lead II if in sinus rhythm) and left atrial dilatation (inverted or biphasic P waves in V_1–V_2 if in sinus rhythm). CXR findings include double right heart border (left atrial enlargement); splaying of the carina (an old sign used to demonstrate a grossly dilated left atrium); pulmonary congestion; and prominent pulmonary arteries (pulmonary hypertension).

Further Reading

Nishimura R, Otto C, Bonow R, et al. (2014). AHA/ACC guideline for the management of patients with valvular heart disease: a report of the American College of Cardiology/American Heart Association Task Force on Practice Guidelines. *Journal of American College of Cardiology* 63(22): e57–185.

23. D) RBBB with right axis deviation

There is a step up in oxygen saturation at the level of the mid RA, suggesting a left-to-right shunt at this level. The diagnosis is ostium secundum ASD. A step up in oxygen saturation in the high RA would suggest a sinus venosus atrial septal defect and in the low RA would suggest an ostium primum atrial septal defect. The ECG in ostium primum defects shows partial or complete RBBB with left axis deviation, whereas in ostium secundum defects there is partial or complete RBBB with right axis deviation. Right ventricular hypertrophy occurs secondary to elevated RV systolic pressures and pulmonary hypertension but is absent in this case. Biatrial enlargement is often present on the ECG in patients with ASD, but this is not a universal finding, and often occurs in the setting of long-standing shunts, the associated presence of mitral and tricuspid regurgitation (as with ostium primum defects), or pulmonary hypertension (right atrial enlargement).

Tutorial

See question 18.

24. B) Eisenmenger's complex

This patient presents with cyanosis and clubbing, indicating cyanotic congenital heart disease. The cardiac catheter data demonstrate a number of findings: (a) large V wave in the right atrial pressure, suggesting tricuspid regurgitation; (b) severe pulmonary hypertension with elevated PA and RV systolic pressures; (c) no gradient across the RVOT (RV systolic pressure—PA systolic pressure), thus excluding pulmonary stenosis or Fallot's; furthermore, Fallot's tetralogy is associated with elevated RV pressures and normal PA pressures; (d) a low PA diastolic pressure, suggesting pulmonary regurgitation; and (e) a marked reduction in saturations in the LV, thus suggesting a right-to-left shunt at the level of the ventricular septum. If the PCWP (left atrial pressure) were elevated, then this would suggest a right-to-left shunt at the level of the interatrial septum. Thus, the diagnosis in this case is Eisenmenger's syndrome with an underlying ventricular septal defect—this is termed Eisenmenger's complex.

Tutorial

Eisenmenger's syndrome results from pulmonary hypertension with reversal of left-to-right shunts (ASD, VSD, PDA, or aortopulmonary window). When due to an underlying VSD, it is termed 'Eisenmenger's complex'. An aortopulmonary window is an uncommon congenital cardiac defect resulting from loss of the septum between the aorta and pulmonary artery, giving rise to a communication between the two arteries. In half the cases, this occurs in isolation, whereas in the remaining half it occurs in conjunction with more complex heart disease.

Complications of Eisenmenger's syndrome include: haemoptysis; right ventricular failure; paradoxical embolism; infective endocarditis; sudden death; polycythaemia; thrombosis (hyperviscosity); hyperviscosity symptoms (myalgia, headaches, visual disturbances, dizziness, and paraesthesia), and bleeding (due to dysfunctional platelets; bleeding complications include mucocutaneous bleeding, epistaxis, menorrhagia, haemoptysis, and pulmonary haemorrhage).

The management of Eisenmenger's syndrome includes: (a) avoiding dehydration and hot/humid conditions—these increase right-to-left shunting; (b) contraception, pregnancy, and genetic counselling; (c) oxygen therapy; (d) anticoagulation; (e) diuretic therapy for right heart failure; (f) phlebotomy for polycythaemia and hyperviscosity symptoms—phlebotomy is recommended if there are symptoms of hyperviscosity or if the haematocrit is greater than 65%; (g) pulmonary vasodilator therapy; (h) surgical repair of primary cardiac defect (selected cases); and (i) heart-lung transplantation. Repair of the primary defect is contraindicated in the setting of established severe *irreversible* pulmonary hypertension. However, corrective surgery may be possible, if the pulmonary hypertension is *reversible*. This can be done by demonstrating either evidence of pulmonary reactivity with a pulmonary vasodilator challenge, or lung biopsy findings consist with *reversible* pulmonary arterial changes.

Further Reading

Vongpatanasin W, Brickner M, Hillis L, Lange R (1998). The Eisenmenger syndrome in adults. *Annals of Internal Medicine* 128(9): 745–755.

25. B) Fallot's tetralogy

The cardiac catheter data demonstrate two key findings: (a) elevated RV pressures and normal PA pressures excluding pulmonary hypertension—however, there is a significant gradient (70 mmHg) across the RVOT (RV systolic pressure—PA systolic pressure) which could be in keeping with pulmonary stenosis (subvalvular, valvular, or supravalvular); and (b) a step down in oxygen saturation in the ascending aorta but not in the left ventricle itself, suggesting a right-to-left shunt 'above' the left ventricle. This is due to an overriding aorta. Thus, the unifying diagnosis is Fallot's tetralogy. A history of appetite suppressant usage in a young patient raises the possibility of primary pulmonary hypertension—this is unlikely given normal pulmonary artery pressures. Eisenmenger's syndrome is unlikely given normal pulmonary artery pressures and the fact that right ventricular pressure hasn't yet equalled left ventricular pressure. A persistent ductus arteriosus is associated with a left-to-right shunt between the aorta and pulmonary artery—this would manifest as a step up in oxygen saturation in the pulmonary artery.

Tutorial

Fallot's tetralogy is characterized by a VSD (with a right-to-left shunt), right ventricular outflow tract obstruction (infundibular stenosis), right ventricular hypertrophy, and overriding aorta (with respect to the ventricular septum). The pulmonary valve is normal and the obstruction is subvalvular. The aortic valve is positioned as to lie over the ventricular septum, thus overriding both the right and left ventricles. Symptoms generally progress secondary to hypertrophy of the infundibular septum, and acute cyanotic spells develop with infundibular spasms. Infundibular spasm and/or decreased systemic vascular resistance increase right ventricular outflow obstruction. This increases right ventricular pressures, resulting in increased right-to-left shunting and cyanosis. The murmur lessens in intensity as the outflow gradient increases. Causes of Fallot's tetralogy include foetal hydantoin syndrome, foetal carbamazepine syndrome, foetal alcohol syndrome, and maternal phenylketonuria. Precipitants of cyanotic spells include exercise, fever, catecholamines (stress), hypoxia, dehydration, and acidosis. Other complications include endocarditis, right heart failure, polycythaemia, thrombosis, paradoxical embolism, and cerebral abscess formation.

The ECG will show right ventricular hypertrophy, right axis deviation, and right atrial enlargement. The CXR will show a boot shaped heart (due to uplifting of the cardiac apex due to right ventricular hypertrophy and the absence of a normal main pulmonary artery segment), decreased pulmonary vasculature, and right-sided aortic arch (present in 20–25% of cases).

Total correction can be performed under cardiopulmonary bypass. A Blalock-Taussig shunt is a palliative procedure not performed routinely nowadays due to the availability of total correction procedures. However, this shunt may be performed if the anatomy is unfavourable for total correction and involves an anastomosis between the subclavian artery (usually the left) to the pulmonary artery, thus bypassing right ventricular outflow obstruction. A modified Blalock-Taussig shunt is the interposition of a tubular graft between the two arteries. Other palliative procedures include Waterston shunt, Potts shunt, and the Glenn operation. The Waterston shunt involves anastomosis of the back of the ascending aorta to the pulmonary artery. This is often performed before the age of three months when the subclavian artery is too small for a Blalock-Taussig shunt. The Potts shunt involves anastomosis of the descending aorta to the back of the pulmonary artery. Finally, the Glenn operation involves anastomosis of the superior vena cava to the right pulmonary artery. A bidirectional Glenn procedure involves anastomosis to both pulmonary arteries.

Further Reading

Starr JP (2010). Tetralogy of Fallot: yesterday and today. *World Journal of Surgery* 34(4): 658–668.

26. E) Add ramipril 2.5 mg od

Cardiac catheter data show a wide pulse pressure which has many causes (see Box 1.7). The most common cardiac causes include aortic regurgitation and patent ductus arteriosus. A patent ductus arteriosus is associated with a left-to-right shunt, and this would be associated with a step up in oxygen saturation in the pulmonary artery. The most likely cause in this case is aortic regurgitation. This question tests the knowledge of vasodilator therapy in the management of chronic aortic regurgitation. A pulse pressure of >100 mmHg suggests severe aortic regurgitation. The left ventricle is dilated and hyperdynamic, but with preserved left ventricular systolic function. This hypertensive patient has asymptomatic severe aortic regurgitation. The most appropriate therapy is initiation of vasodilator therapy. Current evidence exists for the use of ACE inhibitors and calcium antagonists (nifedipine) in patients with aortic regurgitation and hypertension/left ventricular dilatation. This patient would require further investigations to determine suitability for aortic valve surgery.

Tutorial

The role of vasodilator therapy is to reduce systolic BP. Hypertension can increase wall stress and reduce the forward stroke volume. Current trial data exists for vasodilator therapy with nifedipine and ACE inhibitors in patients with severe aortic regurgitation. Vasodilator therapy is recommended for patients with asymptomatic severe aortic regurgitation and left ventricular dilatation. Patients with severe aortic regurgitation without left ventricular dilatation and who have normal BP should not be on long-term vasodilator therapy. Vasodilator therapy is not recommended for asymptomatic patients with mild to moderate aortic regurgitation and normal BP with normal left ventricular size and function. Vasodilator therapy is recommended for patients with hypertension and any degree of aortic regurgitation.

All symptomatic patients with severe aortic regurgitation require aortic valve replacement. Waiting for patients to develop symptoms may result in some degree of irreversible left ventricular dysfunction. Left ventricular dysfunction may preclude optimal surgical results. Therefore, current guidelines recommend aortic valve replacement in asymptomatic aortic regurgitation where there is evidence of left ventricular dysfunction or dilatation (Box 1.8). A left ventricular end-systolic

---

Box 1.7 Causes of a wide pulse pressure

- Persistent ductus arteriosus
- Aortic regurgitation
- Anaemia
- Fever
- Pregnancy
- Thyrotoxicosis
- Arterio-venous fistula
- Severe bradycardia

Box 1.8 Indications for aortic valve replacement in aortic regurgitation

Symptomatic patients
- Severe aortic regurgitation and symptoms of heart failure
- Severe aortic regurgitation with angina

Asymptomatic patients
- Left ventricular systolic dysfunction (ejection fraction <50%)
- Left ventricular dilatation (end-systolic diameter >55 mm or end-diastolic diameter >75 mm)
- Aortic root dilatation ≥50 mm (irrespective of the degree of aortic regurgitation)

---

dimension of 55 mm represents the limit of surgically reversible dilatation of the left ventricle.

Further Reading

Nishimura R, Otto C, Bonow R, et al. (2017). AHA/ACC focused update of the 2014 AHA/ACC guideline for the management of patients with valvular heart disease: a report of the American College of Cardiology/American Heart Association Task Force on Clinical Practice Guidelines. *Circulation* 135(25): e1159–1195.

27. D) Synchronized DC cardioversion

The ECG rhythm strip demonstrates a broad complex tachycardia. All broad complex tachycardias should be regarded as VT until proven otherwise. A history of ischaemic heart disease and impairment of left ventricular systolic function, should further lead one to suspect VT. On analysing the ECG, the QRS complexes are very wide (>140 ms), with a RBBB pattern in the precordial leads. There is extreme left axis deviation. Most VT often has RBBB morphology, as it arises from the left ventricle. Examples of VT which originate from the right ventricle include RVOT tachycardia, ARVC, and congenital heart disease (right-to-left shunt). The combination of RBBB and left axis deviation and QRS width >140 ms in the context of RBBB are also suggestive of VT. An important feature that helps distinguish this as VT is the presence of AV dissociation with independent P waves, seen as notching in the QRS complexes.

Sometimes, independent P waves may not be visible, but this does not necessarily exclude a diagnosis of VT. Although described as a classical feature of VT, the presence of concordance in all the chest leads is also not mandatory for the diagnosis of VT, as demonstrated in this case. The QRS complexes generally appear to have the same morphology, that is, monomorphic VT, as opposed to that in polymorphic VT (torsade de pointes). However, there is beat-to-beat variation, that is, mild irregularities in QRS morphology, which is often seen in VT. This is due to underlying heterogeneity in refractoriness of myocardial tissue and slight changes in rates of ventricular activation. Furthermore, the independent superimposed P waves can further lead to variations in QRS complexes. Often a normal P wave may be conducted through the AV node, when this is not refractory, resulting in ventricular conduction over the normal pathways and a normal appearing (narrow) QRS complex, that is, capture beat. Sometimes this atrioventricular conduction may occur simultaneously with depolarization of the ventricular focus. In this case, the ventricle will be depolarized in part over the normal pathway and in part from the ventricular focus, and the resulting QRS has intermediate morphology between a normal QRS and a QRS of ventricular origin. This is a fusion beat.

This patient is haemodynamically compromised with hypotension and clinical signs of pulmonary oedema. The ECG demonstrates monomorphic VT. Therefore, the best treatment is an emergency synchronized DC cardioversion. Intravenous amiodarone should not be used in patients with haemodynamic compromise due to its mild negative inotropic effect, with potential to precipitate or worsen hypotension. In patients who are haemodynamically stable, initial measures should include correction of electrolyte disturbances, in particular hypokalaemia and hypomagnesaemia. Intravenous amiodarone can be used in such cases, and if this fails then synchronized DC cardioversion should be used. Intravenous magnesium would be indicated for torsade de pointes. Intravenous adenosine would be indicated for supraventricular tachycardia. There is no role for thrombolysis in the management of ventricular arrhythmias, except in the context of acute STEMI, but this has now been superseded by primary percutaneous coronary intervention.

Tutorial

Diagnosing VT can be difficult, especially when differentiation from other causes of broad-complex tachycardia is necessary. Other causes of broad complex tachycardias include supraventricular tachycardia, atrial fibrillation, atrial flutter, or sinus tachycardia with aberrant conduction or pre-excitation. Hyperkalaemia, left ventricular hypertrophy, and cardiomyopathies can result in QRS broadening, and thus tachycardias in these states, will result in broad complex tachycardias. ECG criteria to help diagnose VT are listed in Box 1.9.

Box 1.9 ECG criteria for diagnosing ventricular tachycardia

- Very wide QRS complexes (>160 ms with LBBB pattern or >140 ms with RBBB pattern)
- Beat-to-beat variability of QRS morphology
- Independent P waves (atrial activity)
- Capture beats
- Fusion beats
- Extreme axis deviation
- QRS concordance in precordial leads
- RSr pattern in V_1 (RBBB pattern)
- Combination of RBBB pattern and left axis deviation
- Combination of LBBB pattern and right axis deviation

Further Reading

Gupta A, Thakur R (2001). Wide QRS complex tachycardias. *Medical Clinics of North America* 85: 245.

Vereckei A (2014). Current algorithms for the diagnosis of wide QRS complex tachycardias. *Current Cardiology Reviews* 10(3): 262–276.

28. B) Stop ACE inhibitor

B) Renal angiography

The key feature in the history is a rapid deterioration in renal function on initiation of ACE inhibitor therapy, which is strongly suggestive of renovascular disease. On initiation of an ACE inhibitor or angiotensin II receptor blocker, the serum creatinine should always to be monitored—a rise of >25% suggests underlying renovascular disease. In such cases, ACE inhibitors or angiotensin II receptor blockers must be discontinued until renovascular disease is excluded. Of the investigations listed, renal ultrasound scan, renal angiography, and captopril renogram can be used to investigate renovascular disease (see below), but conventional renal angiography remains the gold standard for the diagnosis of renal artery stenosis. A transrectal ultrasound would be indicated for imaging the prostate. Obstructive uropathy is unlikely to be the cause of acute renal impairment, despite a history of prostate disease, as the patient had been catheterized since admission.

Tutorial

Renal artery stenosis is a major cause of renovascular hypertension, chronic renal failure, and end-stage renal disease. It may present as acute pulmonary oedema (flash pulmonary oedema) in the presence of good left ventricular function. Risk factors include hypertension, smoking, diabetes, age, and the presence of extra-renal atherosclerosis. Renal blood flow is three to five times greater than that of any other organ, because it drives glomerular filtration. In patients with renal artery stenosis, obstruction of renal blood flow results in a state of chronic ischaemia that results in adaptive changes in the kidneys, especially at the tubular level. The GFR is dependent on angiotensin II and other modulators that auto-regulate the afferent and efferent glomerular arteries. The effect of angiotensin II is proportionally increased tone in the efferent arterioles compared to the afferent arterioles, which increases renal perfusion pressure, thus maintaining the GFR. However, when renal perfusion pressure falls below 70 mmHg, there is a reduction in GFR. Impairment of this autoregulation process with resultant reduction in GFR is unlikely to occur until arterial luminal narrowing exceeds 50%.

A renal ultrasound scan is often performed in patients with renal dysfunction. This is an anatomical, rather than functional test. If there is discrepancy in kidney size (>1.5 cm), then significant kidney asymmetry may suggest the diagnosis of renovascular disease. Furthermore, it is useful in detecting the presence of a solitary kidney; in which case, renal artery stenosis of a solitary kidney imposes significant prognostic and therapeutic implications. Duplex ultrasound scanning is a non-invasive technique that is very sensitive and specific. However, it is extremely operator dependent. Radionuclide scanning one hour following a single dose of captopril is more useful in patients with normal renal function in whom fibromuscular disease is suspected. Patients with renovascular disease may have renal parenchymal disease or bilateral renovascular disease. In such cases, captopril renography is unable to distinguish between parenchymal or renovascular disease. Spiral CT angiography involves an intravenous injection of a large dose of iodinated contrast agent and allows 3D reconstructed images of the renal arteries. This avoids arterial catheterization (although there is a risk of contrast nephropathy) and requires significant time to reconstruct the images. Conventional renal angiography is the gold standard for diagnosis of renal artery stenosis but carries risks of arterial catheterization and contrast nephropathy. Low osmolar or carbon dioxide angiography can be used to minimize contrast nephropathy. Magnetic resonance angiography is a non-invasive technique that can demonstrate renal vascular anatomy and detect renal artery lesions without iodinated contrast agents. However, this technique has only been validated for stenosis in the proximal 3–3.5 cm of the renal arteries.

Further Reading

Lao D, Parasher P, Kerry C, et al. (2011). Atherosclerotic renal artery stenosis-diagnosis and treatment. *Mayo Clinic Proceedings* 86(7): 649–657.

29. E) ISDN 10 mg bd and hydralazine 25 mg bd

This patient presents with acute pulmonary oedema and responds well to intravenous diuresis and preload reduction with a nitrate infusion. Echocardiography demonstrates severe impairment of LV systolic function. Beta blockers should be avoided in the acute setting, due to their potential negatively inotropic effects, and should be introduced after 4–8 weeks when heart failure symptoms are stable. All patients with heart failure should be commenced on ACE inhibitors or angiotensin II receptor blockers if there are no contraindications. These agents would be contraindicated in this patient due to renovascular disease. The combination of hydralazine and ISDN has been shown to provide an alternative to ACE inhibitor therapy. Spironolactone should be used for patients in NYHA class III–IV status, after ACE inhibitor/angiotensin II receptor blocker and beta blockers have been introduced and appropriately up-titrated. In this patient, it may be appropriate in due course, but the renal function would need to be closely monitored. A calcium channel antagonist and beta blocker should never be started at the same time due to their potentially synergistic effect in dropping the BP.

Tutorial

Renal impairment is not an absolute contraindication for using ACE inhibitors or angiotensin II receptor blockers. Patients may be initiated on ACE inhibitors/angiotensin II receptor blockers with close monitoring of renal function. A rise in creatinine of >25% would suggest underlying renovascular disease. In such cases, ACE inhibitors/angiotensin II receptor blockers must be discontinued until renovascular disease is excluded. The Vasodilator-Heart Failure Trial (V-HeFT II) demonstrated that a combination of hydralazine and ISDN provided a therapeutic alternative to ACE inhibitors, and both therapeutic regimes improved left ventricular systolic function, although ACE inhibitors were associated with a greater reduction in mortality. Thus, in patients with established renovascular disease where ACE inhibitors/angiotensin II receptor blockers cannot be used, a combination of hydralazine and ISDN provides a suitable and prognostic alternative.

Further Reading

Cohn J, Johnson G, Ziesche S, et al (1991). A comparison of enalapril with hydralazine-isosorbide dinitrate in the treatment of chronic congestive heart failure. *New England Journal of Medicine* 325: 303–310.

National Institute for Clinical Excellence. Chronic heart failure in adults: diagnosis and management [NG106]. September 2018. Available at: http://www.nice.org.uk/guidance/ng106

30. A) IV adenosine

The rhythm strip demonstrates a narrow complex tachycardia in which the complexes are regular (Figure 1.13). Therefore, by definition it is a supraventricular tachycardia (SVT). If patients are haemodynamically compromised, then emergency synchronized DC cardioversion should be performed. In patients who are haemodynamically stable, vagal manoeuvres should initially be used. The treatment strategy in supraventricular tachycardia is to induce AV nodal block. This can be achieved using a number of agents. The safest approach is to use intravenous adenosine. It has an extremely short half-life, and often terminates the arrhythmia. The presence of obstructive airways disease is a relative contraindication for adenosine, though this should only be withheld in advanced cases. The starting dose is often 6 mg, increasing to 12 mg if necessary. Intravenous verapamil is

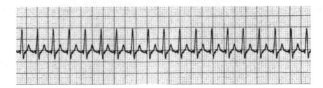

Figure 1.13 ECG rhythm strip.

Reproduced with permission from *Oxford Textbook of Medicine*, Fifth Edition. Edited by David A Warrell, Timothy M Cox, and John D Firth, Fig. 21.5.3, p. 3891. Oxford University Press, Oxford, UK, Copyright © 2010.

also effective but can cause hypotension and bradycardia. It is often an alternative to adenosine in patients with advanced obstructive airways disease but is contraindicated in patients with impaired left ventricular function due to its negative inotropic effects. Amiodarone may be used but is generally not the first-line agent in treating supraventricular arrhythmias. Digoxin has no efficacy in treating supraventricular tachycardia. Although the magnesium is low in this patient, and replacing magnesium is important, the most effective initial therapy that will terminate the arrhythmia is intravenous adenosine. A history of mild asthma as a child, and current infrequent inhaler use should not deter one from using adenosine in this case. Whilst intravenous verapamil may serve as a useful alternative, it is not as effective as adenosine, and there is a risk of hypotension with verapamil administration, given the current BP of 102/70 mmHg.

It is worth noting that both atrial fibrillation and atrial flutter are strictly speaking also SVTs. However, they often have a more characteristic appearance. Atrial fibrillation is usually irregular. In atrial flutter there is a classic 'saw-tooth' pattern. This is because the atrial rate can be very fast, around 300 beats per minute, and if only every other depolarization is conducted through the AV node there will be one QRS complex for every two P-waves (2:1 conduction) giving the characteristic saw-tooth appearance. When the heart rate is very high, however, it can be quite difficult to distinguish between the various SVTs, but giving adenosine remains the correct answer because it will transiently slow the ventricular rate by slowing conduction through the AV node, allowing for the rhythm morphology (e.g. atrial flutter waves) to be distinguished and the correct diagnosis made.

Tutorial

SVT can be broadly classified as atrioventricular nodal re-entrant tachycardia (AVNRT) or atrioventricular re-entrant tachycardia (AVRT). AVNRT may occur in healthy, young individuals, and most patients do not have structural heart disease. Normally, the AV node has a single conducting pathway that conducts impulses in an anterograde manner to depolarize the bundle of His. In certain cases, AV nodal tissue may have two conducting pathways: a relatively slow conducting pathway with a short refractory period and a fast conducting pathway with a long refractory period. These functionally different pathways serve as a substrate for re-entry. Onset of AVNRT is triggered by a premature atrial impulse that may reach the AV node when the fast pathway is still refractory from the previous impulse, but the slow pathway may be able to conduct. The premature impulse then conducts through the slow pathway in an anterograde manner and then travels in a retrograde manner via the fast pathway. If the slow pathway has recovered by the time the impulse completes the retrograde conduction, the impulse can then re-enter the slow pathway and initiate AVNRT. Because the impulse typically conducts in an anterograde manner through the slow pathway and in a retrograde manner through the fast pathway, the PR interval is longer than the RP interval, and the P wave is often seen in the terminal portion of the QRS complex or is buried within the QRS complex. A less common variant is where anterograde conduction is via the fast pathway and retrograde conduction is via the slow pathway, and the P wave occurs relatively late after the QRS complex. In such cases, the RP interval is longer than the PR interval.

AVRT occurs in the presence of accessory pathways, or bypass tracts that connect the atria and the ventricles. AVRT is the result of two or more conducting pathways: the AV node and one or more accessory pathways that form the re-entry circuit. The accessory pathways may conduct impulses in an anterograde manner, a retrograde manner, or both. Conduction through an accessory pathway may be faster, and so anterograde conduction down the accessory pathway results in ventricular pre-excitation. This produces a short PR interval and a delta wave as observed in Wolff-Parkinson-White syndrome. Concealed accessory pathways are not evident during sinus rhythm, and they are only capable of retrograde conduction. Often impulses travel in an anterograde manner through the AV node and in a retrograde manner through the accessory pathway; this is called orthodromic AVRT. Less commonly, an impulse may travel in an anterograde manner through the accessory pathway and in a retrograde manner through the AV node; this is called antidromic AVRT—often producing a broad-complex tachycardia due to pre-excitation.

In patients who are haemodynamically stable, emergency synchronized DC cardioversion is indicated. Vagal manoeuvres are the first-line treatment in haemodynamically stable patients. When SVT is not terminated by vagal manoeuvres, intravenous adenosine, or verapamil can be used. Adenosine is a short-acting drug that blocks AV node conduction and terminates 90% of AVNRT/AVRT. Typical adverse effects of adenosine include flushing, chest pain, and dizziness. These effects are temporary as adenosine has a very short half-life of 8–10 seconds. Verapamil has a longer half-life than adenosine and may help maintain sinus rhythm following the termination of arrhythmia.

Further Reading

Delacrétaz E (2006). Supraventricular tachycardia. *New England Journal of Medicine* 354: 1039–1051.

31. **A 24-year-old man presented with a long-standing rash that was predominantly on his elbows and knees. He had used emollients in the past, but the rash had worsened. He had borrowed a steroid cream from his friend and his rash settled but worsened after he stopped using the cream. He sought help because the rash was itchy and he had noted flakes in his clothes and bleeding from the underlying skin. Examination revealed oval plaques with silvery scaling and occasional bleeding where the silvery scales had been removed. He also had pitting of the nails.**

    Which of the following statements is most accurate?

    A. Arthritis very rarely develops prior to the onset of skin disease
    B. Methotrexate is the best first line therapy for this patient
    C. Nail involvement is associated with an increased risk of arthritis
    D. Newer biologic agents have little role in the treatment of this condition
    E. Systemic corticosteroids should never be used in this condition, because of the risk of significant flare

32. **A 54-year-old man, with no previous medical history, reported an itchy lesion on his back for six months. There was no change during the day or night and it occasionally woke him from sleep. The itchiness did not change with showering or bathing. He had used antihistamines to no avail. On examination he had a small, pigmented lesion measuring 7 mm in diameter with surrounding excoriation on his back. There was crusting on one edge with bleeding. Numerous dysplastic naevi were noted elsewhere on his skin. A suspicion of melanoma was made and an excision biopsy performed.**

    Which aspect of this gentleman's presentation and investigation most affects prognosis?

    A. Age
    B. Bleeding at the edge
    C. Degree of lymphocytes on biopsy (mounted an immune response)
    D. Presence of dysplastic naevus syndrome
    E. Site of the lesion

33. **A 28-year-old male presented with weeping lesions on his hands. He had childhood eczema and suffered from hay fever in the spring and summer, but the lesions on his hands had started 3–4 years previously. He first noticed them on his right little finger and they occasionally spread to his ring finger. Sometimes the lesions bled, but they often settled after a few months with regular application of emollient cream. In the preceding six months the lesions had not settled despite regular emollient and he had noted that his eyelids and the corners of his mouth had started to crack and become dry. Creams and emollients seemed to make things worse. On examination, he had a rash on his right little and ring fingers which particularly affecting the flexures. The lesions were weeping. He had dry skin with cracking on his eyelids and the corner of his mouth.**

    What is the first line of management?

    A. Continue emollients

    B. Low potency topical corticosteroids for both the hands and face

    C. Low potency topical corticosteroids for the face and moderate-high potency topical corticosteroids for the hands

    D. Moderate-high potency topical corticosteroids for both the hands and face

    E. Topical pimecrolimus for the hands and face

34. **A 32-year-old man presented with a week-long history of throat soreness. He subsequently developed severe pain in his ankles and skin lesions on his lower legs. On examination his temperature was 37.9°C and he had erythematous tonsils. His left ankle was swollen and tender, with movement restricted due to pain in all directions. The appearance of his skin is shown in Figure 2.1.**

    ```
    Investigations:
      Hb                       151 g/L
      WCC                      18.2 × 10⁹/L
      Neutrophils              16.4 × 10⁹/L
      Platelets                347 × 10⁹/L
      Sodium                   142 mmol/L
      Potassium                3.8 mmol/L
      Urea                     3.2 mmol/L
      Creatinine               62 µmol/L
      CRP                      117 mg/l
      Urine dipstick           blood++
    ```

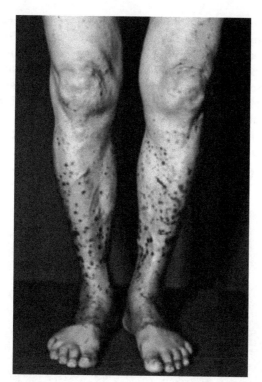

Figure 2.1 Lower-limb rash.

What is the next best management option?

A. Admit the patient for intravenous methylprednisolone 5 mg/kg

B. Commence oral prednisolone 20 mg/day

C. Commence oral prednisolone 40 mg/day

D. Perform a skin biopsy and commence naproxen 500 mg bd

E. Perform a skin biopsy and commence prednisolone 20 mg/day

35. A morbidly obese 59-year-old woman with a past medical history of type II diabetes presented with painful pustules on her leg. She was treated with antibiotics, but the surrounding erythema continued to spread and the blisters soon broke down into a large ulcer. Multiple swabs of the ulcer showed *Staphylococcus aureus*, but despite escalation and optimization of antibiotics she required surgical debridement. After a few days of post-operative care with encouraging signs of healing, she was discharged home with oral antibiotics and ongoing wound dressing with district nurses.

She was admitted to hospital two weeks later with worsening pain and a weeping ulcer. This is shown in Figure 2.2.

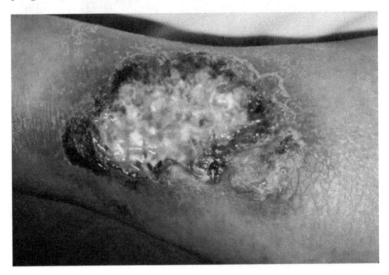

Figure 2.2 Patient's leg ulcer.

Reproduced with permission from *Oxford Handbook of Medical Dermatology*, Second Edition. Edited by S Burge, R Matin, and D Wallis, Fig. 15.5, p. 297. Oxford University Press, Oxford, UK, Copyright © 2016.

What is the most likely diagnosis?

A. Leukocytoclastic vasculitis
B. Necrotizing fasciitis
C. Peripheral arterial disease
D. Pyoderma gangrenosum
E. Squamous cell carcinoma

36. **A 22-year-old woman presented with a painful rash on her shins and difficulty walking. She was usually fit and well but had recently completed a course of amoxicillin for a chest infection. Her only regular medication was the combined oral contraceptive pill. She was also a smoker and drank alcohol at the weekends. On examination, she was mildly febrile at 37.4°C and her cardio-respiratory examination was unremarkable. Examination of her lower limbs revealed very tender bruise-like erythematous lesions and a swollen right ankle (Figure 2.3).**

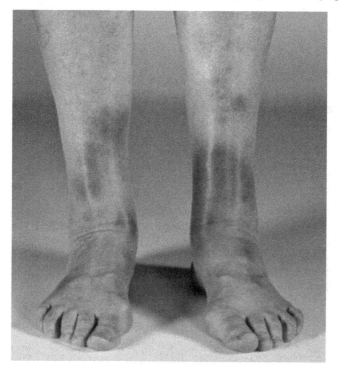

Figure 2.3 Rash on patient's legs.

```
Investigations:
    Hb                      117 g/L
    WCC                     11.4 × 10⁹/L
    Neutrophils             7.8 × 10⁹/L
    Platelets               324 × 10⁹/L
    Sodium                  138 mmol/L
    Potassium               4.6 mmol/L
    Urea                    2.4 mmol/L
    Creatinine              54 µmol/L
    Corrected calcium       2.54 mmol/L
    Phosphate               0.76 mmol/L
    CRP                     84 mg/l
    CXR                     clear lung fields
    She was started on a course of anti-inflammatories but
      re-presented a week later with continuing symptoms.
```

What would the next best step be?

A. Continue non-steroidal anti-inflammatories (NSAIDs)

B. Continue NSAIDs and stop the oral contraceptive pill

C. High-resolution CT chest

D. Request serum ACE level

E. Stop NSAIDs and commence prednisolone 20 mg daily reducing over two weeks

37. A 46-year-old woman presented with a one-week history of cough productive of purulent sputum. She was given a course of antibiotics and seemed to improve. After a few days she developed a rash over her neck and arms, a sore mouth, and joint pains. She became febrile and struggled to cope at home, so she attended the emergency department.

On examination, she was febrile at 38.2°C, but was haemodynamically stable. She had mildly dry mucous membranes. Her systemic examination was unremarkable. Photographs of her skin are shown in Figure 2.4.

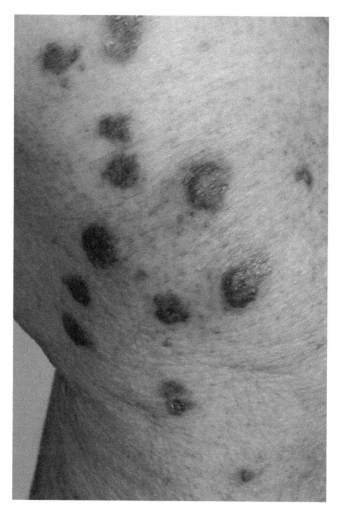

Figure 2.4 Rash on patient's legs.

Investigations:

Hb	123 g/L
WCC	16.4 × 10^9/L
Neutrophils	14.6 × 10^9/L
Platelets	278 × 10^9/L
Sodium	139 mmol/L
Potassium	4.1 mmol/L
Urea	5.8 mmol/L
Creatinine	92 µmol/L
CRP	98 mg/L
ESR	62 mm/hour
ANCA	p-ANCA positive with normal MPO

and PR3 titres

Skin biopsy: dense polymorphonuclear cell infiltrate in the upper dermis and oedema with fragmented neutrophil nuclei. The overlying epidermis is normal.

What is the most likely cause of this presentation?

A. Erythema multiforme minor

B. Leukocytoclastic vasculitis

C. Microscopic polyangiitis

D. Pyoderma gangrenosum

E. Sweet's syndrome

38. **A 29-year-old Chinese female presented with a rash across her cheeks and nose. The rash first occurred during the spring for a few weeks and then returned in the summer. She also had the occasional joint discomfort and oral ulcer. She had acne as an adolescent, but it settled in her early twenties. She was diagnosed with mild Raynaud's disease when she was 14 years old.**

On examination she was apyrexial, with a BP of 112/76 mmHg and heart rate of 64 beats/min. She had erythema across her cheeks with sparing of the nasolabial folds. The rest of her examination was unremarkable.

```
Investigations:
  Hb                      133 g/L
  WCC                     9.2 × 10⁹/L
  Neutrophils             7.6 × 10⁹/L
  Platelets               424 × 10⁹/L
  Sodium                  142 mmol/L
  Potassium               3.9 mmol/L
  Urea                    2.3 mmol/L
  Creatinine              61 µmol/L
  CRP                     12 mg/L
  ESR                     62 mm/hour
  ANA                     1:640
  dsDNA                   13 IU/ml
  ENA                     undetected
  C3                      0.24 g/L (0.8-1.6 g/L)
  C4                      0.97 g/L (0.16-0.48 g/L)
  Urine dipstick: no abnormalities
  Serum protein: polyclonal band in the gamma region
     electrophoresis
```

What is the next best step in her management?

A. High potency topical steroids short term followed by low potency topical steroids

B. Hydroxychloroquine 200 mg daily

C. Low potency topical steroids

D. Methotrexate 10 mg weekly

E. Prednisolone 10 mg daily

39. **A 24-year-old woman presented with all over body pruritus for the preceding eight months. Symptoms came and went rather than being persistent. Occasionally she had raised lumps all over her body and had difficulty sleeping at night due to the pruritus. She took intermittent antihistamines but found them to be of little help. Sometimes emollient baths were helpful in cooling down the pruritus. Consulting online literature, she had made numerous lifestyle changes, including changing washing detergents, soaps, cutting out certain foods, changing mattresses an even using a mattress cover.**

    She had a background of asthma and thought she was allergic to peaches, since her mouth stung when she ate peaches. She had been diagnosed with Raynaud's disease when she was in her teens and was on the oral contraceptive pill but did not take any other medications. Her maternal aunt had rheumatoid arthritis. She did not smoke and drank occasional alcohol. She was a keen runner.

    Examination of her skin revealed occasional scratch marks and she had some raised wheal-like itchy lesions.

    What is the most appropriate course of action?

    A. Advise on regular use of emollients and topical corticosteroids if lesions reappear
    B. Commence hydroxychloroquine 200 mg daily
    C. Commence prednisolone 40 mg daily
    D. Request a patch test
    E. Start regular antihistamines including a night-time sedating antihistamine

40. **A 24-year-old woman attended the dermatology clinic. She had severe acne vulgaris that affected her face. In the past, topical therapies and doxycycline had been ineffective. She was advised to commence isotretinoin and was warned of its teratogenic effects.**

    What other precautions should be taken prior to commencing isotretinoin?

    A. A menstrual history
    B. Hormonal levels and discussion of contraception
    C. Nothing else is required
    D. Referral for insertion of IUCD
    E. Use of both hormonal and barrier contraception and regular pregnancy test

41. **A 34-year-old primary schoolteacher presented with a rash on her hand which over the course of few days had begun to spread. She reported that it was initially vesicular and blistered but had since ruptured. She was otherwise well in herself and had no past medical history. Her rash is shown in Figure 2.5.**

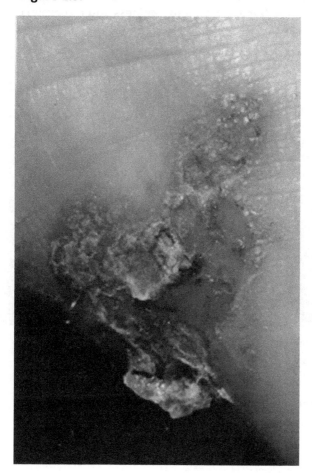

Figure 2.5 Patient's rash.
© Perth Royal Infirmary.

What is the next best course of action?

A. Commence oral aciclovir
B. Commence oral erythromycin
C. Commence oral penicillin V
D. Commence topical mupirocin
E. Take a swab of one of the lesions and await result

42. **A 64-year-old diabetic and hypertensive gentleman was treated for an episode of gout. As this was his second attack, following treatment with anti-inflammatories and symptom resolution, he was started on allopurinol 300 mg once daily. A week later he presented feeling generally unwell and feverish. He reported developing a rash on his hands and arms (Figure 2.6), and itchiness and discomfort around his eyes and mouth.**

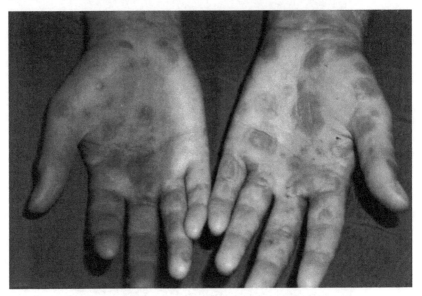

Figure 2.6 Patient's rash.

What is the next best course of action?

A. Ask the patient to stop allopurinol and admit for observation

B. Ask the patient to stop allopurinol and request skin patch testing

C. Ask the patient to stop allopurinol and review the patient in 72 hours

D. Check for anti-allopurinol antibodies

E. Stop allopurinol; commence prednisolone and antihistamines

43. **A 48-year-old male presented to clinic with a rash on his lower limbs. He had trialled a course of oral antibiotics which did not help. He also reported occasional itchiness and irritation around his eyes. On examination, he had erythema around the eyes and blinking appeared to cause discomfort. He had some redness in the mouth, but no blisters. There were some healed lesions on the arms and ankles with some bleeding. There were some tense blisters around the ankles.**

What is the most likely diagnosis?

A. Bullous pemphigoid
B. Cicatricial pemphigoid
C. Pemphigus
D. Stevens-Johnson syndrome
E. Varicella zoster

44. **A 38-year-old man developed an itchy and stinging rash over both arms (Figure 2.7). He was otherwise systemically well and denied any other symptoms. Despite a trial of multiple emollients and topical steroids over many weeks, the rash continued. Aside from a mild microcytic anaemia, blood tests were unremarkable.**

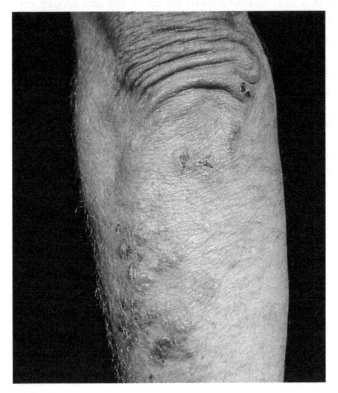

Figure 2.7 Patient's rash.

Reproduced with permission from *Mayo Clinic Internal Medicine Board Review*, Eleventh Edition. Edited by CM Wittich, Fig. 26.10, p. 302. Oxford University Press, Oxford, UK, Copyright © 2016.

What is the best course of action to reach the underlying diagnosis?

A. Anti-endomysial antibodies

B. Biopsy of the lesion

C. Immunoglobulin levels

D. Jejunal biopsy

E. Urine dipstick

45. A 54-year-old man with a history of asthma presented with an itchy rash on his wrists, worse on the left than the right. For the preceding two months he had also been experiencing recurrent oral ulcers for which he had tried mouthwashes and analgesia without response. His wrists are shown in Figure 2.8.

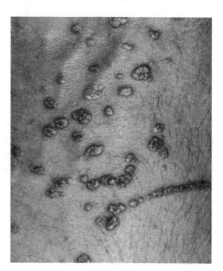

Figure 2.8 Patient's wrists.

Reproduced with permission from *Paediatric Dermatology*. Edited by S Lewis-Jones, Fig. 19.5, p. 311. Oxford University Press, Oxford, UK, Copyright © 2010.

What is the most likely diagnosis?

A. Atopic dermatitis

B. Contact dermatitis

C. Lichen planus

D. Nummular eczema

E. Psoriasis

31. C) Nail involvement is associated with an increased risk of arthritis

This patient has a rash that is predominantly on the extensor surfaces, nail pitting, possible rebound phenomenon on cessation of topical corticosteroid, and demonstration of Auspitz's sign (pinpoint bleeding when plaques are removed). These findings are consistent with a diagnosis of psoriasis.

In psoriasis, there is a close association with nail involvement, whether that is onycholysis or nail pitting, and arthritis. Nail involvement occurs in 20–40% of uncomplicated psoriasis, compared with 60–80% of patients with psoriatic arthritis. Notably, 10–20% of patients with psoriatic arthritis develop arthritis prior to the onset of skin disease.

Although corticosteroids ought to be avoided, in some cases this is not possible, particularly in patients with a severe flare of erythrodermic psoriasis. In erythrodermic psoriasis, corticosteroids can be used with caution and weaned appropriately while avoiding a flare. Often steroid weaning will be in conjunction with the introduction of an alternative systemic therapy. However, in this case, it would be preferable to commence the patient on topical therapy rather than systemic therapy, since he has limited disease. Newer biologic agents have been used with great success in psoriasis but are limited to more severe disease.

Tutorial

Psoriasis is a chronic, inflammatory, multisystem disease that affects 2% of the world's population. The hallmark of this condition is a rash and there are various types of psoriasis. Plaque psoriasis is the most common type accounting for 85–90% of cases. It is characterized by oval plaques with silvery scaling, occurring on the elbows, knees, scalp, and natal cleft. Erythrodermic psoriasis is characterized by widespread inflammation and exfoliation. This usually occurs as a result of rapid withdrawal of systemic therapy for plaque psoriasis and can be fatal. Pustular psoriasis consists of non-infectious pustules surrounded by erythema. There are palmo-pustular and acrodermatitis continua suppurativa varieties, the latter characterized by acropachy.

Arthritis occurs in 5–10% of patients with psoriasis and is more common in patients with nail involvement. There are a variety of different types of psoriatic arthritis:

- DIP arthritis
- Rheumatoid type, but seronegative
- Spondyloarthropathy or sacroiliitis
- Asymmetrical oligoarthritis
- Arthritis mutilans, which leads to 'telescoping' of the small joints of the hands

The CASPAR (ClASsification of Psoriatic ARthritis) study group have come up with criteria to help with the successful diagnosis of psoriatic arthritis. At the time of diagnosis, a patient must have inflammatory articular disease (joint, spine, or entheseal) at time of examination or previously documented by a rheumatologist with ≥3 points from the five categories listed in Box 2.1.

Box 2.1 CASPAR criteria for diagnosing psoriatic arthritis
___

1. Evidence of current psoriasis, a personal history of psoriasis, or a family history of psoriasis: *(2 points)*
   - Current psoriasis is defined as psoriatic skin or scalp disease present today as judged by a rheumatologist or dermatologist.[†]
   - A personal history of psoriasis is defined as a history of psoriasis that may be obtained from a patient, family physician, dermatologist, rheumatologist, or other qualified health care provider.
   - A family history of psoriasis is defined as a history of psoriasis in a first- or second-degree relative according to patient report.
2. Typical psoriatic nail dystrophy including onycholysis, pitting, and hyperkeratosis observed on current physical examination. *(1 point)*
3. A negative test result for the presence of rheumatoid factor by any method except latex. *(1 point)*
4. Either current dactylitis, defined as swelling of an entire digit, or a history of dactylitis recorded by a rheumatologist. *(1 point)*
5. Radiographic evidence of juxta-articular new bone formation appearing as ill-defined ossification near joint margins (but excluding osteophyte formation) on plain radiographs of the hand or foot. *(1 point)*

[†] Current psoriasis is assigned a score of 2; all other features are assigned a score of 1.
Reproduced with permission from W Taylor et al., Classification criteria for psoriatic arthritis: Development of new criteria from a large international study, *Arthritis & Rheumatology*, 54, 8, pp. 2665–2673. Copyright © 2006 by the American College of Rheumatology.

Management of psoriasis is based around the extent and complications of disease. For limited plaque psoriasis, low to mid-potency corticosteroid topical therapy may be adequate in treating these symptoms. However, such therapies suffer from loss of effectiveness and side effects, such as thinning of the skin. Topical vitamin D analogues and retinoids have superseded other therapies such as coal tar. Ultraviolet light therapy remains effective, especially in combination with psoralen, for widespread psoriasis.

For more severe psoriasis, systemic therapy is indicated. Methotrexate, oral retinoids, and ciclosporin are used. Methotrexate is effective in treating psoriasis, but it is particularly useful in treating psoriatic arthritis. Those taking methotrexate are required to have regular blood tests to monitor for liver or haematological disturbances. Oral retinoids and methotrexate are known to be teratogenic. Ciclosporin can cause renal dysfunction, gum hypertrophy, and hypertension.

Biologic therapies have been recommended by NICE when patients have failed, or are intolerant of, ciclosporin, methotrexate, and UV therapy. The particular agents are anti-TNF agents, such as etanercept, infliximab, adalimumab, and ustekinumab. Ustekinumab is a monoclonal antibody against IL-12 and IL-23. Between 66 and 76% of patients with moderate to severe psoriasis treated with ustekinumab will achieve PASI75 (75% reduction in their psoriasis activity and severity index).

Further Reading

Helliwell P, Taylor W (2005). Classification and diagnostic criteria for psoriatic arthritis. *Annals of the Rheumatic Disease* 64, ii3–ii8.

Nestle F, Kaplan D, Barker J (2009). Psoriasis. *New England Journal of Medicine* 361, 496–509.

32. C) Degree of lymphocytes on biopsy (mounted an immune response)

Pruritic lesions often settle with showering or bathing, so this is a little unusual. It is a pigmented lesion with crusting on the edge and some bleeding, with a background of possible dysplastic naevus syndrome. The diagnosis is likely to be melanoma, and it appears to have an inflammatory response.

There are a number of factors that contribute to prognosis in patients with melanoma. The most important factor is stage at the time of presentation. The revised staging for melanoma includes depth (Breslow's thickness), ulceration, nodal involvement, microscopic satellites, and presence of metastases. It is fortunate that most melanomas are diagnosed at stage I or II.

Favourable sites are on the limbs and unfavourable sites include the hands, feet, scalp, and mucous membranes. Women with stage I or II disease tend to do better than men with similarly staged disease. It is likely that earlier presentation and a tendency towards lower limb lesions explains this difference. Older patients do worse than younger patients due to a later presentation and an increased frequency of palmo-plantar lesions.

This question is asking about what most affects prognosis. Breslow's thickness: the depth of the lesion, has the most significant prognostic value. The age of the patient is not a prognostic factor per se, but the delay in presentation is likely to lead to a poorer outcome and delays are more frequent in older age groups. Bleeding at the edge of the lesion is more suggestive of melanoma rather than a pigmented naevus but does not inform prognosis of the melanoma. Dysplastic naevus syndrome is defined as the presence of greater than 100 pigmented naevi. This increases the risk of conversion to melanoma but does not affect prognosis of melanoma.

The degree of lymphocytes on biopsy most affects prognosis, because it suggests there has already been an immune response to melanoma. As a result of the immune response, the melanoma may not be as deep at diagnosis as it was prior to mounting the immune response and thus the staging of melanoma is underestimated.

Tutorial

Diagnosis of melanoma is difficult since many people have multiple pigmented lesions. Melanomas originate from neural crest-derived melanocytes, which are pigmented cells normally present in the dermis and epidermis. The main risk factors for development of melanoma are a positive family history, dysplastic naevus syndrome, and previous melanoma. Exposure to ultraviolet radiation and immunosuppression are additional risk factors. Melanoma occurs when ultraviolet radiation causes genetic changes in the skin that impair immune function and this is most common after sun exposure that leads to sunburn. This is different to tanning, which is a protective response that does not lead to sunburn.

Although it only accounts for 4% of all skin cancers, it accounts for 80% of all skin cancer deaths. The five-year survival has steadily improved to 85%, but it causes a disproportionate amount of deaths before middle age. An average of 18.6 years of life is lost for each melanoma death in the USA. Since the 1960s, the incidence of melanoma has increased by 3–8% per year in Caucasians, such that the lifetime risk will reach ≥1%.

Family history greatly increases the risk of developing melanoma. Less than 2% of melanoma is due to heritable mutations in highly penetrant genes. CDKN2A and CDK4 are the genes known to cause melanoma and the locus on chromosome 1p22 is strongly linked with melanoma susceptibility. Mutations in CDKN2A confer a risk of 50–80% of melanoma by 80 years of age. This mutation is present in 30–40% of families with three or more members with melanoma.

Outcome is much improved by early diagnosis, which is aided by increased clinical suspicion. Non-pigmented melanoma constitutes 5% of the total and can present similarly to basal cell carcinomas. If they arise in those with dysplastic naevus syndrome or out of a pigmented naevus, then the diagnosis of melanoma should be considered. If doubt remains, then an excision biopsy should be taken. Dermatoscopy or skin microscopy is often used to examine pigmented naevi. In addition, computerized monitoring systems are often used to monitor changes in lesions.

If in doubt, the whole lesion should be excised with a clear margin of 2 mm. Management of melanoma is dependent on accurate histopathological diagnosis. If uncertainty remains, then a second opinion should be sought. Not only should the tumour thickness and ulceration be documented, but other features such as desmoplasia, neurotropism, tumour mitotic rate, growth phase, lymphatic invasion, and vascular invasion are also considered.

Prognosis depends mainly on thickness of the lesion and presence or absence of metastases to regional lymph nodes. However, other factors such as patient gender, ulceration, mitotic rate, regression, and site of tumour also need to be taken into account. Initially, primary tumours are managed surgically, with the main issue being resection margins. General consensus is that 1 cm margins are adequate for tumours ≤1 mm deep and 2 cm for between 1 and 2 mm deep. For those greater than 2 mm it is unclear whether excision margins should be 2 or 3 cm. Often the sentinel node is assessed. This can be by lymph node mapping or by biopsy; however, the latter remains controversial due to risk of in transit metastatic spread.

More than 80% of patients who develop melanoma will die from other causes. Those with tumour depths ≥4 mm and lymph node spread are at greatest risk of death. These patients may be candidates for therapy other than surgery. A number of agents are used, but the most commonly used is high-dose interferon α. Other agents being investigated include bevacizumab which selectively binds to VEGF; ipilimumab which is a monoclonal antibody against CTLA-4; interleukin-2; and PARP inhibitors.

Further Reading

Dickson P, Gershenwald J (2011). Staging and prognosis of cutaneous melanoma. *Surgical Oncology Clinic North America* 20, 1–17.

Miller A, Mihm M (2006). Melanoma. *New England Journal of Medicine* 355, 51–65.

33. C) Low potency topical corticosteroids for the face and moderate-high potency topical corticosteroids for the hands

This patient has atopic dermatitis. The supportive features are a history of eczema as a child and the pattern of the rash. Atopic dermatitis commonly affects the flexures, but also affects the face, particularly around the eyes. The age of the patient is not against the diagnosis, since there is a bimodal pattern of peak incidence between ages 0–5 years and 21–25 years.

The patient has had these symptoms for a few years but has not regarded the rash as serious enough to warrant intervention until now. Thus, continuing emollients is not adequate in this case. Although it is important to relieve the patient's symptoms, high potency topical steroids can cause significant thinning of the skin and extensive use can lead to hypoadrenalism. It is best to avoid using high-potency topical corticosteroids, at least in the first instance, on the face.

Dermatitis on his hands is relatively localized. It seems to be appropriate to use a higher potency on these areas to resolve his symptoms quickly, since his lesions are weeping. It is important to note that there are no open cracks or bleeding. High potency topical corticosteroids ought to be avoided in that instance.

The most appropriate option for therapy is high potency corticosteroids for his hands and low potency corticosteroids for his face. Although topical calcineurin inhibitors would be an option, these can only be prescribed once he has failed or proven intolerant to topical corticosteroids.

Tutorial

Atopic dermatitis is a chronic relapsing inflammatory skin condition characterized by pruritus and erythema. It often occurs in the skin flexures, but can occur elsewhere, including the face. It is part of the atopic state and up to 70% have a family history of hay fever, asthma, or dermatitis. It is increasingly common, with the point prevalence in a Norwegian study being 23%. This condition tends to be more common in western countries, but this may be due to reporting bias. The hygiene hypothesis is thought to explain this increased frequency but remains controversial. To note, those with atopic dermatitis tend to have more allergies, for example eggs or cat hair. Up to 80% develop allergic rhinitis or asthma.

Diagnostic criteria are not reflective of severity, since they tend to describe the difference between acute and chronic disease. Erythema, exudate, papules, and vesiculopapules characterize acute disease. Chronic disease results in indurated erythema, lichenification, and prurigo. Scales and crusts feature in both. The distribution tends to be symmetrical, but in adults it tends to be more severe in the upper half of the body, particularly the neck and face.

Stepwise treatment is recommended and varies with acuteness, chronicity, and side effects of therapy. Emollients can be used, as well as other conservative measures, such as soap substitutes and avoidance of precipitating allergens such as dairy products and lanolin. Topical corticosteroids have a role and recent guidelines recommend they be used twice daily. Creams or ointments can be used, depending on skin dryness, with patients often using cling film over applied ointment to maintain its effect.

There are a variety of different strengths of topical corticosteroids, ranging from hydrocortisone 0.5% to mometasone 0.1%. In general, they should be applied thinly to affected areas only, with open sores avoided. Low potency corticosteroids ought to be used initially, but it is not unreasonable to use more potent corticosteroids in short bursts in more localized areas. Occasionally, these are used in more widespread disease with caution due to side effects, including thinning of the skin and, rarely, developing Cushingoid features.

Topical calcineurin inhibitors, namely pimecrolimus and tacrolimus, are new steroid sparing agents. These are recommended by NICE for more severe disease refractory to topical corticosteroids or requiring prolonged therapy. It is also advisable to use these products on the face and neck with more severe disease, since they do not cause thinning of delicate skin.

Further Reading

Bieber T (2008). Atopic dermatitis. *New England Journal of Medicine*, 358, 1483–1494.

Saeki H, Furue M, Furukawa F, et al. (2009). Guidelines for management of atopic dermatitis. *Journal of Dermatology*, 36, 563–577.

34. D) Perform a skin biopsy and commence naproxen 500 mg bd

This gentleman has presented with the sequelae of a preceding illness—likely a streptococcal sore throat. Subsequent to this he has developed fever, arthritis, and a painful rash. The picture shows purpura distributed over the lower limbs. His full blood count demonstrates a neutrophilia, but it is notable that he does not have thrombocytopaenia or anaemia, so this is not a haematological disorder. His inflammatory markers are raised and his renal function is normal, but he has microscopic haematuria on dipstick. This makes it more likely to be a vasculitic condition. The diagnosis is Henoch-Schönlein purpura (HSP), due to the painful purpuric rash, normal platelet count, and arthritis. Although he is pyrexial and in discomfort, he is not haemodynamically unstable and his renal function is normal and would not require inpatient admission. Histology, whilst not always necessary for diagnosis, as discussed in the tutorial, is very helpful and so a punch biopsy of the rash should be performed. In terms of treatment, corticosteroids are often used, but there is little evidence that outcome is improved or that the duration or symptoms are significantly shortened versus the use of non-steroidals. The best first-line therapy is NSAIDs. It is likely he will respond to them and corticosteroids can be reserved for second-line therapy. The natural history of the disease suggests that the symptoms will settle.

Tutorial

HSP is leukocytoclastic vasculitis involving the small vessels, with deposition of immune complexes containing IgA. It classically presents as purpura on the buttocks and back of the legs, but can present with purpura elsewhere, as in this case. The clinical features are listed in Table 2.1.

Table 2.1 Clinical features of Henoch-Schönlein purpura

Clinical feature	% at onset	% during course
Purpura	50	100
Subcutaneous oedema	10–20	20–50
Arthritis (large joints)	25	60–85
Gastrointestinal	30	85
Renal	—	10–50
Genitourinary	—	2–35
Pulmonary (DLCO)	—	95
Pulmonary haemorrhage	—	Rare, may be fatal
CNS (headache, seizures)	—	Rare, may be fatal

It is more common in children than adults and affects 10–22 persons in 100,000 per year. In adults, HSP is more severe and more likely to cause long-term renal disease. Biopsies of patients with renal involvement usually show IgA mesangial deposits. Crescents found on biopsy are predictive of progressive renal involvement and correspondingly poor outcome. There is no relationship between the extent of purpura and prognosis.

There is no definitive test to diagnose HSP and its diagnosis remains clinical, although classically a triad of purpura, abdominal pain, and arthritis. The most up-to-date criteria are from EULAR. Patients must have palpable purpura and any one of the following:

• Diffuse abdominal pain
• Any biopsy showing predominantly IgA deposition
• Arthritis or arthralgia
• Renal involvement (haematuria or proteinuria)

Since there are no diagnostic serological tests, the purpose of laboratory evaluation is to determine alternative causes to the presentation and complications. Consideration of other causes of purpura, abdominal pain, and arthritis is an important aspect of the diagnostic work-up. It is imperative that a full blood count is taken to rule out thrombocytopaenia. All patients should have their urine dipped for blood and protein and have their renal function checked. Other investigations such as ASO titres, renal biopsy, and search for infectious causes are dependent on clinical presentation. All patients should have their BP checked at presentation and subsequent follow-up visits.

The management of HSP is mainly supportive, since 94% of children and 89% of adults spontaneously remit. In general, most patients can be managed with supportive care and pain relief, using either paracetamol or NSAIDs. Corticosteroids are used in patients with more severe arthritis, abdominal discomfort, or mild renal involvement; however, there is no evidence that they alter the course of the condition. Those patients who develop progressive renal disease or pulmonary haemorrhage should be treated by the appropriate speciality and receive additional immunosuppression.

Further Reading

Ozen S, Ruperto N, Dillon MJ, Bagga A (2006). EULAR/PReS endorsed consensus criteria* for the classification of childhood vasculitides. *Annals of Rheumatic Diseases* 65(7): 936–941.

35. D) Pyoderma gangrenosum

The most likely diagnosis is pyoderma gangrenosum because the key feature in this case is the return of the ulcer after debridement. In addition, the patient initially had pustules on presentation, which can precede ulcers in pyoderma gangrenosum. Often pyoderma gangrenosum occurs in areas of trauma and does not respond to antibiotics. Whilst she had positive swabs for S. *aureus*, this often represents either a superimposed infection or skin flora colonization.

Given the location of the ulcer is in the gator region and there was initial good healing following the debridement, peripheral arterial disease is unlikely, though assessment of peripheral vasculature patency is often necessary in these patients if pulses are faint on examination. Squamous cell carcinomas can be ulcerative and these are known as Marjolin's ulcers, but this is very unlikely given the short natural history. Usually these occur associated with chronically traumatized skin, such as venous ulcers, chronic osteomyelitis, or burns.

Necrotizing fasciitis is rapidly progressive and often the area of skin affected increases in size. It is severely painful and crepitus can be found on examination due to the causative organisms being gas forming (e.g. *Clostridium perfringens*).

The lesion does not look like leukocytoclastic vasculitis. Although this would not respond to antibiotics or anticoagulation, the condition is not normally ulcerative. Leukocytoclastic vasculitis is a pathological diagnosis associated with other conditions such as HSP, urticarial vasculitis, or cryoglobulinaemic vasculitis.

Tutorial

Pyoderma gangrenosum is a rare condition, which consists of four types:

   a) Classic (ulcerative)

     Most commonly this type occurs on the lower extremities but can occur elsewhere. The lesions often start as painful nodules or sterile pustules. These then expand laterally over days, developing an ulcerated centre and erythematous to violaceous border. Twenty-five per cent have a history of trauma prior to onset. The borders are well demarcated and raised, but these become less prominent with healing.

   b) Bullous

     This variant is characterized by painful vesicles and bullae. These coalesce quickly and then form an erosive central lesion. Seventy per cent of these patients have an underlying haematological malignancy, so appropriate investigations should be performed.

   c) Pustular

     This is described as painful pustules on an erythematous base that do not ulcerate. There is an association with inflammatory bowel disease.

   d) Vegetative

     This is also known as superficial granulomatous pyoderma and patients present with erythematous furunculoid lesions or plaques that slowly ulcerate. The borders are not undermined as in classical pyoderma gangrenosum. The lesions are typically on the trunk and are not usually associated with an underlying disease.

Patients with pyoderma gangrenosum tend to have underlying inflammatory or haematological conditions. Twenty-five per cent of patients have arthritis, particularly seropositive rheumatoid arthritis, whilst 2% have inflammatory bowel disease. Occasionally, patients can present with pyoderma gangrenosum prior to the onset of inflammatory bowel disease. Haematological malignancies tend to be myeloid rather than lymphoid in origin, most commonly being acute myeloid leukaemia.

The differential diagnoses for pyoderma gangrenosum are wide; as a result 15% of patients are misdiagnosed and there is a delay in the introduction of therapy. These are listed in Box 2.2.

Box 2.2 Differential diagnosis of lower limb ulceration

Vascular ulceration
- Venous or arterial ulceration
- Antiphospholipid syndrome
- Calciphylaxis (end-stage kidney disease patients)

Systemic conditions
- Systemic lupus erythematosus
- Rheumatoid arthritis
- Behçet's syndrome
- Wegener's granulomatosis
- Sweet's syndrome

Infections
- Bacterial
- Fungal
- Viral
- Mycobacterial

Parasitic

Malignancy

Squamous cell carcinoma

Cutaneous lymphoma

Management can be topical or systemic. Topical therapy includes corticosteroids and topical pimecrolimus. Topical therapy is rarely used in isolation, since pyoderma gangrenosum can progress rapidly and lead to significant morbidity. Systemic corticosteroids, either 1–2 mg/kg oral prednisolone or pulsed methylprednisolone, are used. If this is ineffective than the next steps include ciclosporin, azathioprine, or anti-TNF therapy. Often infliximab is used, since it has a more rapid onset of action compared to the other anti-TNF agents. Azathioprine is used in conjunction to limit the formation of anti-infliximab antibodies.

Further Reading

Dabade T, Davis M (2011). Diagnosis and treatment of the neutrophilic dermatoses (pyoderma gangrenosum, Sweet's syndrome). *Dermatologic Therapy* 24, 273–284.

Miller J, Yentzer B, Clark A, Jorizzo J, Feldman S (2010). Pyoderma gangrenosum: a review and update on new therapies. *Journal of the American Academy of Dermatology* 62, 646–654.

36. B) Continue NSAIDs and stop the oral contraceptive pill

The patient is a young woman with no significant past medical history and is only on the oral contraceptive pill. She has presented to her GP with a painful rash on her legs and ankle swelling following a recent respiratory tract infection. The most likely explanation for the painful rash on her shins is erythema nodosum and indeed the clinical findings are consistent with this. Erythema nodosum can occur on its own, often precipitated by an infection, but is also common in other conditions, such as sarcoid and Behçet's syndrome. Sarcoid can present with respiratory symptoms, arthritis, and erythema nodosum. Most commonly, sarcoid causes an interstitial pneumonitis, which leads to shortness of breath and a non-productive cough. Her investigations show normal calcium and no hilar lymphadenopathy on the chest radiograph. It is not necessary to request a serum ACE level or HRCT chest for this patient currently. The hallmark of Behçet's is oro-genital ulceration, but it is also characterized by uveitis, arthralgia, and vascular involvement. There is an increased frequency of venous thrombi and pulmonary artery aneurysms. There is rarely lung involvement.

In many cases the cause of erythema nodosum is unknown, but the most likely cause in this case is the combined oral contraceptive pill. Amoxicillin is a known cause, but she has only been taking amoxicillin for a couple of days. In this case, corticosteroids are not necessary. She would benefit from a longer course of NSAIDs. It is also important to alter her contraception and stop the combined oral contraceptive pill, which is the likely trigger for her erythema nodosum.

Tutorial

Erythema nodosum is the most frequent panniculitis and manifests as a painful violaceous rash, which is nodular in nature and can be 1–6 cm. Ninety-eight per cent of lesions are found in the pretibial regions, and 85% are bilateral. If lesions are present elsewhere, they are usually found on the lower limbs, but can also be found on the trunk. The incidence is 5 cases per 100,000 persons/year, with a male to female ratio of 1:6 and a peak incidence in the third decade.

Erythema nodosum is mostly a self-limiting condition, but it can recur in up to one third of patients, usually as smaller less tender nodules. For the most part, the rash resolves with bruise-like colour changes and without atrophy or ulceration. Histopathology does not show vasculitis and there is no immune complex deposition, but biopsy is rarely required for diagnosis. There are many different causes of erythema nodosum, but the majority (approximately a third) are idiopathic (Box 2.3).

The diagnosis of underlying conditions or aetiology is dependent on history and clinical examination. Although patients often present with systemic symptoms, such as fever, myalgia, arthralgia, and malaise, this may also represent the underlying condition, such as infection or sarcoidosis. Investigations should be tailored to the clinical presentation.

Since the 1960s, it has been noted that pregnancy and oestrogen-containing contraceptives are associated with erythema nodosum. Up to 5% of erythema nodosum cases are in pregnant women. This may partially explain why erythema nodosum is more common in women than men and the observed increased frequency in childbearing years. Although oestrogens are not thought to be causative, it is interesting that the frequency of erythema nodosum has decreased with the reduction of oestrogen content of contraceptives over the last couple of decades.

The management of erythema nodosum is dependent on the cause. If an underlying cause is found that should be treated. The local treatment of erythema nodosum is often analgesia. NSAIDs are helpful and occasionally patients receive intra-lesional corticosteroid injections. Although the latter can be very effective, side effects include localized fat atrophy and hypopigmentation. If required, 10–40 mg prednisolone daily is adequate, with rapid dose reduction once symptoms start to resolve. Use of additional immunosuppression should be tailored if there is an underlying autoimmune cause.

Box 2.3 Differential diagnosis for erythema nodosum

Idiopathic

Infections

- Epstein Barr Virus
- Cytomegalovirus
- Streptococcus*
- Mycoplasma
- Leprosy
- Tuberculosis
- Salmonellosis
- Enteroviruses

Autoimmune

- Sjögren's syndrome
- Behçet's syndrome
- Sarcoid
- Inflammatory bowel disease

Hormonal

- Combined oral contraceptive pill
- Pregnancy

Drugs

- Sulphonamides
- Amoxicillin

* Most common cause

Further Reading

Papagrigoraki A, Gisondi P, Rosina P, Cannone M, Girolomoni G (2010). Erythema nodosum: etiological factors and relapses in a retrospective cohort study. *European Journal of Dermatology* 20, 773–777.

37. E) Sweet's syndrome

The patient's initial chest infection seems to respond to a course of antibiotics. Her subsequent illness, the features of which are, rash, sore mouth, fever, and arthralgia, is unlikely to be related. Figure 2.4 shows well-demarcated irregular erythematous macules. The lesions are paler in the centre, but there is no ulceration. Blood tests show an inflammatory process, with raised CRP, ESR, and neutrophils. This is likely to be acute since the patient is not anaemic and there is no other biochemical abnormality. The ANCA screen is positive, but the MPO and PR3 titres are normal.

Based on the picture and the biopsy result, the most likely cause is Sweet's syndrome. The clinical presentation and biopsy are not consistent with leukocytoclastic vasculitis. The rash in leukocytoclastic vasculitis is often papular and coalesces but does not consist of macules. This is also true for microscopic polyangiitis. A positive p-ANCA with normal MPO and PR3 levels is a non-specific finding, and although 10–20% of small vessel vasculitides have negative ANCA serology, the time course of the illness is not consistent with a small vessel vasculitis and there are no other supporting clinical features. Erythema multiforme minor classically produces target lesions and is different to the described rash.

Pyoderma gangrenosum can present in a variety of ways, but classically presents as an ulcerative condition on the background of trauma. Non-ulcerative forms have pustules or an irregular granulomatous surface, neither of which are present here. Although the biopsy findings are similar, the combination of clinical presentation and biopsy are more consistent with Sweet's syndrome than pyoderma gangrenosum.

Tutorial

Dr Robert Douglas Sweet first described an acute febrile neutrophilic dermatosis in 1964. Sweet's syndrome is characterized by pyrexia, neutrophilia, painful red papules, plaques, and an infiltrate consisting predominantly of mature neutrophils that are diffusely distributed in the upper dermis.

Sweet's syndrome most commonly occurs in women between the ages of 30–50 years, but it can occur in younger adults and children. Patients can appear dramatically unwell and the fever can precede the skin disease by several days to weeks, or be present concurrently with dermatosis. The skin lesions are tender red papules or nodules and frequently occur on the face, upper limbs, and neck. The lesions tend to enlarge over a period of days and weeks, and coalesce, forming irregular, sharply bordered plaques. Usually the lesions resolve without scarring following therapy but can recur in up to two thirds of patients. Occasionally, patients can have a pustular variant which tends to occur on the dorsum of hands. Sweet's syndrome has a number of extracutaneous manifestations which are described in Table 2.2.

Table 2.2 Extracutaneous manifestations of Sweet's syndrome

Site	Manifestations
Bone	Arthritis, arthralgia, focal aseptic osteitis, sterile osteomyelitis
CNS	Aseptic meningitis, brain stem lesions, encephalitis, Guillain-Barré syndrome, idiopathic bilateral sensorineural hearing loss, psychiatric symptoms
Eyes	Blepharitis, conjunctivitis, conjunctival haemorrhage, episcleritis, glaucoma, iritis, scleritis, uveitis
Kidneys	Mesangiocapillary glomerulonephritis
Abdomen	Diffuse neutrophil infiltration, culture-negative pancolitis, hepatic portal triad with neutrophilic inflammation, LFT abnormalities, hepatomegaly, splenomegaly
Heart	Aortic stenosis, aortitis, cardiomegaly, myocarditis, vascular dilatation
Lung	Bronchi with red pustules and neutrophilic inflammation, pleural effusion with neutrophilia, pulmonary tissue with neutrophil infiltrates
Mouth	Aphthosis, bullae and vesicles, necrotizing ulcerative periodontitis, nodules, papules, pustules, glossitis
Muscles	Myalgia, neutrophilic myositis

Although Sweet's syndrome is a benign condition it has multiple associations (not listed here), including haematological malignancy, recurrent malignancy, drugs, and autoimmune conditions. In those with an underlying malignant cause, 85% of patients have a haematological malignancy, usually acute myeloid leukaemia. In the majority of cases, the lesions appear concurrently or prior to the diagnosis of malignancy.

The main laboratory findings are a raised ESR and peripheral leukocytosis with a predominant neutrophilia. The latter is not always present with biopsy-confirmed Sweet's syndrome. Other haematological abnormalities can occur, such as anaemia, a low neutrophil count, or thrombocytopaenia, if malignancy is the underlying cause. If there is involvement of other organs then the corresponding tests can be deranged, such as renal and liver function.

A biopsy is often required for definitive diagnosis. The histopathological features are a diffuse infiltrate of mature neutrophils in the superficial dermis and oedema of the dermal papillae and papillary dermis. Sometimes, there can be lymphocyte and eosinophil infiltrates, but there is sparing of the epidermis. There are no disease-specific findings on immunofluorescence.

Treatment may be directed at the underlying condition, which could be surgery to remove a solid tumour or chemotherapy. Systemic and local corticosteroids are often the treatment of choice. Oral corticosteroids are commenced at 1 mg/kg/day and tapered over 4–6 weeks, but may be given for 2–3 months. If these fail, then pulsed methylprednisolone can be given. Occasionally ciclosporin or dapsone are used as second-line agents. These patients may also respond to colchicine.

Further Reading

Cohen P, Kurzrock R (2002). Sweet's syndrome: a review of current treatment options. *American Journal of Clinical Dermatology* 3, 117–131.

Cohen P, Kurzrock R (2003). Sweet's syndrome revisited: a review of disease concepts. *International Journal of Dermatology* 42, 761–778.

38. B) Hydroxychloroquine 200 mg daily

This patient has systemic lupus erythematosus (SLE). The question is examining how severe her SLE is and what therapy she requires. Her major symptom is a classic butterfly rash with nasolabial sparing and evidence of photosensitivity, since her rash was worse in the summer than in the spring. She also has other features of SLE such as recurrent oral ulceration and Raynaud's, although it should be noted that a third of young women have primary Raynaud's.

Examination confirms she has a butterfly rash, but she has no features of severe SLE. Importantly, she is normotensive. Blood tests show her full blood count and biochemistry is normal. The CRP and ESR are raised, but the ESR is out of proportion with the CRP. The polyclonal rise in immunoglobulins found on the serum protein electrophoresis explains the raised ESR. This is a common finding in patients with SLE and Sjögren's syndrome. She has a moderately raised ANA, but normal complement levels (C3 and C4) and negative ENAs. She has a negative urinary dipstick, indicating at low risk of renal involvement in the future.

The management issues in this patient are her butterfly rash and oral ulceration. Her Raynaud's is not much of an issue and she has no other features requiring therapy. There is therefore no requirement for her to commence methotrexate or azathioprine. She also has no history to suggest serositis or arthritis, so she does not require oral prednisolone.

Topical corticosteroids are a reasonable treatment option for butterfly rash. If given, it is best to use low potency topical corticosteroids on the face rather than high potency, even for a short duration. This patient's rash is not severe enough to merit high potency corticosteroids.

Hydroxychloroquine is a better option than topical corticosteroids. Hydroxychloroquine is very useful in SLE and is used to treat rash, arthralgia, hair loss, and fever in SLE. It is effective in treating the butterfly rash, and this patient's rash does not require any other intervention.

Tutorial

Approximately 50% of patients with SLE suffer from skin photosensitivity, but there are other skin manifestations of SLE as well as subtypes of lupus. The best-recognized cutaneous feature of SLE is the malar or 'butterfly' rash, which is more prevalent when exposed to the sun. It classically spares the nasolabial folds and can last from days to weeks. Although it can be the sole clinical feature of SLE, it is often accompanied by other inflammatory features. Histology on immunofluorescence classically shows immune deposits at the dermal-epidermal junction.

Subacute cutaneous lupus erythematosus is a non-fixed and non-scarring lesion that remits and worsens. This is a distinct cutaneous lesion separate to malar rash. Often this lesion is seen as in between a malar rash and the scarring lesion of chronic lupus. These lesions are usually in sun-exposed regions. The lesions originate as papules or small plaques, with a slight scale that further evolves into lesions that look more psoriasiform in nature.

Discoid lesions can present either as an entity in itself, termed discoid lupus, or as part of SLE. The lesions start as erythematous papules or plaques, then thicken and become adherent, before developing a hypopigmented central area. Eventually the lesions scar with central atrophy. These lesions can occur in sun-exposed areas in the malar region and scalp, and in the latter area can cause permanent alopecia.

Corticosteroids are the cornerstone of SLE management and thus have a key role in the management of the cutaneous manifestations of SLE. Typically, low potency topical corticosteroids are used to manage facial lesions and peripheral lesions. Higher potency topical and oral corticosteroids are occasionally used if there is concern that lesions will scar.

Hydroxychloroquine is used in all manifestations of SLE, but is typically used to treat rash, fever, arthralgia, and hair loss. It appears to work by increasing intracytoplasmic pH and thereby altering the molecular assembly of a-e-peptide complexes of class II MHC molecules. This leads to decreased antigen processing and presentation by both macrophages and lymphoid dendritic cells. As a result, there is decreased stimulation of CD4+ T cells with decreased production of IL-1, IL-2, IL-4, IL-5, IL-6, and TNF-α. Many patients can be managed solely with hydroxychloroquine without recourse to corticosteroids.

Further Reading

Kuhn A, Ruland V, Bonsmann G (2011). Cutaneous lupus erythematosus: update of therapeutic options: part I. *Journal of the American Academy of Dermatology* 65, e179–e193.

Kuhn A, Ruland V, Bonsmann G (2011). Cutaneous lupus erythematosus: update of therapeutic options: part II. *Journal of the American Academy of Dermatology* 65, e195–e213.

39. E) Start regular antihistamines including a night-time sedating antihistamine

This patient presents with a generalized prurigo characterized by intermittent raised wheal-like lesions, which come and go. There is no psoriasiform quality to the lesions. Of note she has a stinging sensation in her mouth when she eats peaches, but has no localized swelling anywhere either in the face or the hands. This is likely to represent oral allergy syndrome, which is a self-limiting condition and is not related to type I hypersensitivity and is not angioedema.

Her background includes Raynaud's, which occurs in up to 30% of women at her age and is not likely to represent an underlying connective tissue disorder. The oral contraceptive pill can be used to treat recurrent angioedema and there have been case reports documenting angioedema associated with progesterone containing contraceptives. The oral contraceptive is not relevant in this case.

Chronic urticaria can be a symptom of hypocomplementaemia. Classically, hereditary angioedema occurs as a consequence of C1 esterase inhibitor deficiency, which causes hypocomplementaemia. As noted, she does not have psoriasiform lesions, which can occur in hypocomplementaemic vasculitis and can be confused with psoriasis.

The most likely cause of her symptoms is chronic urticaria, which is a condition that can persist or occur intermittently. The best therapy is regular antihistamines, in particular a sedating antihistamine to help her sleep. It is not appropriate to commence moderate dose corticosteroids, since she is likely to require long-term therapy, and this would lead to significant side effects. Hydroxychloroquine might have been useful if she had a hypocomplementaemic disorder, which is part of the lupus spectrum.

Tutorial

Chronic urticaria is characterized by the appearance of urticarial wheals, which last 4–36 hours; the duration of the lesion is what differentiates it from dermatographism. Dermatographism can occur in up to 4% of people, and describes the phenomenon when a wheal is induced with trauma or 'writing' on the skin. Sometimes this can remain for days or weeks.

Chronic urticaria can be a manifestation of an underlying disorder. In fact, up to 40% of patients with idiopathic chronic urticaria have a circulating IgG to the α subunit of the IgE receptor, which can activate mast cells and basophils to release histamine. There is also an association with hypocomplementaemia, which may explain urticaria occurring in hypocomplementaemic disorders. Hashimoto's thyroiditis is the only disorder with a clear and common association with chronic urticaria. Graves' disease is not as commonly associated.

In general, the evaluation of patients with chronic urticaria yields very little. Full blood count, biochemistry, and autoimmune serology are invariably normal. It is not useful to check the complement levels of patients with chronic urticaria. Hereditary angioedema due to C1 esterase inhibitor deficiency causes isolated angioedema and is not associated with hives. It is useful to check thyroid function and test for antithyroglobulin and antimicrosomal antibodies, since 19% will have disordered thyroid function and 27% will have antibodies. Patch testing is not useful, since a trigger is invariably not found.

Non-sedating H1-receptor antagonists such as cetirizine, desloratadine, or fexofenadine are the mainstay of therapy in chronic urticaria, and higher than standard doses are often needed. Sometimes, it is necessary to also give a sedating antihistamine, in particular if sleep is affected. The best option in this case is doxepin at 10–20 mg nightly. It is a psychotropic agent with tricyclic antidepressant and anxiolytic properties and is also a very potent H1- and H2-antagonist to the extent it is more potent at blocking H1 receptors than the other antihistamines mentioned.

Leukotriene antagonists have been used, but tend to be an adjunct to antihistamine therapy, rather than used in isolation. Corticosteroids are avoided due to the side effects of chronic use. Immunosuppressive drugs are very rarely used, with only case reports documented in the literature, so there are no recommendations for their use in chronic urticaria.

Further Reading

Kaplan A (2002). Chronic urticaria and angioedema. *New England Journal of Medicine* 346, 175–179.

40. E) Use of both hormonal and barrier contraception and regular pregnancy test

It is well known that isotretinoin causes birth defects. Even taking it for a few days during pregnancy can lead to central nervous system, cardiac, facial, and skull abnormalities. As a result, isotretinoin can only be prescribed by a dermatologist in a consultant-led service and patients are entered into a pregnancy prevention programme.

Guidelines drawn up by the British Association of Dermatologists carefully describe the process by which acne sufferers of childbearing age should be counselled and screened prior to commencing isotretinoin. A detailed menstrual and sexual history must be taken and contraception should be discussed in detail. Two forms of contraception should be used regularly, which are hormonal and barrier. Patients should be using regular contraception for one month prior to commencing treatment and then have a supervised pregnancy test to measure β-human chorionic gonadotropin either in the blood or urine. Once the pregnancy test returns negative, the patient signs a form confirming they understand the risks of using isotretinoin and that they will continue to use two forms of contraception. Using an IUCD is a more long-term form of contraception and dependent on the patient and whether there are any concerns with other forms of contraception.

Tutorial

Acne is a common skin condition of adolescence and frequently continues into adulthood until the fourth decade of life. The social, psychological, and emotional impact of acne is akin to that of arthritis, diabetes, and epilepsy. Acne is a follicular disease that is characterized by the impaction and distension of the pilosebaceous unit. Inflammation is often a feature and is caused by *Propionibacterium acne* colonization.

Acne is characterized by the presence of open and closed comedones, that is, blackheads and whiteheads, which often present with pustules and patches of erythema, but can present on their own. It is readily diagnosed by this presentation alone, so a skin biopsy is not necessary. The intensity of therapy is dependent on the presence of or the potential for scarring. The commonly used definition is highlighted in Table 2.3.

Table 2.3 Classification of acne in terms of potential for scarring

Severity	Description
Mild	Comedones are the main lesion, and papules and pustules number fewer than ten.
Moderate	There are 10–40 papules and pustules as well as 10–40 comedones. Maybe some truncal involvement.
Moderately severe	There are 40–100 papules and pustules as well as 40–100 comedones with up to five larger deeper nodular inflamed lesions, affecting the face, trunk, and back.
Severe	Nodulocystic acne and acne conglobate with many large, painful nodular or pustular lesions present and many smaller papules, pustules, and comedones.

There are topical and oral agents used for treatment. Topical therapy is only active where it is applied and used to prevent further lesions so should be applied daily to prevent recurrence. The two main classes of topical agents are:

1. Topical retinoids

These work by correcting abnormalities in follicular keratinocytes, treating and preventing comedones whilst limiting inflammatory lesions. They also appear to improve penetration of other topical therapies and may reduce hyperpigmentation on darker skin on resolution of inflammatory lesions. The maximal response to topical retinoids occurs over 12 weeks.

2. Topical antimicrobials

Topical antimicrobials are effective first-line agents. Benzoyl peroxide is notable for its rapid effect, but often leads to skin irritation. Topical macrolides are useful, but more so with other topical therapies.

Oral therapy is recommended for those with moderate-severe disease. The types of commonly used oral therapies are:

1. Oral antibiotics

Oral tetracyclines are the most commonly used antibiotics. Studies show that a 50–60% improvement in inflammatory lesions can be expected. It is often necessary to commence at a higher dose before reduction. If there is a lack of response this may be due to an inadequate duration of therapy, resistance, or infection by Gram-negative bacteria. Tetracyclines can cause gastrointestinal upset, especially at higher doses.

2. Hormonal therapy

Women with hyperandrogenism (irregular menses, hirsutism) who have acne resistant to conventional therapy, or have acne that quickly relapses after isotretinoin, ought to have an evaluation for androgen excess. These patients may benefit from oestrogen-containing hormonal contraceptives or spironolactone.

3. Isotretinoin

This should be confined to severe cases that have not responded to combination topical and oral therapy, with particularly severe inflammatory lesions. Isotretinoin reduces the size and secretion of sebaceous glands, prevents comedogenesis, and inhibits the growth of *Propionibacterium acnes* and inflammation. Forty per cent remain free of acne after one course; 40% have a less severe further eruption, which responds to less intensive therapy; and 20% require further isotretinoin. Isotretinoin has a number of other side effects including:

- Mood change: commonly manifests as depression, but also encompasses anxiety, mood swings, aggression, suicidal ideation, and psychosis. This also has to be discussed with the patient.
- Facial erythema, eczema, hair loss, photosensitivity, skin fragility.
- Variable dryness of the skin and mucous membranes.
- Myalgia and erythema.
- Photophobia, keratitis, and impaired night vision that can persist despite withdrawing the medication.
- Abnormal liver function tests, including hepatitis.
- Nausea, colitis, and pancreatitis (in those with hypertriglyceridaemia).
- Dyslipidaemia.
- Acne flare.
- Cutaneous vasculitis.
- Benign intracranial hypertension.

Due to the ocular complications, isotretinoin is contraindicated in those who require good night vision for their occupation, such as pilots, taxi and coach drivers.

Further Reading

Albert E (2008). Acne scarring: a review and current treatment modalities. *Journal of the American Academy of Dermatology* 59, 659–676.

Goodfield M, Cox N, Bowser A, et al. (2010). Advice on the safe introduction and continued use of isotretinoin in acne in the UK 2010. *British Journal of Dermatology* 162, 1172–1179.

41. D) Commence topical mupirocin

In this question, the patient's occupation is key to diagnosis. She has dry crusted lesions on her face, which is consistent with a diagnosis of impetigo. The rash is not typical of eczema, because it is neither weeping nor excoriated as a result of scratching. The question is specifically asking about management. Oral aciclovir is used to treat herpes simplex, so would not be useful in this case. The most likely organisms to cause impetigo are *Staphylococcus aureus* and β-haemolytic streptococci, thus an antibiotic would need to treat both organisms. The updated Cochrane review showed that in six studies consisting of 575 patients, topical antibiotics were superior to topical placebo. In ten studies of 440 patients neither topical mupirocin nor fusidic acid were superior to topical placebo. In ten studies, topical mupirocin was shown to be slightly superior to oral erythromycin, whilst oral penicillin has been shown to be inferior to both erythromycin and flucloxacillin. Overall, the best course of action is to commence topical mupirocin. There is no need to take a swab once the diagnosis of impetigo is made.

Tutorial

It is important to be aware of the common skin infections encountered in the community. These include impetigo, erysipelas, folliculitis/furunculosis, abscesses, and cellulitis.

1. Impetigo

This is the most common skin infection in children, but often occurs in adults especially those in close contact with children. It consists of superficial, non-follicular pustules, which are often crusted over with a yellow exudate. Most commonly it occurs in people of low socio-economic status, but it can occur in all communities. Ecthyma is a deeper form of impetigo caused by the same organisms but infiltrating deeper into the dermis. Like impetigo, it is characterized by crusting, but over ulcers that can scar. Studies have shown that topical antibiotics are the treatment of choice for impetigo, as compared with placebo and oral antibiotics. Antibiotics are required to cover the most common organisms, namely *Staphylococcus aureus* and β-haemolytic streptococci. Those with repeated episodes or extensive spread may benefit from oral antibiotics.

2. Folliculitis/furunculosis and abscesses

Folliculitis and furunculosis are infections of the hair follicle. Furunculosis is deeper than folliculitis, such that suppuration infiltrates into the deep dermis. Folliculitis can still cause suppuration, but more superficially. There tends to be a correlation between *Staphylococcus aureus* carriage and frequency of folliculitis and furunculosis in a population. This may be due to increased frequency of contact with those with infections and *Staphylococcus aureus* carriage. Folliculitis tends to be more common in patients with impaired immunity, such as diabetics, organ transplant recipients, or others on immunosuppressants. Chronic furunculosis tends to be difficult to treat, and sometimes requires sequential topical and oral antibiotics, as well as other conservative measures. Sometimes it requires the eradication of *Staphylococcus aureus* carriage, in particular from the nasal nares. Folliculitis is simply treated with oral flucloxacillin. Abscesses often require incision and drainage to treat effectively.

3. Erysipelas and cellulitis

Erysipelas is an acute, superficial, non-necrotising dermal/hypodermal infection most often caused by streptococci. The diagnosis is made when a patient presents with a sudden onset sharply demarcated shiny erythematous plaque accompanied by pain, swelling, and fever. It differs from cellulitis, because it does not spread. Erysipelas tends to be caused by β-haemolytic streptococci group A and rarely by staphylococci, which tends to cause spreading cellulitis. Risk factors include chronic lymphoedema, venous insufficiency, and toe-web intertrigo. The latter is the most common portal of entry. Other risk factors include diabetes mellitus and immunosuppression. Antibiotic choice for erysipelas must cover β-haemolytic streptococci and can be given parenterally depending on severity. Penicillin is usually adequate. The main issue in therapy is recurrence, which occurs in 20% of cases. Treating toe-web intertrigo and chronic lymphoedema can reduce recurrence. Treatment of cellulitis is again based upon clinical severity and often requires antibiotics to cover staphylococci.

Further Reading

Bernard P (2008). Management of common bacterial infections of the skin. *Current Opinion in Infectious Diseases* 21, 122–128.

Koning S, van der Sande R, Verhagen A, et al. (2012). Interventions for impetigo. *Cochrane Database Systematic Reviews* 1, CD003261.

42. A) Ask the patient to stop allopurinol and admit for observation

After commencing allopurinol the patient has developed a rash consistent with Stevens-Johnson syndrome (SJS). This can be life-threatening and is thought to be part of the spectrum of erythema multiforme. There are two types of erythema multiforme: major and minor. The frequency of erythema multiforme due to allopurinol is 1 in 300. To reduce the risk of this occurring, allopurinol ought to be commenced gently, increasing by 50–100 mg increments 2–4 weekly, until reaching a dose compatible with the patient's calculated creatinine clearance. The dose of allopurinol can be increased further at the same rate aiming for a urate level <0.36 mmol/L. Since SJS can be life-threatening, progress rapidly, and the patient already reports symptoms of the mouth and eyes, the appropriate action is for the patient to stop allopurinol and be admitted to hospital for observation and supportive therapy. It is dangerous to wait 72 hours, since there is a chance that the patient's condition will worsen. Skin patch testing is used when the cause of the reaction is not known. It is clear that allopurinol is the cause in this case, so is not useful in this case. There is no clinical utility to testing anti-allopurinol antibodies. Although erythema multiforme is not a type I hypersensitivity reaction, many would treat with prednisolone and antihistamines, but the evidence is unclear. However, this alone is not sufficient to treat SJS.

Tutorial

Erythema multiforme is a delayed type hypersensitivity reaction to infections or drugs. Classically it has been categorized into minor and major, with the major category encompassing SJS and toxic epidermal necrolysis (TEN), which are both life-threatening variants. Erythema multiforme minor differs from SJS and TEN in that it is confined to the mucosa. Exfoliation characterizes SJS and TEN, with <10% exfoliation in SJS and >30% in TEN. The causes of erythema multiforme are listed in Table 2.4.

Table 2.4 Common causes of erythema multiforme major and minor

Infections	Medications
Herpes simplex virus 1 and 2	Barbiturates
Mycoplasma pneumoniae	Hydantoins
Fungal infections	NSAIDs
Varicella zoster	Penicillins
Hepatitis C	Phenothiazines
Cytomegalovirus	Sulphonamides
HIV	Immunizations
	Ciprofloxacin
	Allopurinol

Herpes simplex virus accounts for 50% of cases and accounts for the majority of recurrent erythema multiforme. Otherwise, erythema multiforme is usually a self-limiting eruption that is mild and has no prodromal features. Occasionally there is itchiness and burning at the site of the rash, which is a characteristic target lesion. The lesions start as macules and become papules, which can gradually enlarge before becoming plaques over a few days. The lesions commence distally and progress proximally. Usually the lesions resolve within five weeks.

SJS and TEN share many of the same causes as erythema multiforme, but they tend to be triggered more by medications and an upper respiratory tract infection rather than herpes simplex virus. Both tend to commence 1–3 weeks following the introduction of the medication or the onset of infection. Within three days, mucous membranes of the eyes, mouth, nose, and genitalia become involved in almost 90% of cases. Exfoliation occurs in the next 3–5 days, at which point the process becomes life-threatening with extensive loss of skin function, which causes fluid and protein loss, barrier function, and hypothermia.

Treatment of erythema multiforme, SJS, and TEN first involves identification of the triggering factor, and if it is a medication this must be stopped. In the case of erythema multiforme, if it is suspected that herpes simplex is the cause, then it is reasonable to commence anti-viral therapy. Histamine and prednisolone can be given for symptom relief.

SJS and TEN have significant mortality rates at 1–3% and 30–50% respectively. To improve outcome, there should be early transfer to a dedicated burns unit and introduction of supportive care, such as fluid resuscitation and mechanical ventilation. Systemic corticosteroids remain a mainstay of therapy in SJS and TEN, but their use in TEN is more controversial. There have been conflicting reports of increased mortality with corticosteroid use in TEN, particularly with increased rates of infection. Other studies using immunosuppressive therapies, such as cyclophosphamide and intravenous gammaglobulin have proved inconclusive, although some centres advocate the use of intravenous gammaglobulin since it is less likely to cause infections.

Further Reading

Gerull R, Nelle M, Schaible T (2011). Toxic epidermal necrolysis and Stevens-Johnson syndrome: a review. *Critical Care Medicine* 39, 1521–1532.

Lamoreux M, Sternbach M, Hsu W (2006). Erythema multiforme. *American Family Physician* 74, 1883–1888.

43. B) Cicatricial pemphigoid

This middle-aged gentleman has presented with a rash on his legs as well as pronounced eye symptoms and corneal irritation as denoted by discomfort blinking. The patient also has oral involvement and blisters are present on his ankles.

From the history and presentation, it is unlikely to be due to antibiotics. SJS can occur following administration of medications or following infections. There is no significant history of a preceding infection and the timing of the lesions is not consistent with SJS caused by antibiotics. The pattern of involvement crosses the midline and is not dermatomal which makes reactivation of varicella zoster unlikely, though it can be generalized in the immunosuppressed.

The most likely cause of this patient's symptoms is an autoimmune blistering skin condition. In pemphigus, blisters are less commonly present on examination. Those that are present tend to be flaccid, which is not typical of the ulcers in this case. Blisters in bullous pemphigoid tend to be present at examination and are tenser than in pemphigus. This patient seems to have bullous pemphigoid in view of the presence of blisters; however, eye and oral mucosal involvement is key in this question. There is a subset of bullous pemphigoid patients that tend to have more mucocutaneous involvement, especially oral and ocular mucous membranes, called cicatricial pemphigoid. The patient fits this clinical picture the best.

Tutorial

Pemphigus and bullous pemphigoid are two autoimmune skin diseases characterized by acantholysis and blister formation. Both occur as a result of autoantibodies directed at specific skin components, eventually leading to blister formation.

In pemphigus, autoantibodies are directed against components of desmosome structures involved in cell adhesion. The disruption of these cause blister formation. There are several types of pemphigus, but the two major types are: foliaceous and vulgaris. Vulgaris is characterized by a flaccid bulla due to separation in the deep part of the epidermis. It can involve solely the mucosa or have extensive involvement with mucosal and cutaneous lesions with acantholysis deep in the epidermis. The foliaceous variant causes blister formation by detachment at the granular layer in the superficial epidermis. The pathogenesis of pemphigus is not fully understood, but common precipitants include infections, especially herpes simplex, thiol drugs, penicillins, stress, neoplasms, thermal burns, and ionizing radiation are known environmental triggers.

Classically, pemphigus affects patients in middle age, aged 40–60 years. It is a rare condition, with an incidence of approximately two cases per 100,000 person years. It presents with painful oral lesions in 50–70%, with deeper involvement causing hoarseness and dysphagia. It can also involve the eyes, genitalia, and anus. Diagnosis is based on histology, with gold standard being indirect immunofluorescence demonstrating IgG autoantibodies directed against keratinocyte structures.

Bullous pemphigoid is a blistering condition that tends to affect older people with a peak incidence in the seventh decade. Autoantibodies are directed against hemidesmosomes, a basement membrane apparatus that promotes adhesion between the basal cell and basement membrane. In bullous pemphigoid, tenser sub-epidermal blisters form, rather than the more flaccid blisters found in pemphigus. When these tense blisters rupture, they leave shallow ulcers. Although oral involvement is more common in pemphigus, up to a third of patients with pemphigoid can have oral involvement. Cicatricial pemphigoid is a subset of bullous pemphigoid, which is characterized by predominant mucous membrane involvement, particularly of the oral and ocular mucous membrane. It causes scarring and can lead to blindness.

Pemphigoid tends to have a chronic course with exacerbations and remissions. Like pemphigus, diagnosis is based on histopathology with indirect immunofluorescence demonstrating circulating IgG that binds to the basement membrane of normal stratified squamous epithelium.

Both pemphigus and pemphigoid are treated with immunosuppressants, with corticosteroids and dapsone used earlier in disease. Dosing and delivery of corticosteroids are dependent on severity of diseases. If there is substantial body surface area or extensive oral and ocular mucous membrane involvement, then a more aggressive corticosteroid and immunosuppressive regimen is undertaken. Azathioprine or mycophenolate mofetil are the immunosuppression drugs of choice. Rituximab has also been used in treatment, following a four-weekly regimen similar to that found in the treatment of lymphoma. The concern with aggressive immunosuppression is the risk of infection, particularly in elderly patients, so they require close monitoring whilst on treatment.

Further Reading

Lawrence S (2012). Ocular and oral mucous membrane pemphigoid (cicatricial pemphigoid). *Clinics in Dermatology* 30, 34–37.

Parker S, MacKelfresh J (2011). Autoimmune blistering diseases in the elderly. *Clinics in Dermatology* 29, 69–79.

44. D) Jejunal biopsy

The patient has a papular rash with evidence of excoriations consistent with scratching. It is notable that the rash does not respond to emollients and corticosteroid creams. The most likely cause of this rash is dermatitis herpetiformis (DH). This is often characterized by intense itchiness and stinging and is often associated with coeliac disease, which is likely the cause of his microcytic anaemia. It is worth noting, that often patients with coeliac disease may have no gastrointestinal symptoms at all.

A skin biopsy or urine dipstick is not useful in diagnosing coeliac disease. A urine dipstick would be useful if the patient had Henoch-Schönlein purpura, since renal involvement is a known complication of this condition. A skin biopsy is useful in diagnosing DH, but would not identify the cause of the condition.

Immunoglobulin levels are not useful in the diagnosis of coeliac disease. IgA levels are 10–15 times more likely to be lower in coeliac disease than in the general population, but this is not diagnostic.

Anti-endomysial antibodies are sensitive, but not specific, for coeliac disease and are not the gold standard for diagnosis. They are found in inflammatory bowel disease and arthritis. It is useful to screen for coeliac disease and would be the first test to do in this instance. The best test to diagnose coeliac disease is a jejunal biopsy. This would show flattened villi, which is pathognomonic of coeliac disease.

Tutorial

DH is an itching, blistering skin condition first described in 1884 and its association with coeliac disease (CD) was first described in 1967. This was confirmed when the enteropathy in the bowels of patients with CD and DH were found to be similar, with increased fat excretion, low serum folate levels, low iron stores, and low serum IgM.

CD is five times more common than DH. However, it is thought that asymptomatic CD is five times more common than symptomatic CD. DH typically consists of papules on urticarial plaques and is most often present on the extensor surfaces of the elbows, forearms, knees, and buttocks. In severe disease, lesions can occur on the scalp and face. Biopsy demonstrates granular IgA deposits in the papillary dermis by direct immunofluorescence. Without the presence of IgA, DH cannot be diagnosed, so serial sections may be required for diagnosis.

IgA tissue transglutaminase (TTGA) and anti-endomysial (AEA) antibodies can also be used in the diagnosis of DH and CD. In CD, IgA-TTGA and IgA-AEA have been shown to be positive in untreated CD in 93–97% and 89–100% of patients respectively. These are lower for DH in both IgA-TTGA and IgA-AEA, at 75% and 66% respectively. Thus, antibodies are less sensitive in DH than in CD.

To confirm the diagnosis of CD in DH, a jejunal biopsy is necessary. Two-thirds of patients will show villous atrophy consistent with a diagnosis of CD, whilst one third will show raised intra-epithelial lymphocyte counts and/or an increase in T-cell receptor gamma delta intraepithelial lymphocytes.

Although DH is primarily associated with CD, it is also associated with other autoimmune conditions, such as pernicious anaemia, type I diabetes, and inflammatory bowel disease. There is also an increased risk of lymphoma in this group of patients, and as in CD, a gluten-free diet is protective.

Dapsone, sulphapyridine, and sulphamethoxypyridazine can be used to treat the rash in DH. The dose should be titrated to the lowest dose required for symptomatic control. Relapse occurs within a week of stopping this medication and it should be commenced at the same time as gluten withdrawal. This is done within the first six months of therapy. Gluten withdrawal is the mainstay of management of both DH and CD, but there are a number of issues with the gluten-free diet:

1. The diet needs to be strict to be effective.
2. It takes an average of 6–9 months before dose reduction of oral therapies can be achieved.
3. It takes an average of two years for the diet to be effective at controlling DH.

The gluten-free diet is difficult to maintain for many patients, so it is important that patients are instructed and supervised by a dietician.

Further Reading

Kárpáti S (2012). Dermatitis herpetiformis. *Clinical Dermatology* 30(1): 56–59.

45. C) Lichen planus

The presentation is most akin to lichen planus (LP). The picture demonstrates a papulosquamous rash. The lesions are pruritic, polygonal, flat-topped violaceous papules. On the surface is a network of grey lines called Wickham's striae. The lesions are often symmetrical and oral involvement is common. There is a predilection for the wrists, as demonstrated in the picture and there is also often oral ulceration as is the case here.

Whilst one may have considered psoriasis to be the diagnosis, it is important to remember that psoriasis classically consists of oval plaques with silvery scaling on the elbows, knees, hairline, and natal cleft in particular. It does not affect oral mucosa.

Contact dermatitis is usually the result of an exogenous agent or agents that causes injury. It usually occurs in two forms. The first is due to an irritant, such as an acid; or second, as a manifestation of delayed-type hypersensitivity, such as exposure to plants or metals. There is no history of exposure and contact dermatitis normally presents as hand eczema, which is not consistent with the above picture.

The pattern does not follow atopic dermatitis, which normally affects the flexures. Occasionally it can affect the wrist, but more typically affects the elbows, back of the knees, neck, and face. Although patients often have a history of asthma and eczema, it does not always occur.

Nummular eczema is characterized by circular or oval 'coin like' lesions. Initially the lesions consist of oedematous papules that become crusty and scaly. This tends to occur on the trunk or extensor surfaces of the extremities, particularly the dorsum of the hands and the pretibial areas. It most commonly occurs in middle-aged men. The cause of it is unknown.

Tutorial

LP is an inflammatory dermatosis that affects mucocutaneous surfaces. LP tends to affect the young or the middle-aged, with an incidence of 20–30 per 100,000 in the young. There is an equal incidence in men and women. It is a self-limiting condition that can last anywhere between one month and seven years. The pathogenesis of LP is not fully understood but thought to be T-cell mediated.

Classically, LP presents as polygonal, flat-topped violaceous papules and plaques, with superimposed greyish lines called Wickham's striae. Most commonly it affects the extremities, particularly the wrists and ankles. It also exhibits Köebner's phenomenon, whereby lesions arise at the site of trauma. The clinical features are relatively specific, but a biopsy can be taken for diagnosis. The characteristic finding is lymphohistiocytic infiltration at the dermal-epidermal junction with hydropic degeneration of the epidermis.

There are various types of LP:

1. Oral involvement

This is the most common autoimmune involvement of the oral mucosa and occurs in 30–70% of patients with LP. They can be non-tender white reticulated patches or tender erosions or ulcers.

2. Genital involvement

The most common type in this area is erosive, and can affect the vulva and glans penis. Often there is superimposed infection, which should be investigated and treated.

3. Oesophageal involvement

This is a rare variant, which is heralded by dysphagia and can lead to stricture formation.

4. Lichen planopilaris

This affects the hair follicles and can lead to alopecia, with women more commonly affected than men. The alopecia is scarring in nature and affects frontal, parietal, and occipital areas. Lesions tend to be pruritic and painful.

5. Nail involvement

There are several nail changes occurring in LP. The most specific type is a wedge-shaped deformity of the nail bed, causing a dorsal pterygium.

It is generally recommended that patients with LP should continue to be monitored due to the risk of developing cutaneous malignancy. Cutaneous involvement does not appear to increase risk, but penile and vulval involvement may. It is also notable that LP is associated with other autoimmune conditions, such as alopecia areata, vitiligo, and discoid lupus. Hepatitis C is also associated with the condition and the prevalence of LP correlates positively with background rates of hepatitis C. LP is also part of Good's syndrome, which consists of combined variable immunodeficiency, thymoma, and LP.

Treatment of cutaneous LP is usually topical medium- to high-potency corticosteroids and occasionally oral corticosteroids are used. Oral retinoids are not often used. With oral involvement, topical calcineurin inhibitors are also used. First-line therapy for genital involvement is potent topical corticosteroids.

Further Reading

Lehman J, Tollefson M, Gibson L (2009). Lichen planus. *International Journal of Dermatology* 48, 682–694.

46. **A 68-year-old male attended for his annual diabetes review. His past
medical history included hypertension, ischaemic heart disease
complicated by a myocardial infarction three years previously, stage II
diabetic retinopathy, and proteinuric chronic kidney disease—presumed
to be due to diabetes. His medications included metformin 1g bd,
gliclazide 40 mg bd, ramipril 10 mg od, bisoprolol 5 mg od, atorvastatin
40 mg od, and sodium bicarbonate 500 mg bd. He reported good
compliance with his medication and no symptoms of hypoglycaemia.
Unfortunately, blood tests demonstrated that his renal function had
continued to decline over the previous year and his eGFR had fallen from
30 ml/min.1.73 m² to 24 ml/min/1.73 m². His HbA1c was 56 mmol/mol.**

    **Given the drop in renal function, a decision was made to stop his
metformin due to risk of adverse effects.**

    How should his diabetes regimen be best managed?

    A. Continue gliclazide 40 mg bd monotherapy

    B. Increase dose of gliclazide to 80 mg bd

    C. Start a dipeptidylpeptidase-4 (DDP4) inhibitor

    D. Start a SGLT2 inhibitor

    E. Start insulin

47. **A 38-year-old male attended his GP surgery and reported that he often suffered from tension type headaches and passed a lot of urine. Three weeks previously, he had had loin to groin pain which settled after a few days. He had smoked 30 cigarettes a day since childhood. He had a past medical history of meningitis in his early twenties; pulmonary tuberculosis as a child; and bipolar depression for which he took lithium. On examination he had a BP of 130/80 mmHg, a heart rate of 70 beats per minute with normal skin turgor and moist mucous membranes with a normal JVP.**

```
Investigations:
   WCC 12 × 10⁹/L
   CRP                       <10 g/L
   Sodium                    129 mmol/L
   Potassium                 4.4 mmol/L
   Urea                      3.4 mmol/L
   Creatinine                86 µmol/L
   Fasting glucose           4.6 mmol/L
   HbA1c                     37 mmol/mol     (20-42 mmol/mol)%
   AST                       20 iU/L
   ALT                       28 iU/L
   ALP                       120 iU/L
   Bilirubin                 14 µmol/L
   Albumin                   32 g/L
   Corrected calcium         2.38 mmol/L
   Lithium level             1.0 mmol/L      (0.6-1.2 mmol/L)
   24-hour urine volume      4.3 litres
   Urine dipstick            negative for all abnormalities
   Plasma osmolality         274 mOsm/kg
   Urine osmolality          150 mOsm/kg
   Overnight                 fluid deprivation test: morning
                             urine osmolality 880 mOsm/kg
```

Which of the following is the diagnosis?

A. Diabetes insipidus secondary to pituitary tuberculosis

B. Diabetes mellitus

C. Lithium induced nephrogenic diabetes insipidus

D. Polyuria post obstructive nephropathy secondary to calculus

E. Primary polydipsia

48. **A 16-year-old female presented with a ten-month history of amenorrhoea after previously having irregular menstrual cycles. She was also troubled by significant facial hair. She had a past medical history of multiple UTIs during infancy. On examination she had hirsutism, a lying BP of 115/70 mmHg and a standing BP of 100/50 mmHg. Her heart sounds were normal and her JVP was not raised. She had normal and equal breath sounds. Abdominal examination does not reveal organomegaly or masses and her neurological examination was entirely normal.**

```
Investigations:
  Sodium                           138 mmol/L
  Potassium                        4.8 mmol/L
  Urea                             5 mmol/L
  Creatinine                       71 µmol/L
  AST                              30 iU/L
  ALT                              28 iU/L
  ALP                              180 iU/L
  Bilirubin                        14 µmol/L
  Albumin                          39 g/L
  Corrected calcium                2.39 mmol/L
  Blood glucose                    4.0 mmo/L
  9 am 17-OHprogesterone           30 nmol/L (normal <5 nmol/L)
  Dehydroepiandrostenedione        25 nmol/L (normal <12 nmol/L)
  Androstenedione                  20 nmol/L (normal 5-12 nmol/L)
  Testosterone                     5.1 nmol/L (0.8-3.1 nmol/L)
  Prolactin                        200 miU/L (normal 100-550 miU/L)
  Recumbent and ambulant           normal
  renin levels
```

Which of the following is true?

A. Autonomic function testing should be carried out

B. Fludrocortisone is the only treatment needed

C. The patient has 11β-hydroxylase deficiency

D. The patient has partial 21-hydroxylase deficiency

E. The patient should be commenced on furosemide

49. **A 22-year-old male presented with a complaint of bilateral breast enlargement. On direct questioning he also reported reduced libido and erectile dysfunction. He had no past medical history and was on no medication. On examination he had absent pubic and axillary hair, gynaecomastia, and small firm testes with around 6 ml volume. He had a height of 2.0 metres and his BP was 125/80 mmHg with normal heart sounds. His respiratory examination revealed normal breath sounds with no chest wall deformities. Abdominal and neurological examination was entirely normal.**

```
Investigations:
  Sodium                    140 mmol/L
  Potassium                 4.1 mmol/L
  Urea                      4.9 mmol/L
  Creatinine                87 µmol/L
  Testosterone              6 nmol/L (11-36 nmol/L)
  LH                        42 iu/L (1.8-12 iu/L)
  FSH                       26 iu/L (1.5-12.4 iu/L)
  Oestradiol                200 pmol/L (20-100 pmol/L)
  Prolactin                 112 miU/L (<450 miU/L)
```

What is the most likely diagnosis?

A. Congenital adrenal hypoplasia

B. Cryptorchidism

C. Kallmann syndrome

D. Klinefelter's syndrome

E. Prolactinoma

50. **A 32-year-old male presented with numbness and tingling of the lips and fingers, and cramps. He had no past medical history. On examination he had a BP of 130/80 mmHg with normal heart sounds and a JVP at +1 cm. He exhibited positive Chvostek's and Trousseau's signs. His fourth and fifth fingers were shortened bilaterally. His height was 1.4 metres with a BMI of 34. His breath sounds were normal with no added sounds. There were no abdominal masses. Neurological examination was normal.**

```
Investigations:
   Hb                       141 g/L
   MCV                      89 fL
   WCC                      10 × 10⁹/L
   Platelets                400 × 10⁹/L
   CRP                      <10 g/L
   Sodium                   146 mmol/L
   Potassium                3.8 mmol/L
   Urea                     3.0 mmol/L
   Creatinine               72 µmol/L
   Corrected calcium        1.35 mmol/L
   Magnesium                0.79 mmol/L
   Phosphate                1.4 mmol/L
   Blood glucose            4.1 mmol/L
   PTH                      18 pmol/L
   CXR                      normal
   Hand X-rays              shortened fourth metacarpals
```

What is the most likely diagnosis?

A. DiGeorge syndrome

B. Idiopathic hypoparathyroidism

C. Pseudohypoparathyroidism type Ia

D. Pseudohypoparathyroidism type Ib

E. Pseudopseudohypoparathyroidism

51. **A 43-year-old male presented with episodes of pallor, sweating, tremor, and irritability which were relieved by eating. He had no previous medical history. On examination his BMI was 32, heart rate was 72 beats per minute, and BP was 110/80 mmHg. His cardiovascular, respiratory, abdominal, and neurological examinations were completely normal. The patient was given a blood glucose monitor, which measured a glucose of <2.2 on three separate occasions when he was experiencing the above symptoms.**

```
Investigations:
  Sodium                   136 mmol/L
  Potassium                4.8 mmol/L
  Urea                     5.0 mmol/L
  Creatinine               94 µmol/L
  AST                      30 iU/L
  ALT                      28 iU/L
  ALP                      180 iU/L
  Bilirubin                13 µmol/L
  Albumin                  35 g/L
  Corrected calcium        2.84 mmol/L
  Magnesium                0.99 mmol/L
  Phosphate                0.7 mmol/L
  Random blood glucose     4.5 mmol/L
```

What is the likely underlying diagnosis?

A. Insulinoma

B. MEN type I

C. MEN type II

D. POEMS syndrome

E. Primary hyperparathyroidism

52. **A 50-year-old female presented with a 14-month history of dry cough, night sweats, and gritty eyes following an episode of tender lesions on her shins. She also reported a history of arthralgia, galactorrhoea, and menstrual disturbance. Her medical history included type II diabetes. She was a non-smoker. On examination she had cervical and axillary lymphadenopathy, enlarged parotid glands, and lupus pernio. On examination her heart sounds were normal, her BP was 120/80 mmHg and auscultation of her chest revealed fine crackles bilaterally. Her abdominal examination was unremarkable apart from bilateral inguinal lymphadenopathy. Neurological examination was normal.**

```
Investigations:
    Hb                        136 g/L
    MCV                       92 fL
    WCC                       10 × 10⁹/L
    Platelets                 310 × 10⁹/L
    CRP                       <10 g/L
    Sodium                    136 mmol/L
    Potassium                 4.6 mmol/L
    Urea                      5.0 mmol/L
    Creatinine                74 µmol/L
    Corrected calcium         2.39 mmol/L
    Blood glucose             5.6 mmol/L
    Serum ACE                 220 units/L (8–53 u/L)
    Serum                     βHCG Negative
    TSH                       2.5 mU/L (0.4–5.0 mU/L)
    LDH                       150 iU/L (10–250 iU/L)
    ECG                       normal sinus rhythm
    CXR                       bilateral hilar lymphadenopathy
                              and fibrosis
    Lymph node biopsy         non-caseating granulomata
```

Which of the following blood tests should next be performed based on endocrine history?

A. Serum oestradiol and gonadotrophins
B. Serum prolactin
C. Sex hormone binding globulin
D. Testosterone and androstenedione
E. Thyroid function tests

53. **A 32-year-old female presented to her GP stating that she had become pregnant. This was subsequently confirmed. Her previous medical history included meningococcal sepsis during which she experienced bilateral adrenal haemorrhage. Subsequently she had been treated for adrenal insufficiency with hydrocortisone 5 mg tds and fludrocortisone 50 μg od. On examination her BP was 118/80 mmHg lying and 125/80 mmHg on standing.**

   Which of the following is correct with regard to her pregnancy?

   A. Her current medication doses should be continued throughout her pregnancy

   B. Her current medication should remain unchanged until the third trimester when her hydrocortisone should be decreased by 50% and the fludrocortisone dose should be guided by BP and serum potassium

   C. Her current medication should remain unchanged until the third trimester when her hydrocortisone should be increased by 50% and the fludrocortisone dose should be guided by BP and serum potassium

   D. Renin levels can be used to guide her hydrocortisone dosing

   E. Two days before labour the hydrocortisone should be stopped

54. **A 27-year-old male presented to clinic with intermittent episodes of visual blurring. The patient reported experiencing headaches, palpitations, abdominal pains, and nausea, with the episodes of visual disturbance. He had no past medical history and took no regular medications. He was a smoker and drank 5–10 units of alcohol per week. He worked in a stressful occupation as a financial analyst. On examination, the pulse rate was 88 beats per minute and BP was 160/98 mmHg. Auscultation of the heart sounds revealed a mid-systolic click, but no murmurs. The chest was clear to auscultation. Abdominal examination revealed no palpable masses. Neurological examination was unremarkable. Direct slit lamp ophthalmoscopy demonstrated retinal angiomas.**

```
Investigations:
   Hb                    140 g/L
   MCV                   90 fL
   WCC                   10 × 10⁹/L
   Platelets             300 × 10⁹/L
   CRP                   <10 g/L
   Sodium                136 mmol/L
   Potassium             4.8 mmol/L
   Urea                  5.0 mmol/L
   Creatinine            102 µmol/L
   Corrected calcium     2.42 mmol/L
   Magnesium             0.99 mmol/L
   ECG                   sinus rhythm; S in V₁ + R in V₆ ≥ 35 mm
   Abdominal USS         bilateral renal cysts
```

Which investigation should be performed to biochemically confirm the diagnosis?

A. 24-hour urine for catecholamines/metanephrines or plasma metanephrines

B. MRI of adrenal glands

C. Renal biopsy

D. Thyroid function tests

E. Urinary VMAs

55. **A 28-year-old male presented with recurrent episodes of diarrhoea associated with flushing. On direct questioning he also reported trouble swallowing. He had no past medical history. On examination he had a dominant thyroid nodule and cervical lymphadenopathy. He also had a high arched palate, painless nodules on his lips, pectus excavatum, and scoliosis. Heart sounds were normal, and his chest was clear on auscultation. Abdominal and neurological examination was normal.**

```
Investigations:
   Hb                        139 g/L
   MCV                       92 fL
   WCC                       12 × 10⁹/L
   Platelets                 400 × 10⁹/L
   CRP                       <10 g/L
   Sodium                    139 mmol/L
   Potassium                 4.8 mmol/L
   Urea                      5.0 mmol/L
   Creatinine                81 µmol/L
   Corrected calcium         2.39 mmol/L
   Magnesium                 0.94 mmol/L
   Calcitonin                95 pg/mL (M5.0 pg/mL)
   Pentagastrin test         stimulated calcitonin of >200 ng/l
                             (normal <80 ng/L)
   Thyroid nodule biopsy     C cell hyperplasia and amyloid
```

Which of the following is the likely diagnosis?

A. Hirschsprung's disease
B. MEN type I
C. MEN type IIa
D. MEN type IIb
E. Primary hyperparathyroidism

56. **A 41-year-old female presented with headaches, sweating, and irregular periods. Her past medical history included a recent admission with renal calculi. On examination she had macroglossia, increased interdental spacing, prognathism, proximal myopathy, and normal heart sounds with displaced apex beat. The chest was clear on auscultation and abdominal examination revealed no masses. Neurological examination was unremarkable.**

Which of the following would confirm the clinically suspected diagnosis?

A. A growth hormone measurement of <1 mU/L (0.3 µg/L) after a 75 g glucose load
B. A growth hormone measurement of 20 mU/L (6.3 µg/L) after a 75 g glucose load
C. MRI revealing a mass in the pituitary
D. Raised IGF-1
E. Random growth hormone measurement of 24 mU/L (8 µg/L)

57. A 45-year-old female presented with tiredness, dizziness, abdominal pain, and weight loss. She was known to have antiphospholipid syndrome complicated by two episodes of pulmonary embolism. Warfarin was her only medication. On examination her heart sounds were normal, BP lying was 110/80 mmHg and on standing was 80/50 mmHg. Chest examination was normal and there were no abdominal masses. Neurological examination was also normal.

```
Investigations:
  Hb                       136 g/L
  WCC                      11 × 10⁹/L
  Platelets                310 × 10⁹/L
  INR                      3.0
  Sodium                   122 mmol/L
  Potassium                5.4 mmol/L
  Urea                     4.9 mmol/L
  Creatinine               86 µmol/L
  Corrected calcium        2.60 mmol/L
  Fasting blood glucose    3.5 mmol/L
  9 am cortisol            105 nmol/L (138–635 nmol/L)
```

Which of the following is correct?

A. A short Synacthen (tetracosactide) test should be performed, along with an MRI of her abdomen

B. Fludrocortisone only should be commenced

C. Her warfarin should be stopped

D. Random cortisol level is always diagnostic

E. She has autoimmune polyglandular syndrome type II

58. A 47-year-old man presented with episodes of flushing for the previous year. These episodes were often precipitated by hot drink and had recently been associated with diarrhoea and wheezing. His medications included aspirin, salbutamol, and omeprazole. He had a history of bipolar disorder and panic attacks, hypertension, and asthma. On examination he had a fixed split-second heart sound, a BP of 125/75 mmHg and occasional bilateral wheeze on respiratory examination. He had normal abdominal and neurological examination. A concern was raised of a possible diagnosis of carcinoid syndrome and he was referred for further investigation.

Which of the following is true?

A. Chromogranin A is a sensitive test for carcinoid tumours but may be falsely positive in this case

B. If the patient's liver function tests are normal then he is unlikely to have carcinoid syndrome, which would involve liver metastases

C. Investigations for MEN type II should also be considered

D. Radio-labelled octreotide scanning can be used for localization of carcinoid tumours in only 20% of cases

E. The finding of thickened mitral and aortic valves on echocardiography would be typical

59. **A 53-year-old female presented with fatigue, weight gain, and easy bruising. She had a past medical history of severe depression. Apart from aspirin, her only medication was an antidepressant, but she reported she had recently stopped taking that. On examination she had three bruises on her upper and lower limbs, a dorsocervical fat pad, a BP of 150/90 mmHg, and purple striae on her abdomen.**

```
Investigations:
   Sodium                        140 mmol/L
   Potassium                     3.2 mmol/L
   Urea                          4.9 mmol/L
   Creatinine                    86 µmol/L
   Albumin                       39 g/L
   Corrected calcium             2.39 mmol/L
   Blood glucose                 12 mmol/L
   Random cortisol               1000 nmol/L
```

To help confirm the diagnosis, which of the following should be done next?

A. Insulin tolerance test

B. Overnight dexamethasone suppression test

C. Spot urinary free cortisol

D. Two further random serum cortisol measurements

E. Urinary 17-ketosteroids

60. **A 38-year-old female presented with painful grittiness of her eyes and new blurred vision. Four months previously, she had been diagnosed with Graves' disease for which she was treated with carbimazole. She had a past medical history of vitiligo. Her only medication was carbimazole 20 mg od. On examination she had eyelid retraction, proptosis and visual acuity of <6/18. Heart sounds were normal with a BP of 140/90 mmHg. Neurological examination was normal.**

```
Investigations:
   Hb                    140 g/L
   WCC                   10 × 10⁹/L
   Platelets             300 × 10⁹/L
   TSH                   <0.01 mU/L (0.3–5.5 mU/L)
   Serum freeT4          25 pmol/L (10–22 pmol/L)
```

What is your next best course of action?

A. Artificial tears and liquid paraffin ointment only

B. Continue current dose of carbimazole

C. Increase carbimazole to 30 mg od and refer to the ophthalmologist urgently

D. Recommend prisms

E. Urgent ophthalmology review

61. **A 36-year-old male was referred for investigation of his hypertension. He had no past medical history. He had a mother and grandmother who were both treated for hypertension. His only medication was atenolol 50 mg od. His BP was 175/95 mmHg and equal in both arms. The remainder of his physical examination was largely unremarkable.**

Investigations:

Hb	145 g/L
MCV	99 fL
WCC	10 × 10⁹/L
Platelets	355 × 10⁹/L
CRP	<10 g/L
Sodium	140 mmol/L
Potassium	3.0 mmol/L
Urea	4.9 mmol/L
Creatinine	86 μmol/L
AST	30 iU/L
ALT	28 iU/L
ALP	180 iU/L
Bilirubin	14 μmol/L
Albumin	37 g/L
Protein	60 g/L
Corrected calcium	2.38 mmol/L
Magnesium	0.99 mmol/L
Blood glucose	4.5 mmol/L
ECG	sinus rhythm; S in V_1 + R in $V_6 \geq 35$ mm

Which of the following would you do next?

A. Increase his atenolol dose only

B. Perform an aldosterone/renin assay

C. Start a calcium channel antagonist

D. Switch his antihypertensive to doxazosin, control hypokalaemia with supplementation and then perform an aldosterone/rennin assay

E. Titrate up the doxazosin dose to maximum

62. **A 25-year-old female was admitted to hospital with seizures, episodes of visual disturbance, and altered mental state. These episodes had been preceded by her experiencing sweating and tremors. Her past medical history included bipolar disorder and hypertension. She had a strong family history of diabetes affecting both of her parents. On examination she was drowsy, clammy, and sweaty. Her BP was 110/70 mmHg. Heart sounds revealed an ejection systolic murmur, normal breath sounds, and normal abdominal examination. Her blood glucose was measured at 1.9 mmol/L. She was treated with intravenous dextrose and her symptoms resolved.**

```
Investigations:
  Hb                     127 g/L
  MCV                    88 fL
  WCC                    12 × 10⁹/L
  Platelets              320 × 10⁹/L
  CRP                    <10 g/L
  Sodium                 140 mmol/L
  Potassium              3.1 mmol/L
  Urea                   10 mmol/L
  Creatinine             100 µmol/L
  Blood glucose          2.1 mmol/L
  Insulin level          1300 pmol/L (normal 21-115 pmol/L)
  C-peptide              0.1 ng/mL (0.27-1.3 ng/mL)
  TSH                    4 mU/L
  Urinary sulphonylurea metabolites: negative
```

What is the next step in management?

A. Arrange calcium stimulation test

B. Arrange mixed meal test

C. Organize an abdominal CT

D. Refer for psychiatric input

E. Start diazoxide

63. A 61-year-old male presented with bilateral breast enlargement and lethargy. He had a history of hypertension and psoriasis. He was on aspirin, atenolol, and doxazocin. On examination he had gynaecomastia without any distinct masses. His BMI was 26 and he had a BP of 130/80 mmHg. The remainder of his physical examination was unremarkable.

```
Investigations:
  Hb                    129 g/L
  MCV                   88 fL
  WCC                   11 × 10⁹/L
  Platelets             340 × 10⁹/L
  CRP                   <10 g/L
  Sodium                136 mmol/L
  Potassium             4.8 mmol/L
  Urea                  5.0 mmol/L
  Creatinine            98 µmol/L
  ALT                   21 iU/L
  ALP                   123 iU/L
  Bilirubin             7 µmol/L
  Albumin               38 g/L
  Serum βHCG            negative
  TSH                   0.3 mU/L        (0.35-5.5 mU/L)
  Serum free T4         10 pmol/L       (10-22 pmol/L)
  Testosterone          6 nmol/l        (8.4-28.7 nmo/l)
  SHBG                  67 nmol/L       (13-71 nmol/L)
  Prolactin             200 mU/L        (<375 mU/L)
  LH                    0.2 U/l         (1-10 U/l)
  FSH                   1.4 U/L         (1.4-18 U/L)
  CXR                   normal
```

What should be done next?

A. Abdominal CT scan
B. Biopsy of the breast
C. MRI of the pituitary gland
D. Stop the doxazocin
E. Testicular ultrasound

64. **A 28-year-old male presented with painless lumps in his neck. He was otherwise asymptomatic. He had a past medical history of polyostotic fibrous dysplasia, which had progressed and been complicated by multiple nerve entrapments and paroxysmal atrial fibrillation. On examination multiple irregular hyperpigmented lesions were seen on his left flank and back, and examination of his thyroid revealed multiple painless nodules. His BP was 120/85 mmHg. His heart sounds were normal with occasional basal crackles on auscultation of the chest. Abdominal and neurological examination was normal.**

    What of the following is true?

    A. He may have a mutation in GNAS4 gene
    B. He may have McCune-Albright syndrome
    C. He may have neurofibromatosis type I
    D. He may have neurofibromatosis type II
    E. His children have a 50% chance of developing the same condition

65. **A 19-year-old man presented with weakness, muscle aches, and cramps. He had not experienced diarrhoea or vomiting. He had a past medical history of asthma and neonatal jaundice but was not on any regular medication. He had a strong family history of hypertension. On examination his BP was 170/95 mmHg, with normal heart sounds and an undisplaced apex beat. Respiratory examination revealed only occasional polyphonic wheeze. Abdominal and neurological examination were normal.**

    ```
    Investigations:
      Hb                        132 g/L
      MCV                       98 fL
      WCC                       12 × 10⁹/L
      Platelets                 180 × 10⁹/L
      Sodium                    140 mmol/L
      Potassium                 2.5 mmol/L
      Urea                      9 mmol/L
      Creatinine                78 µmol/L
      Renin (supine)            0.2 nmol/L/h (normal range lying
                                supine 0.5
                                2.2 nmol/L/h)

      Aldosterone (supine)      50 pmol/L (normal 100–500 pmol/L)
      24-hour urine potassium   80 mmol/L (normal 20–60 mmol/L)
    Arterial blood gas:
      pH 7.47
      pO2 11.4 kPa
      pCO2 6.3 kPa
      HCO3 33 mmol/L
    ```

    Which of the following is true about the patient's likely diagnosis?

    A. Spironolactone should be commenced.
    B. The patient and his family are likely to have mutations in the SLC12A1 gene
    C. The patient has Conn's syndrome
    D. The patient has Liddle's syndrome
    E. The patient's urinary calcium will be low

66. **A 50-year-old man presented with decreased libido and erectile dysfunction. He had a past medical history of diabetes for which he used insulin. He was not taking any other medication. On examination his skin was noted to have a slate-grey pigmentation. His BP was 140/90 mmHg, his pulse rate was 110/min and irregularly irregular with a displaced apex beat. Heart sounds were normal. He had hepatomegaly but his testicles were normal in size without any palpable masses.**

```
Investigations:
   Hb                      170 g/L
   MCV                     99 fL
   WCC                     10 × 10⁹/L
   Platelets               200 × 10⁹/L
   CRP                     <10 g/L
   Sodium                  138 mmol/L
   Potassium               4.9 mmol/L
   Urea                    5.0 mmol/L
   Creatinine              90 µmol/L
   AST                     400 iU/L
   ALT                     280 iU/L
   ALP                     230 iU/L
   Bilirubin               20 µmol/L
   Albumin                 30 g/L
   Protein                 50 g/L
   Corrected calcium       2.20 mmol/L
   Blood glucose           5.5 mmo/L
   Alpha fetoprotein       300 U/ml (normal <10 U/ml)
   HbA1c                   64 mmol/mol (20-42 mmol/mol)
   TSH                     1.2 mU/L
   9 am testosterone       7 nmol/L (normal male range 8.4-28.7
                           nmol/L)
   LH                      2 U/L (3-8 U/L)
   ECG                     atrial fibrillation, rate 105/min
   Echocardiogram          dilated cardiomyopathy
```

Which of the following would be best in diagnosing a unifying underlying diagnosis?

A. Cardiac biopsy
B. CT abdomen
C. Ferritin and transferrin saturation measurements
D. Serum iron and transferrin saturation measurements
E. Testing of the HFE gene for mutations

67. **A 60-year-old male presented with a three-month history of orthopnoea, decreased appetite, and ankle oedema. He had also reported increasing pains in his right lower leg, worse on weight bearing. On examination he had a pulse of 104 beats per minute, a BP of 180/ 90 mmHg and a JVP raised at 6 cm. Auscultation of his chest revealed an ejection systolic murmur and fine bibasal crackles to the mid zones. Pulse oximetry readings revealed saturations of 91% on air with a respiratory rate of 26 breaths per minute. His right tibia was also very tender to touch.**

```
Investigations:
  Hb                      100 g/L
  MCV                     88 fL
  WCC                     14 × 10⁹/L
  Platelets               330 × 10⁹/L
  CRP                     <10 g/L
  Sodium                  140 mmol/L
  Potassium               4.1 mmol/L
  Urea                    4.9 mmol/L
  Creatinine              130 µmol/L
  AST                     30 iU/L
  ALT                     38 iU/L
  ALP                     360 iU/L
  Bilirubin               13 µmol/L
  Albumin                 39 g/L
  Protein                 59 g/L
  Corrected calcium       2.19 mmol/L
  Phosphate               1.0 mmol/L
  Magnesium               0.99 mmol/L
  X-Ray right tibia       increased tibial size and sclerosis
                          with osteolysis
  ECG                     sinus rhythm; S in V₁ + R in V₆ ≥35 mm
```

Which potential diagnosis are his symptoms suggestive of?

A. Aortic dissection
B. Mitral valve prolapse
C. Osteogenic sarcoma of the tibia
D. Paget's disease
E. Severe vitamin D deficiency

68. A 26-year-old female with no past medical history suffered a large post-partum haemorrhage following delivery of her first child. Her **BP** at one point dropped to 60/40 mmHg. She was aggressively resuscitated with six units of blood, seven litres of Gelofusin and normal saline in total, two units of platelets, and four units of FFP. Her **BP** was stabilized at 110/75 mmHg and she underwent an emergency hysterectomy which was performed successfully without further complications and her condition improved. Over the next few days she developed nausea and vomiting associated with a severe frontal headache. On examination she had normal heart sounds and a JVP that was not visible after hepato-jugular reflux was performed. Her **BP** was 110/75 mmHg lying and 85/60 mmHg standing. Respiratory examination revealed occasional bibasal crackles with oxygen saturations of 95% on air. Abdominal examination revealed a diffusely tender abdomen but no guarding, peritonism, or localizing signs. The neurological examination was normal.

```
Investigations:
  Hb                      89 g/L
  MCV                     89 fL
  WCC                     14 × 10⁹/L
  Platelets               290 × 10⁹/L
  CRP                     40 g/L
  Prothrombin time        14s (10–14s)
  Sodium                  133 mmol/L
  Potassium               4.1 mmol/L
  Urea                    4.9 mmol/L
  Creatinine              87 µmol/L
  9 am cortisol           90 nmol/L (180–620 nmol/L)
```

Which of the following would you do next?

A. Check TSH and serum free T4, if serum free T4 is low replace with L-thyroxine

B. Give a further two units of blood

C. IV fluid resuscitation, 100 mg hydrocortisone IV stat and 6-hourly IM afterwards

D. Lumbar puncture after CT head

E. MRI head

69. **A 72-year-old male presented with generalized aches and pains, and pain in his right femur following a recent fall. He had a past medical history of ischaemic heart disease and hypertension, and reported recent weight loss, though was unable to quantify this. On examination he was noted to have a BMI of 22 but revealed no clinical abnormalities. There were no clinical signs of hip fracture. Neurological examination was normal.**

Investigations:

Hb	130 g/L
MCV	89 fL
WCC	14×10^9/L
Platelets	290×10^9/L
CRP	10 g/L
ESR	30 mm/hr
Sodium	140 mmol/L
Potassium	4.1 mmol/L
Urea	4.9 mmol/L
Creatinine	87 µmol/L
AST	30 iU/L
ALT	38 iU/L
ALP	390 iU/L
Bilirubin	13 µmol/L
Albumin	39 g/L
Protein	59 g/L
Corrected calcium	2.00 mmol/L
Phosphate	0.6 mmol/L
Magnesium	0.99 mmol/L
Femur and hip X-rays:	linear areas of decreased opacity

What is the most likely diagnosis?

A. Myeloma

B. Osteomalacia

C. Osteoporosis

D. Paget's disease of bone

E. Sarcoma

70. **A 42-year-old female presented with increasing shortness of breath over two months. She reported no wheezing, cough, or expectoration of sputum. She denied any other symptoms. She had a past medical history of breast cancer which was treated with mastectomy and axillary node clearance followed by radiotherapy five years previously. She took no regular medications and had no allergies. On examination, she was noted to have a hoarse voice. An inspiratory stridor was noted on auscultation and her trachea was deviated to the left with a poorly defined large mass to the right of which the lower margin could not be palpated.**

```
Investigations:
  Corrected calcium      2.39 mmol/L
  Magnesium              0.99 mmol/L
  TSH                    0.5 mU/L (0.4-5.0 mU/L)
  Serum free T4          15 pmol/L (10-22 pmol/L)
  Serum free T3          5 pmol/L (3-7 pmol/L)
  CXR                    mass in the right superior mediastinum,
                         tracheal shift
  99mTC scan             decreased uptake in the right lobe of
                         the thyroid
```

What is the most appropriate next line of investigation?

A. Anti-TPO, anti-thyroglobulin and TSH receptor antibody

B. CT scan chest and neck followed by USS guided FNA (fine needle aspiration) of the right thyroid nodule

C. Flow volume loops

D. Serum calcitonin

E. Serum thyroglobulin

71. **A 72-year-old female was referred following abnormal thyroid function being detected on routine blood tests for which she was completely asymptomatic. She had a past medical history of a breast lump being removed when she was 58 years old, with subsequent histology showing only benign changes; and ischemic heart disease for which she took aspirin, bisoprolol, and simvastatin. She had a bone mineral densitometry measurement undertaken one year previously, which gave a T-score of the spine and total hip -1.8 and -1 respectively. On examination her heart rate was 72 beats per minute and BP was 120/70 mmHg.**

```
Investigations:
Initial thyroid function test:
   TSH                          0.1 mU/L        (0.3-5.5 mU/L)
   Serum free T4                15 pmol/L       (10-22 pmol/L)
   Serum free T3                5 pmol/L        (37 pmol/L)
Repeat thyroid function test (8 weeks later):
   TSH                          0.06 mU/L       (0.3-5.5 mU/L)
   Serum free T4                14 pmol/L       (1022 pmol/L)
   Serum free T3                4.5 pmol/L      (37 pmol/L)
   Thyroid uptake scan: increased uptake unilaterally
       consistent with toxic nodule
```

What will be best next step in the management?

A. Carbimazole should be commenced and continued for 18 months

B. No action needed

C. Refer for radioactive iodine treatment

D. Refer to the surgeon for thyroid lobectomy

E. Thyroid function tests should be checked every 2–3 months only

72. **A 32-year-old male smoker presented with a fatigue and weight gain. He had a history of peptic ulcer disease, epilepsy, and lymphoma treated with both chemotherapy and radiotherapy. His medications included omeprazole and phenytoin. Examination revealed he had dry skin with some hair loss, and he had no palpable goitre. Thyroid function testing was performed:**

```
TSH                        16 mU/L      (0.3-5.5 mU/L)
Serum free T4              4 pmol/L     (1022 pmol/L)
Serum free T3             2 pmol/L      (3-7 pmol/L)
Thyroid peroxidase and TSH receptor antibodies: negative
99mTc scintiscan: decreased uptake throughout the gland
A diagnosis of radiation-induced hypothyroidism was made
  and the patient was commenced on levothyroxine, which was
  titrated up to a dose of 200 micrograms daily.
On follow-up, despite having his dose titrated up to 200
  micrograms daily, his free T4 remained low-normal (9.6 pmol/L)
  and his TSH remained persistently elevated at 10 mU/L.
```

Which of the following would not explain his test results?

A. Calcium carbonate
B. Cholestyramine
C. Hydrocortisone
D. Malabsorption/coeliac disease
E. Omeprazole

73. **A 68-year-old female presented with a one-week history of right temporal headache. She had no past medical history. Her only medication was aspirin 75 mg od which she opted to take herself given a family history of ischaemic heart disease. She did not have hormone replacement therapy during her menopause. On examination she was euvolaemic with a BP of 120/80 mmHg. She had right temporal artery tenderness but fundoscopy was normal. Blood tests were unremarkable except for an ESR of 100 mm/hr. A diagnosis of temporal arteritis was made, and the patient was started on prednisolone 60 mg od.**

Given that she is likely to be on prednisolone for more than three months as pa rt of her treatment, which of the following is true regarding her fracture risk?

A. Hormone replacement therapy (HRT) would be first-line treatment for bone protection whilst on prednisolone
B. She is at increased risk due to loss of bone mineral density due to her age alone
C. She should be recommended lifestyle measures and alendronate
D. She should be recommended lifestyle measures only
E. She should undergo a DEXA scan and be recommended bone protection if her T-score is between 0 and −1.5

46. C) Start a dipeptidylpeptidase-4 (DDP4) inhibitor

With the rising prevalence of diabetes, the scenario presented in this case is not uncommon and physicians are likely to encounter it not just in diabetic or renal clinics, but also on the acute medical take. The patient is clinically well but his diabetic kidney disease is progressing. Metformin is renally excreted and its levels can build up with both acute and chronic renal impairment resulting in a lactic acidosis and symptoms of toxicity, for example nausea, vomiting, or diarrhoea. Whilst some specialists will continue to use metformin at the lower dose of 500 mg bd when the GFR is between 15–30 ml/min/1.73 m^2 due to its benefits of weight reduction and increasing insulin sensitivity, it is licensed only for a GFR >30 ml/min/1.73 m^2.

Continuing gliclazide 40 mg bd monotherapy would be a plausible option if the patient's HbA1c was lower. It is not unusual for patients' HbA1c to fall as their renal impairment progresses for two reasons. First, many hypoglycaemic agents are metabolized by the kidney and excreted and so drug levels can increase with renal impairment. The second is that insulin itself is metabolized by proximal tubular cells, so the insulin release that is often stimulated by hypoglycaemic agents such as gliclazide, or the injected insulin itself, will remain in circulation for longer. For these reasons, patients with significant renal impairment (CKD IV–V) are at greater risk of hypoglycaemia, especially nocturnal, and so the target HbA1c level of 53 mmol/mol can be relaxed somewhat and patients' medication regime may need curtailing as their renal dysfunction progresses. However, given that this patient's current HbA1c is 56 mmol/mol and metformin is going to be stopped, continuing on gliclazide 40 mg bd alone is likely to result in poor control and so may not be the best strategy. Increasing the dose of gliclazide to 80 mg bd is an option, but this would risk potential hypoglycaemic episodes.

Adding on a low dose DDP4 inhibitor, such as sitagliptin 25 mg od, would be the ideal choice here as it is licensed in renal impairment, does not cause hypoglycaemia, and will lead to weight reduction. The latter is especially important as it is useful in reducing insulin resistance which is important in this case as metformin is now being stopped.

SGLT2 inhibitors are effective at weight loss and controlling blood sugars but are not licensed or efficacious in CKD (as their mechanism of action is reliant on adequate glomerular filtration to cause a glycosuria). Thiazolidinediones (not listed as an option), whilst safe in CKD, as they are principally metabolized by the liver, are generally avoided in CKD due to the risk of fluid retention and exacerbation of heart failure which is often co-existing to a greater or lesser degree in patients with CKD stage IV and V. Due to the limited number of available hypoglycemic agents that are safe in CKD, many patients do end up being on insulin, but this should only be the next stage after the appropriate oral hypoglycaemic agents have been tried and utilized.

Tutorial

The various classes of hypoglycaemic agents themselves often have different mechanisms of action, as well as being metabolized in different ways, and thus some are safe and efficacious in renal impairment whilst others are not. These are discussed in more detail in Table 3.1. Even those that are safe in renal impairment, should be used with caution and dose titration should be performed in small steps because of the greater risk of hypoglycaemia (because of the potentiated endogenous insulin release). Generally, non-hypoglycaemia causing agents (e.g. DPP-4 antagonists) are preferred to those that cause hypoglycaemia for safety reasons.

Insulin itself is licensed in end-stage renal impairment, but it is important to remember that patients will need a lower dose and, if on haemodialysis, may need adjustment of their regimen as glucose is cleared by dialysis membranes whereas insulin is not, thus precipitating peri-dialysis hypoglycaemic episodes.

The common hypoglycaemic agents, their mechanisms of action, and suitability in renal impairment is detailed in Table 3.1. It is worth familiarizing oneself with the NICE guidelines on oral hypoglycaemic agents as this is a common source for MRCP questions (see Further Reading section).

Table 3.1 Hypoglycaemic agents used in CKD and their characteristics

Agent	Mechanism of action	Use in renal impairment
Biguanides, for example metformin	• Inhibits hepatic gluconeogenesis • Increased peripheral insulin sensitivity (especially in skeletal muscle)	Renally excreted so not licensed for eGFR <30 ml/min due to risk of lactic acidosis. NB: recent studies have shown that a lower dose of metformin (500 mg bd) can still be used safely in patients until they reach CKD stage V (eGFR of 15 ml/min).
Thiazolidinediones, for example pioglitazone	PPAR (peroxisome proliferator-activated receptors) agonist which results in decreased release of fatty acids into circulation thereby increasing tissue dependence (sensitivity) to insulin.	Metabolized by the liver so renal impairment not a contraindication but due to risk of fluid retention, exacerbation of heart failure, and risk of fractures, are generally avoided in CKD IV and V.
Sulphonylureas, for example gliclazide	Increase insulin secretion by inhibiting pancreatic K_{ATP}^+ channels.	Metabolized by the liver but breakdown metabolites of certain sulphonylureas, for example glimeperide are renally excreted and thus accumulate in CKD. Gliclazide is suitable at any GFR but others may be contraindicated when eGFR <30 ml/min.
Glucagon-like peptide-1 (GLP-1) agonists, for example exenatide	• Increases pancreatic insulin secretion in response to meals • Delays gastric emptying thus reducing post-prandial hyperglycaemia • Is an appetite suppressant, thus reducing weight and overall improving peripheral insulin sensitivity	Renally excreted so not licensed for eGFR <30 ml/min due to unpredictable pharmacokinetics in this group of patients. However, some centres are using lower doses in patients with CKD IV–V given its benefits and low side-effect profile. Thus, guidance may change in the future.
Dipeptidyl peptidase-4 (DPP-4) inhibitors, for example sitagliptin	Inhibit DPP4, the enzyme responsible for breakdown of endogenous GLP-1. The resulting mechanism of action is thus the same as GLP-1 agonists, listed above.	Renally excreted but licensed for use at small doses with an eGFR <30 ml/min.
SGLT2 inhibitors, for example empagliflozin	Inhibit proximal tubule sodium-glucose transporter 2 (SGLT2) thereby promoting glycosuria and reducing blood sugar.	Its mechanism of action, and thus excretion, depends upon secretion into urine. Its efficacy decreases and potential toxicity increases with declining function, and it is thus not licensed for an eGFR <45 ml/min.

Further Reading

Hahr A, Molitch M (2015). Management of diabetes mellitus in patients with chronic kidney disease. *Clinical Diabetes Endocrinology* 1: 2.

National Institute for Clinical Excellence (2019). Type 2 diabetes in adults: management [NG28]. December 2015, updated August 2019. Available at: https://www.nice.org.uk/guidance/ng28

47. E) Primary polydipsia

Lithium-induced diabetes insipidus is unlikely to respond to water deprivation. The patient's fasting glucose and HbA1c are normal, which excludes diabetes mellitus. Polyuria following obstructive nephropathy will resolve earlier than three weeks. Overnight water deprivation test resulted in appropriate concentration of urine, which makes the diagnosis of psychogenic polydipsia most likely. Pituitary tuberculosis may cause diabetes insipidus (DI) though it is very rare. If DI was the answer, plasma Na^+ and osmolality would be high or in the upper normal range, urine osmolality would remain low despite overnight water deprivation; and continuation of water deprivation will be required until plasma osmolality reaches more than 305 mOsm/kg or there is more than 5% weight loss. After this desmopressin would be administered and would result in concentration of the urine (osmolality >800 mOsm/kg).

Tutorial

Primary polydipsia is much more common in the general population than idiopathic DI, and describes excessive compulsive (behavioural) water drinking and consequent polyuria. It is associated with abnormal thirst perception even in the setting of low plasma osmolality. Overnight water deprivation with supervision will normalize urine osmolality in most patients, while some will require continuation of water deprivation for an extra 2–6 hours to achieve this. Plasma sodium and osmolalities will normalize with reduction of fluid intake to around 2 L/24 hours. Counselling or an input of a psychiatrist maybe required.

The polyuria seen in DI results in a low urine osmolality (<300 mOsm/kg). Polyuria, polydipsia, and nocturia are predominant symptoms. The daily urine volume is variable (3–28 L/day). Neurological symptoms vary with the patient's access to water and ability to keep hydrated. Such patients may appear dehydrated if they are not able to match their fluid intake with the volume of urine output, which may be up to 30 litres in extreme cases. After excluding diabetes mellitus, hypercalcaemia, and diuretic use, a water deprivation test can be used to differentiate the causes as summarized in Figure 3.1. If after eight hours of water deprivation, the urine remains diluted, 2 µg of desmopressin (DDAVP®) IM is given to assess the response. In cranial DI, the urine will concentrate, which will not be the case with nephrogenic DI, when resistance to desmopressin is causing polyuria and much higher doses of DDAVP are needed to overcome it.

Treatment is then aimed at removing any possible reversible causes and patient education with regard to maintaining adequate fluid intake, especially during exercise and periods where insensible losses are high, for example in hot weather or with episodes of vomiting and diarrhoea. In cranial DI, if hydration remains difficult to achieve then enhancing vasopressin action with an analogue such as desmopressin is used. Nephrogenic DI may be more difficult to manage if there is no reversible aetiology. In some cases, high dose desmopressin may help, as can thiazides or NSAIDs, particularly indomethacin, as last resort. The treatment for lithium-induced nephrogenic DI is discussed further in the tutorial of question 189.

Further Reading

British Medical Journal (2017). Best Practice. Diabetes Insipidus (2017). Available at: http://bestpractice.bmj.com/best-practice/monograph/288.html

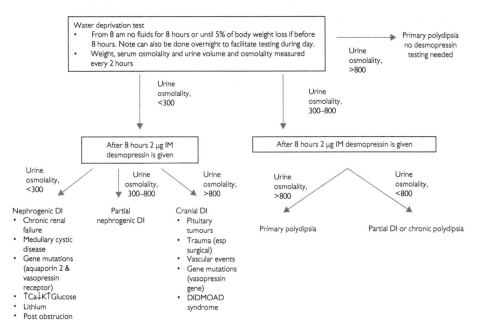

Figure 3.1 The water deprivation test and causes of diabetes insipidus.

48. D) The patient has partial 21-hydroxylase deficiency

The clinical picture with raised 17-hydroxyprogesteorone levels is suggestive of congenital adrenal hyperplasia (CAH) secondary to 21-hydroxylase deficiency. The presentation at the age of 16 rather than at birth suggests partial 21-hydroxylase deficiency, which is supported by the lack of features of mineralocorticoid loss. There is no indication for furosemide and even if there was mineralocorticoid deficiency this would only worsen volume depletion. Glucocorticoid replacement is needed and fludrocortisone is only required if mineralocorticoid deficiency is present. Autonomic function testing would be useful in the investigation of a postural BP drop in the absence of mineralocorticoid deficiency. Patients with 11β-hydroxylase deficiency have increased 11-deoxycortisol and deoxycorticosterone levels with hypertension, suppressed renin activity, and salt retention with hypokalaemia.

Tutorial

The different phenotypes seen in congenital adrenal hyperplasia relate to the point of enzyme deficiency in the adrenal cortical steroid pathways as detailed in Figure 3.2. The amount and type of precursors which build up and the increased shunting down alternative pathways ultimately dictate the phenotype. In general, an increase in androgens and a decrease in cortisol and aldosterone is seen. Whichever syndrome is present, patients may present with the full house of symptoms (classical CAH) or partial syndromes (non-classical CAH). Classical form tends to present earlier in infancy and the non-classical form tends to present in adulthood. Non-classical presentations in females usually involve menstrual irregularities, hirsutism, and infertility. Symptoms in males are more non-specific. The most common deficiency is 21-hydroxylase deficiency, which in its classical form presents at birth or in neonatal period with virilization in females and salt wasting in both females and males. Non-classical

21-hydroxylase deficiency also occurs, presenting later with androgen excess but not features of mineralocorticoid loss. 11β-hydroxylase deficiency leads to androgen excess. As opposed to mineralocorticoid deficiency they exhibit hypertension with sodium retention due to the build-up of deoxycorticosterone, which whilst it is not as potent as aldosterone at salt retention, builds up to much higher levels due to loss of feedback loops. 3β-hydroxysteroid dehydrogenase deficiency and 17α-hydroxylase deficiency are much rarer syndromes that tend to present classically.

Diagnosis of CAH involves demonstration of cortisol and aldosterone deficiency as well as increased levels of relevant precursors in the presence of clinical features. A 24-hour urine steroid profile will allow detection of precise enzymatic defect. In terms of precursors 21-hydroxylase deficiency will lead to increased serum levels of 17-hydroxyprogesterone and 17-hydroxypregnenolone, which will be converted to adrenal androgens: DHEAS and androstenedione. Low serum aldosterone, increased renin, hyponatraemia, and hyperkalaemia will be seen in those with salt wasting forms.

An excess of 11-deoxycortisol and deoxycorticosterone is seen in 11β-hydroxylase deficiency, and these patients, who are hypertensive, will have a suppressed renin and hypokalaemia

Management involves glucocorticosteroid replacement in the form of hydrocortisone or prednisolone with the feedback effect of decreased ACTH normalizing androgen levels. Fludrocortisone is needed if mineralocorticoid deficiency is present.

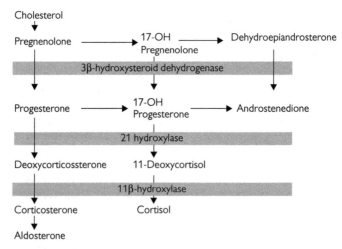

Figure 3.2 Adrenal cortical steroid biosynthetic pathways and the three most common CAH deficiencies.

Further Reading

Merke D (2008). Approach to the adult with congenital adrenal hyperplasia due to 21-hydroxylase deficiency. *Journal of Clinical Endocrinology Metabolism* 93(3): 653–660.

Witchel S (2012). Nonclassic congenital adrenal hyperplasia. *Current Opinion Endocrinology and Diabetes and Obesity* 19(3): 151–158.

49. D) Klinefelter's syndrome

The patient has hypogonadism as evidenced by the low testosterone. The increased LH and FSH indicate that the hypothalamic-pituitary axis is intact. Thus, this is primary hypogonadism, and the most common congenital cause is Klinefelter's syndrome. It is believed a significant number of males with Klinefelter's are undiagnosed. Karyotyping reveals 47XXY in the majority, with higher grade aneuploidy or mosaicism in the rest. Azoospermia is also seen. Treatment involves lifelong androgen replacement and fertility treatment may be successful with intracytoplasmic sperm injection. Surgical correction of gynaecomastia may also be required. Kallmann syndrome, congenital adrenal hypoplasia, and prolactinoma are causes of secondary hypogonadism, with low or normal LH and FSH. Both testes have descended and so cryptorchidism is ruled out as a cause of primary hypogonadism and is uncommon as a post-pubertal cause.

Tutorial

Male hypogonadism is an inadequate gonadal function, as manifested by failure of the testes to produce adequate amounts of testosterone and/or spermatozoa. The differential diagnosis is discussed in Table 3.2. Onset before puberty leads to small genitalia (testes <5 ml) and prostate with scanty pubic and axillary hair. The lack of the usual tonal drop in voice may also be seen. Onset after puberty may manifest as erectile dysfunction, loss of libido, and lethargy. Whilst penile length may be normal, the testes may be small with a volume <15 ml. Primary hypogonadism describes testicular failure with normal hypothalamic and pituitary function (hypergonadotrophic hypogonadism) and secondary hypogonadism is a result of hypothalamic or pituitary dysfunction (hypogonadotrophic hypogonadism).

Table 3.2 Causes of hypogonadism

Primary hypogonadism	Secondary hypogonadism
• Klinefelter's syndrome • XX Males, X/XO, XYY, Y chromosome microdeletion • Chemotherapy/radiotherapy • Cryptorchidism usually resolves in first few years of life • Infective or autoimmune orchitis • Chronic renal/liver failure • Trauma • Alcohol	• Kallmann syndrome/idiopathic hypogonadotrophic hypogonadism • Congenital adrenal hypoplasia • Infiltration of pituitary/hypothalamus (tumours, haemochromatosis*, sarcoid) or trauma or radiotherapy • Prader-Willi syndrome • Hyperprolactinaemia • Laurence-Moon-Biedl syndrome (severe obesity, gonadotrophin deficiency, polydactyly, learning disability, retinal disorders) • Fertile eunuch syndrome (normal testicular growth but inadequate virilization due to decreased GnRH)

*Haemochromatosis my also rarely lead to primary hypogonadism.2

Serum testosterone exhibits diurnal variation and so standard practice is to measure it at 9 am. Sex hormone binding globulin (SHBG) should also be assessed as the majority of testosterone is bound to SHBG and albumin, though most laboratories now measure total testosterone. Raised FSH and LH are seen in primary hypogonadism and low levels are seen in secondary hypogonadism. A raised oestradiol would raise suspicion of testicular tumours or testicular failure, but has a limited value and may also be seen with adrenal tumours, liver disease and hepatomas, thyrotoxicosis, androgen resistance syndromes, anti-androgen therapy, and obesity. It may be decreased in Kallman syndrome.

Kallmann syndrome is characterized by secondary hypogonadism and anosmia or decreased smell due to absence or malformation of the olfactory bulb, with the rest of the pituitary function being normal. Mutations have been found in several genes, leading to X-linked, autosomal dominant and recessive types. It is associated with a higher incidence of cleft palate/lip, ichthyosis, and neurological findings such as synkinesia and ataxia. Idiopathic hypogonadotrophic hypogonadism has the same features of Kallman syndrome but with normal sense of smell.

Further Reading

Isidori A, Giannetta E, Lenzi A (2008). Male hypogonadism. *Pituitary* 11: 171–180.

50. C) Pseudohypoparathyroidism type Ia

The hypocalcaemia in association with a raised phosphate, normal ALP and high PTH, along with the features of Albright's hereditary osteodystrophy (AHO) are in keeping with pseudohypoparathyroidism type Ia. The osteodystrophic features are not seen in type Ib. Idiopathic hypoparathyroidism would lead to a low PTH. Pseudopseudohypoparathyroidism involves the osteodystrophic features but no disorder in PTH/calcium metabolism. DiGeorge syndrome would be associated with a low PTH and features of thymic aplasia, immunodeficiency, and cardiac abnormalities.

Tutorial

Resistance to parathyroid hormone action results in pseudohypoparathyroidism (PHP) leading to hypocalcaemia, hyperphosphataemia, and increased serum PTH. The classic type is PHP type Ia which is due to a defect in the GNAS1 gene leading to deficiency in the alpha subunit of stimulatory G proteins and to defective signalling of PTH action via the cell membrane receptor. The skeletal abnormalities originally described by Fuller Albright (Box 3.1) are then seen. Whether the biochemical features are also seen is dependent on genetic imprinting. Paternal transmission of the gene defect results in features of AHO only and causes pseudopseudohypoparathyroidism. On the other hand, maternal transmission causes pseudohypoparathyroidism type Ia with PTH resistance. Both can therefore be found in the same family. In PHP type Ia and b, raised phosphate and normal ALP are present. The PTH level is normal or raised as opposed to the low PTH level seen in primary hypoparathyroidism secondary to gland destruction (autoimmune, surgical, radiation) or maldevelopment. The diagnosis is confirmed with no response in urinary cAMP and phosphate to a PTH infusion (Ellsworth-Howard test). Hypothyroidism and reproductive dysfunction may also be seen with GNAS1 mutations as TSH, LH, FSH, and GH signalling may also be aberrant.

The mainstay of treatment is calcium replacement. This may initially need to be intravenously if symptomatic hypocalcaemia is present, followed by maintenance of low normal calcium levels with oral calcium supplements and 1-alpha-hydroxylated vitamin D metabolites. Treatment should entail titrating dosage to suppress PTH levels to a normal range to avoid iatrogenic hypercalcaemia which can precipitate renal stone formation.

Patients with PHP type Ib do not have Albright's hereditary osteodystrophy but have PTH resistance which is usually limited to certain organs. For example, resistance in the kidneys but normal bone response to PTH results in hyperparathyroid-like bone lesions. It is due to a mutation in a *STX16* gene encoding syntaxin 16.

PHP type Ic has similar clinical and biochemical features to 1a but without deficiency in the alpha subunit of stimulatory G proteins.

Patients with PHP type II do not have the Albright's phenotype but express a normal response to PTH in the Ellsworth-Howard test in terms of urinary cAMP but a blunted phosphaturic response, distinguishing them from 1b.

> **Box 3.1** Clinical features of pseudohypoparathyroidism (Albright's hereditary osteodystrophy)
>
> Pseudohypoparathyroidism (AHO)
> - Short stature
> - Round face
> - Short metacarpals (classically fourth and fifth)
> - Obesity
> - Other short bones of hands and feet
> - Dental hypoplasia
> - Soft tissue calcifications and ossification

Further Reading

British Medical Journal (2016). Best Practice. Pseudohypoparathyroidism (Aug 2016). Available at: http://bestpractice.bmj.com/best-practice/monograph/1150.html

51. B) MEN type I

The patient is experiencing symptoms of episodic hypoglycaemia, which is supported by the glucose readings. The demonstration of an inappropriately elevated insulin with the episodes of hypoglycaemia and elevated C-peptide would provide a laboratory diagnosis of insulinoma. Exogenous insulin use should be ruled out and urine should be checked for sulphonylurea metabolites, as these drugs cause a hypoglycaemia by increasing endogenous insulin release which would also cause elevated C-peptide. The patient also has raised calcium. Although the initial manifestation of MEN type I is usually primary hyperparathyroidism, insulinoma may be identified prior to hypercalcaemia. The clinical manifestation of MEN-I is a composition of: (1) parathyroid tumours or hyperplasia; (2) anterior pituitary adenomas; and (3) pancreatic neuroendocrine tumours. A clinical diagnosis is reached if two out of three of these are present or one in the context of a family history. MEN IIa syndrome usually presents with familial thyroid medullary cell carcinoma, although 50% of patients have phaeochromocytoma and 20–30% have parathyroid neoplasia at presentation. The acronym POEMS is a syndrome of the following features P: polyneuropathy (progressive), O: organomegaly, E: endocrinopathy (often more than one of the of the following: hypothyroidism, hypogonadotrophic hypogonadism, hypoadrenalism, and diabetes mellitus), M: monoclonal gammopathy, and S: skin changes (many changes have been associated with POEMS but particularly hyperpigmentation and thickening). The multi-organ involvement is a paraneoplastic phenomenon and is usually due to a plasma cell dyscrasia.

Tutorial

Primary hyperparathyroidism is the most common clinical presentation in patients with MEN-I and occurs in more than 90% of cases. The parathyroid lesions may be adenomas or hyperplasia. Pancreatic tumours associated with MEN-I in decreasing order of frequency are gastrinoma, insulinoma, non-functioning tumours, PPoma, and glucagonoma. The pituitary associations in decreasing order of frequency are prolactinoma, acromegaly, and non-functioning tumours. Phaeochromocytomas are only seen in about half a per cent of MEN-I cases. Adrenal cortical tumours are more common. Genetic analysis of this highly penetrant autosomal dominant syndrome has revealed a mutation in menin on chromosome 11q13. Mutational analysis of suspected cases or relatives is performed in tertiary centres, with a mutation found in around 80% of families. Screening of asymptomatic mutation carriers involves examination and assessment of relevant endocrine and biochemical parameters as well as MRI. Screening can lower the age of detection of the syndrome and decrease morbidity. The penetrance of MEN-I should be remembered in that at age 10 only 7% have the phenotype, increasing to 98% at age 40.

Treatment of tumours associated with MEN-I is mainly surgical: three and a half glands or total parathyroidectomy; partial or total pancreatectomy for neuroendocrine tumours of the pancreas; and transsphenoidal adenomectomy for pituitary lesions. Medical therapies and radiotherapy are limited except in certain cases of pituitary tumours.

There is also a related condition MEN-II which is discussed further in the tutorial to question 55.

Further Reading

Brandi M, Gagel R, Angeli A, et al. (2001). Consensus: guidelines for diagnosis and therapy of MEN type 1 and type 2. *Journal of Clinical Endocrinology & Metabolism* 86: 5658–5671.

Thakker R, Newey P, Walls G, et al. (2012). Clinical practice guidelines for multiple endocrine neoplasia type 1 (MEN1). *Journal of Clinical Endocrinology and Metabolism* 97(9): 2990–3011.

52. B) Serum prolactin

The patient has a diagnosis of sarcoidosis. The symptoms of galactorrhoea and menstrual irregularities may be due to hyperprolactinaemia, which may be secondary to infiltrative involvement of the pituitary stalk disrupting the negative effect of hypothalamic dopamine that usually inhibits prolactin secretion. Clinical suspicion of hyperprolactinaemia needs to be demonstrated on serum testing. Normal prolactin levels in women and men are usually quoted as below 31 μg/L (620 mIU/L) and 19 μg/L (375 mIU/L) respectively. The normal ranges should be adjusted to the specific assay used locally. Oestradiol and gonadotrophins will be suppressed in presence of hyperprolactinaemia and could be checked after confirming hyperprolactinaemia. Elevated testosterone/adrenal androgens can cause dysmenorrhoea but not galactorrhoea. Hypothyroidism may cause mild hyperprolactinaemia and irregular periods but again not galactorrhoea.

Tutorial

Neurosarcoidosis can rarely involve pituitary and/or hypothalamus, with optic nerve infiltration occurring in 60% of patients. Growth hormone and gonadotrophin production are most commonly affected. Approximately 20–50% of patients may develop DI and 30% develop hyperprolactinaemia. Pituitary/hypothalamic involvement can be confirmed by MRI scan with gadolinium, which shows contrast enhancement. CSF angiotensin converting enzyme (ACE) levels will confirm neuroendocrine sarcoidosis. Immunosuppressive treatment of sarcoidosis usually fails to improve hormonal deficiencies.

Hyperprolactinaemia leads to galactorrhoea, secondary hypogonadism, and osteopenia. If the cause is due to a pituitary or hypothalamic tumour then the mass effect of the tumour may also lead to symptoms of headache, visual field defects, and cavernous sinus syndrome. Prolactinomas are rarely malignant and are normally benign pituitary adenomas. Microprolactinomas are more common and are also seen as part of MEN-I. Macroprolactinomas tend to lead to very high prolactin levels. Non-functioning macroadenomas may lead to hyperprolactinaemia due to stalk compression. MRI with gadolinium is more effective than CT at revealing microprolactinomas.

Dopamine agonists (bromocriptine or cabergoline) are the first line of treatment for prolactinomas, if there are no absolute surgical indications, usually leading to a decrease in prolactin secretion and tumour shrinkage. If the tumour is resistant to dopamine agonists or side effects are intolerable then transsphenoidal adenomectomy should be considered. Oestrogen replacement may be appropriate in females with idiopathic hyperprolactinaemia or microprolactinomas where fertility and galactorrhoea are not a problem. Follow-up monitoring of tumour size by imaging in case of macroprolactinomas and prolactin levels in any prolactinoma is required although the surgical cure rate for macroprolactinomas is poor and for microprolactinomas runs a significant risk of hypopituitarism.

The causes of hyperprolactinaemia are listed in Box 3.2. If no cause is found and a diagnosis of idiopathic hyperprolactinaemia is made, follow-up is required as a very small microprolactinoma may be the cause.

Box 3.2 Causes of hyperprolactinaemia

Physiological
- Pregnancy
- Breast stimulation
- Can occur in neonates

Pituitary/hypothalamic
- Prolactinomas (micro and macro)
- Stalk compression or trauma
- Infiltrative disease, for example sarcoidosis
- Increased thyroid releasing hormone, for example hypothyroidism

Chronic diseases
- Chronic liver failure
- Chronic renal failure*

Drugs
- First-generation antipsychotics, for example haloperidol and chlorpromazine
- Dopamine antagonists
- Tricyclic antidepressants
- Antihypertensives: verapamil, methyldopa, atenolol
- H2 antagonists, omeprazole
- Oestrogens
- Opioids

Other
- Thoracotomy
- Herpes zoster
- Burns
- Mastectomy

* Prolactin is cleared by the kidneys

Further Reading

Casanueva F, Molitch M, Schlechte J, et al. (2006). Guidelines of the pituitary society for the diagnosis and management of prolactinomas. *Clinical Endocrinology* 65: 265–273.

Mancini T, Casanueva F, Giustina A (2008). Hyperprolactinaemia and prolactinomas. *Endocrinology Metabolism Clinic North America* 37: 67–99.

Murialdo G, Tamagno G (2002). Endocrine aspects of neurosarcoidosis. *Journal of Endocrinological Investigation* 25(7): 650–662.

53. C) Her current medication should remain unchanged until the third trimester when her hydrocortisone should be increased by 50% and the fludrocortisone dose should be guided by BP and serum potassium

The foetal adrenal glands have a large capacity for cortisol production and near term produce more than an unstressed adult. Very little maternal cortisol enters the foetal compartment and the placenta is not known to produce steroid. Although there is increased demand during pregnancy there is also increase in levels of cortisol as well as oestrogen. The rate of secretion of cortisol from the adrenals is not increased but clearance is decreased. Thus, hydrocortisone dosing is not increased until the third trimester. Pregnancy leads to many effects on the renin-angiotensin system. For example, despite increase in plasma volume, renin production increases and the pressor effects of angiotensin II are reduced. Clinically, postural BP and electrolytes are the best guide for mineralocorticoid dosing. In case of intercurrent illness, regardless of pregnancy or its stage, hydrocortisone dose should be doubled or if oral intake impossible/decreased absorption parenteral treatment should be instigated (e.g. in cases of hyperemesis gravidarum). Steroids must not be discontinued at any point. During labour and for 24–48 hours after delivery parenteral hydrocortisone should be given (100 mg IM/IV six hourly).

Tutorial

The causes and investigation of adrenal insufficiency are discussed in a separate question. The management of adrenal insufficiency can be divided into emergency management of an acute adrenal crisis and maintenance therapy for adrenal insufficiency. In the acute situation aggressive volume replacement with normal saline and strict fluid balance are required. A dose of 100 mg of hydrocortisone should be given immediately and continued six hourly. Any likely biochemical disturbances particularly hypoglycaemia, hyperkalaemia, and hypercalcaemia should be addressed. Of particular note is hyponatraemia which may be chronic due to the underlying pathology. This may complicate fluid management as rapid correction may lead to pontine myelinolysis. If there are features such as seizures or a sodium of <120 mmol/l then sodium levels should only be increased by 10 mmol/l per 24 hours at the most, with close monitoring. Blood tests should not delay hydrocortisone treatment in the acute situation and there is no time for a Synacthen test. Serum cortisol and ACTH can be tested on a blood sample while treatment is in progress. Once the patient recovers from the acute illness hydrocortisone dose should be decreased to double normal dose for the patient and back to a maintenance oral dose of 15–25 mg daily in divided doses (usually 10/5/5 mg).

Over or under replacement can be assessed with serum cortisol day curve. A mineralocorticoid is also needed and fludrocortisone dose is adjusted according to postural BP and renin level (except pregnancy). Patients should also be informed that any intercurrent illness or operations can precipitate an Addisonian crisis and an increase in hydrocortisone will be needed. This is guided by the severity of the illness or procedure but if in doubt it is always better to over replace than not to give enough. Uncontrolled hyperthyroidism also requires higher glucocorticoid requirements as cortisol clearance is increased.

Further Reading

Ambrosi B, Barbetta L, Morricone L (2003). Diagnosis and management of Addison's disease during pregnancy. *Journal of Endocrinological Investigation* 26(7): 698–702.

54. A) 24-hour urine for catecholamines/metanephrines or plasma metanephrines

The patient presents with *intermittent* symptoms of visual blurring, headache, palpitations, and nausea. On examination he is hypertensive, and there are clinical signs of mitral valve prolapse. The ECG demonstrates left ventricular hypertrophy, indicating established hypertension. The presence of renal cysts on abdominal USS and clinical finding of mitral valve prolapse may lead the candidate to consider the diagnosis of polycystic kidney disease. However, this would not be associated with intermittent symptoms. Mitral valve prolapse may be an incidental finding. The intermittent symptoms in a young hypertensive patient raise the possibility of phaeochromocytoma. The presence of retinal angiomas and renal cysts should alert to a possible rare diagnosis of Von Hippel-Lindau disease (VHL). The 24-hour urine metanephrines or plasma metanephrines are preferred tests to biochemically confirm phaeochromocytoma. If not available 24-hour urine catecholamines could be used. Urinary VMAs are no longer recommended. Adrenal imaging should not be performed before biochemical diagnosis as 10% of the population have adrenal adenomas/incidentalomas. This patient should also undergo a cerebral MRI (to look for CNS haemangioblastomas associated with VHL) and abdominal MRI (for renal, adrenal, and pancreatic lesions associated with VHL).

Tutorial

Phaeochromocytomas have been termed a 'tumour of tens': 10% are bilateral, 10% are malignant, 10% are found in asymptomatic patients, 10% are hereditary, 10% are extra-adrenal (which arise from sympathetic and parasympathetic neural crest cells and are termed paragangliomas). They are seen in up to a fifth of VHL families and it is an important association not to miss. Syndromes associated with phaeochromocytoma and paragangliomas are listed in Box 3.3. Episodic headache, sweating, and palpitations are considered the classic triad of presentation with hypertension. However, a wide range of non-specific symptoms may be associated. Phaeochromocytomas should be first biochemically confirmed by demonstration of increased catecholamines or metanephrine (their metabolites) secretion, and then the tumour localized by specific imaging. The adrenal incidentaloma picked up on a CT or MRI performed for another reason should also first have a secure biochemical diagnosis before more specific imaging tests are performed. Plasma/urine metanephrines offer the most sensitive screening test but if not available then urinary 24-hour urine collection for catecholamines should be used. Ideally the above tests should be performed in a period when symptoms are occurring. It is worth noting that a large number of medications can interfere with the results, such as alpha and beta blockers, levodopa, and ACE inhibitors. Suppression tests, for example clonidine may be helpful in borderline cases.

Before surgery alpha and beta blockade must be achieved. To prevent a catastrophic hypertensive crisis secondary to unopposed alpha blockade, alpha blockade should be achieved first, typically with phenoxybenzamine, which is titrated gradually to BP and heart rate. Propranolol can then be added. If surgery is not curative this treatment may need to be lifelong.

Box 3.3 Syndromes associated with phaeochromocytoma MEN-IIa and MEN-IIb

- Von Hippel-Lindau syndrome
- Neurofibromatosis
- Succinate dehydrogenase mutations

Further Reading

Adler J, Meyer-Rochow G, Chen H, et al, (2008). Phaeochromocytoma: current approaches and future directions. *Oncologist* 13: 779–793.

Kudva Y, Sawka A, Young W Jr (2003). The laboratory diagnosis of adrenal pheochromocytoma: the Mayo Clinic experience. *Journal of Clinical Endocrinology and Metabolism* 88: 4533–4539.

55. D) MEN type IIb

The histology confirms medullary thyroid carcinoma, which is also indicated by the pentagastrin test result. The high-arched palate, scoliosis, and pectus excavatum suggest Marfanoid habitus and the lip nodules may be mucosal neuromas. This would be consistent with MEN type IIb rather than MEN type IIa. Hirschsprung's disease is due to absence of the ganglionic cells of the neural plexus of the colonic wall, with most cases presenting in early childhood with acute intestinal obstruction or chronic constipation. Metastatic disease from medullary thyroid carcinoma is more likely to present with diarrhoea. Intestinal neuromas can lead to diarrhoea or constipation in MEN-IIb. The normal calcium is against primary hyperparathyroidism. Medullary carcinoma is not a feature of MEN type I.

Tutorial

Multiple endocrine neoplasia type II (MEN-II) is an autosomal dominant disorder classified into MEN-IIa, MEN-IIb, and familial medullary thyroid carcinoma (FMTC) as in Table 3.3. MEN-II is caused by activating mutations in the RET proto-oncogene (chromosome 10q11.2) which lead to increased tumour formation. Inactivating mutations in the same gene are involved in the aetiology of Hirschsprung's disease. Table 3.3 details the features of MEN-IIa, MEN-IIb, and FMTC. Medullary thyroid carcinoma usually develops during childhood and begins as thyroid parafollicular C-cell hyperplasia, progressing to a multifocal tumour associated with high calcitonin levels. It is generally more aggressive in MEN-II and presents earlier in MEN-IIb compared to MEN-IIa. However, neuromas are still often the earliest feature in MEN-IIb. The pentagastrin test may be useful in those with borderline calcitonin levels. The level of stimulated calcitonin correlates with likelihood of MTC. Total thyroidectomy is the treatment of choice and prophylactic surgery in a young age should be considered in known cases of MEN-II. Hypercalcaemia from hyperparathyroidism involves multiple glands due to either diffuse hyperplasia or multiple adenomas and treatment follows the same pathway as in primary hyperparathyroidism.

The features and diagnosis of MEN-I are discussed further in the tutorial to question 51.

Table 3.3 Shared and differentiating features of MEN-IIa, MEN-IIb, and FMTC

	MEN2a	MEN2b	FMTC
Medullary thyroid carcinoma	✓	✓	✓
Phaeochromocytoma	✓	✓	✗
Primary Hyperparathyroidism	✓	✗	✗
Neuromas (mucosal and intestinal)	✗	✓	✗
Marfanoid features	✗	✓	✗

Further Reading

Brandi M, Gagel R, Angeli A, et al. (2001). Consensus: guidelines for diagnosis and therapy of MEN type 1 and type 2. *Journal of Clinical Endocrinology and Metabolism* 86: 5658–5671.

56. B) A growth hormone measurement of 20 mU/L after a 75 g glucose load

This is the classical presentation for acromegaly. However, the question is testing the correct investigation to confirm the clinical diagnosis. The correct method is to carry out an oral glucose tolerance test, which entails giving a 75 g oral glucose load and then assessing the growth hormone (GH) response. In normal individuals the GH will become undetectable but a cut-off of <1 mU/L is used. A high random GH level cannot be diagnostic as pulses of GH release occur in normal cases. IGF-1 levels are raised in acromegaly and can be suggestive of the diagnosis but not used to make a diagnosis. They may be useful for assessing response to treatment.

Tutorial

The majority of cases of acromegaly are due to a pituitary adenoma (macro- more common than microadenomas) which may also secrete prolactin. It may be seen with GH release from pancreatic islet cell tumours, lymphoma, and excess GHRH release from the hypothalamus or an ectopic source, for example bronchial carcinoma. Acromegaly may also be part of inherited syndromes (Box 3.4). Once confirmed biochemically, MRI of the pituitary confirms a pituitary tumour in 98% of patients. If this is not seen then assessment for an ectopic source of GH or GHRH should be carried out. In cases of a pituitary tumour, levels of all pituitary hormones should also be assessed.

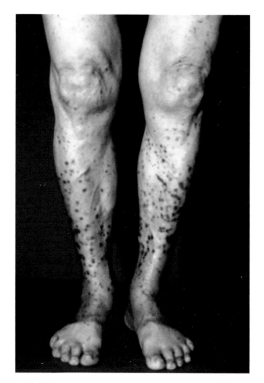

Figure 2.1 Lower-limb rash.

Reproduced with permission from *Oxford Textbook of Vasculitis*, Third Edition. Edited by GV Ball, BJ Fessler, and SL Bridges, Fig. 39.3, p. 530. Oxford University Press, Oxford, UK, Copyright © 2014.

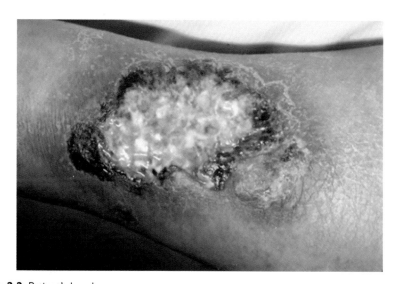

Figure 2.2 Patient's leg ulcer.

Reproduced with permission from *Oxford Handbook of Medical Dermatology*, Second Edition. Edited by S Burge, R Matin, and D Wallis, Fig. 15.5, p. 297. Oxford University Press, Oxford, UK, Copyright © 2016.

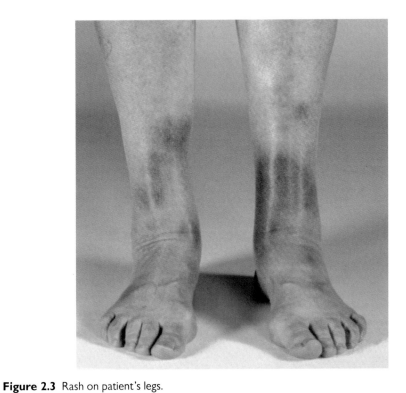

Figure 2.3 Rash on patient's legs.

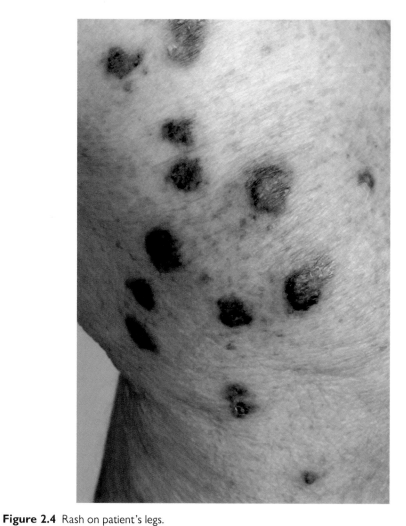

Figure 2.4 Rash on patient's legs.

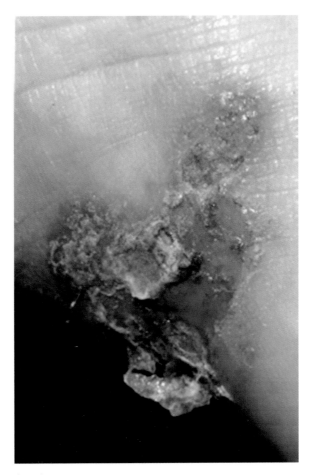

Figure 2.5 Patient's rash.

Reproduced from Lewis-Hones S. *OSH Paediatric Dermatology*. Oxford University Press. 2010. Chapter 26: Crusts, scabs and eschars. Figure 26.1(a).

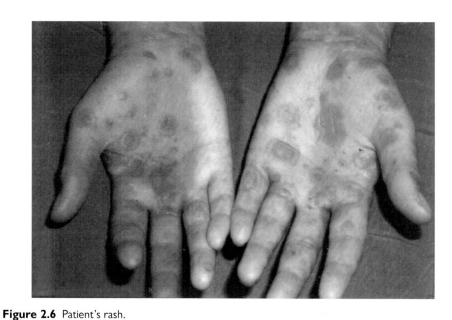

Figure 2.6 Patient's rash.

Reproduced with permission from *Adverse Syndromes and Psychiatric Drugs: a clinical guide*. Edited by P Haddad, S Dursun, and B Deakin, Fig. 15.1 Plate 1 p. 272. Oxford University Press, Oxford, UK, Copyright © 2004.

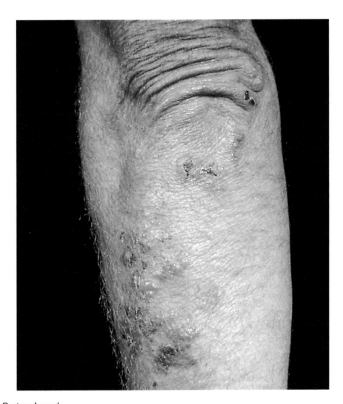

Figure 2.7 Patient's rash.

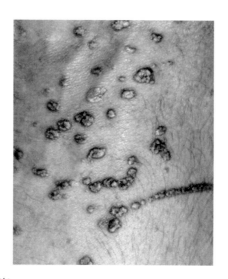

Figure 2.8 Patient's wrists.

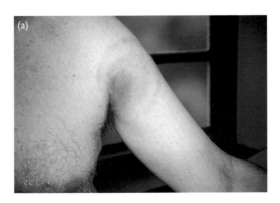

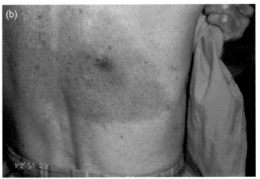

Figure 6.2 Patient's rash.

Surgery, usually transsphenoidal, to remove the pituitary tumour is the management of choice if the patient is able to undergo the procedure. Radiotherapy is reserved for unsuccessful surgical or medical management. Assessment of GH through a 24-hour period (GH day curve) as well as IGF-1 levels are used to assess the success of surgery/radiotherapy or medical treatment and are required on an annual basis.

The role of medical therapy in acromegaly is to shrink the tumour preoperatively or if surgery has failed or is inappropriate. The three classes of drugs used are somatostatin analogues (octreotide, lanreotide), dopamine agonists (cabergoline, bromocriptine) and GH receptor antagonists (pegvisomant). Somatostatin analogues are most effective at tumour shrinkage but dopamine agonists may be useful as an adjuvant or in cases where prolactin secretion is also seen. The complications of acromegaly are listed in Box 3.5.

Box 3.4 Familial syndromes associated with acromegaly

- MEN type I
- McCune-Albright syndrome
- Carney's syndrome
- Familial acromegaly

Box 3.5 Complications of acromegaly

- Hypertension
- Left ventricular hypertrophy
- Ischaemic heart disease
- Diabetes mellitus
- Hypercalciuria and renal stones (GH stimulates renal 1α-hydroxylase)
- Local mass effects of pituitary tumour (visual field defects, cranial nerve palsy, hypopituitarism)
- Carpal tunnel syndrome
- Increased risk of colonic polyps and carcinoma
- Obstructive sleep apnoea
- Goitre

Further Reading

Melmed S (2006). Medical progress: acromegaly. *New England Journal of Medicine* 355(24): 2558–2573.

57. A) A short Synacthen test (tetracosactide) should be performed, along with an MRI of her abdomen

Unlike the general population, where 80% of adrenal failure is due to autoimmune adrenalitis, the pathogenesis of adrenal failure in patients with antiphospholipid syndrome is most commonly haemorrhagic infarction after adrenal vein thrombosis or secondary to anticoagulant therapy (either of which may be possible in this case and would be seen on MRI of the adrenal glands). As concentrations of ACTH and cortisol vary throughout the day, usefulness of random samples is limited. However, a cortisol above 500 nmol/l rules out the diagnosis of adrenal insufficiency. Morning cortisol below 100 nmol/L is diagnostic of adrenal insufficiency, but the basal cortisol is usually in the normal range. Therefore, most of patients require a short Synacthen test to demonstrate insufficient response to stimulation. Warfarin should be continued in context of a therapeutic level of INR, remembering that the underlying pathology in antiphospholipid syndrome is thrombosis. High doses of hydrocortisone IM is the main treatment of acute adrenal failure and fludrocortisone needs to be added when total daily dose of hydrocortisone decreases to less than 40 mg. Autoimmune polyglandular syndrome type II includes Addison's disease and other autoimmune endocrinopathies, which the above case scenario does not suggest. The mild hyponatraemia, hyperkalaemia, and hypercalcaemia are in keeping with primary adrenal insufficiency.

Tutorial

Adrenal insufficiency may be either: (a) primary (Addison's disease), due to adrenal destruction or enzymatic defects secondary to genetic disorders; or (b) secondary, due to disordered pituitary or hypothalamic function, as summarized in Box 3.6. The clinical features can be deduced from the pathophysiology of glucocorticoid deficiency, adrenal androgen deficiency in both primary and secondary adrenal insufficiency, and mineralocorticoid deficiency in primary adrenal insufficiency only. It should also be remembered that skin hyperpigmentation due to deficiency of pro-opiomelanocorticoids in primary adrenal insufficiency usually occurs with exception of patients with very fair skin with low pigment (blue eyes and freckles). Thyroid function may also be affected due to associated autoimmune hypothyroidism or direct inhibitory action of cortisol on TRH.

An early morning (9 am) cortisol and ACTH (an elevated ACTH with low cortisol) is a sensitive first-line test. To confirm adrenal insufficiency a short Synacthen test is performed. This involves measuring serum cortisol before and after (at 30 and 60 mins) injection of 250 μg of ACTH IM (e.g. Synacthen®). In healthy individuals, this challenge leads to a physiological increase in serum cortisol usually to >500 nmol/L (cut-off value depends on local assay) with a lack of response seen in adrenal failure. If ACTH level is equivocal then a long Synacthen test is needed to differentiate primary from secondary adrenal insufficiency. A depot injection of Synacthen® 1 mg IM and serum cortisol measured 30, 60, 120 minutes, 4, 8, 12, and 24 hours. In secondary adrenal insufficiency the levels will gradually rise by 24 hours. There is no response in primary adrenal insufficiency.

Box 3.6 Causes of adrenal insufficiency

Primary adrenal insufficiency

Autoimmune (isolated or as part of autoimmune polyglandular syndrome type I and II)

Infiltration (metastatic, lymphoma, amyloid, haemochromatosis)

Infarction and/or haemorrhage (including Waterhouse-Friderichsen syndrome)

Infection (especially TB and fungal infections)

Bilateral adrenalectomy

Genetic (e.g. congenital adrenal hyperplasia, leukodystrophy)

Drugs (fluconazole, mitotane, phenytoin)

Secondary adrenal insufficiency

Pituitary tumours (other signs of panhypopituitarism may be seen)

Tumours in the region of the hypothalamus-pituitary (craniopharyngioma, meningioma, ependymoma, intrasellar, or suprasellar metastases)

Pituitary infiltration or infection (especially TB, sarcoidosis, and lymphocytic hypophysitis)

Pituitary trauma or radiation

Pituitary apoplexy (including Sheehan's syndrome)

Previous chronic glucocorticoid excess (glucocorticoid use or Cushing's disease

Extending the test out to three days allows even better differentiation of primary and secondary adrenal insufficiency. Once adrenal insufficiency is diagnosed, the cause should be identified. As from Box 3.6 it can be seen that adrenal imaging and/or biopsy will usually be required. In about three quarters of autoimmune causes 21-hydroxylase antibodies are seen.

Further Reading

Charmandari E, Nicolaides N, Chrousos G (2014). Adrenal insufficiency. *Lancet* 383: 2152–2167.

58. A) Chromogranin A is a sensitive test for carcinoid tumours but may be falsely positive in this case

Plasma chromogranin A is a very sensitive marker for neuroendocrine tumours (NETs) but less specific for midgut NETs than urinary 5HIAA. False positives occur with omeprazole use (also with renal and liver failure). Chromogranin A can also be used to monitor response to treatment. Metastatic disease to the liver does not always lead to a derangement of LFTs so this is not a reliable indicator of metastatic disease in these tumours. Octreotide scan is usually very helpful in localizing and monitoring secreting neuroendocrine tumours as the majority express somatostatin receptors. Signs of tricuspid regurgitation may be seen on examination as the right side of the heart is usually affected. Carcinoid syndrome may be seen in the setting of MEN type I, von Hippel-Lindau syndrome, type I neurofibromatosis, and tuberous sclerosis.

Tutorial

Carcinoid tumours are currently named neuroendocrine tumours (NETs) and hence the term 'carcinoid tumour' is no longer recommended, though the terms 'carcinoid syndrome' and 'carcinoid heart disease' still remain in use. NETs constitute a group of neoplasms with common biological features, which can secrete tachykinins, prostaglandins, and bradykinins. The carcinoid syndrome (flushing, diarrhoea, wheezing, intermittent abdominal pain, and/or scale-like skin lesions) occurs only in around 20% of cases with NETs and only when vasoactive substances from the tumours are able to enter the circulation in significant amounts; that is when liver is unable to deactivate excess of serotonin/tachykinins (liver metastases) or if the tumour is able to circumvent the liver circulation, as occurs with some ovarian, pulmonary, and retroperitoneal neuroendocrine tumours.

Biochemical diagnosis rests on demonstration of raised urinary 5HIAA (a serotonin metabolite) and serum chromogranin A. The former is more specific but only seen in excess in midgut tumours and the latter is more sensitive. Proton pump inhibitors, inflammatory bowel disease, and renal and liver failure may lead to false positive chromogranin A and some foods (e.g. cheese, pineapple, bananas, plums, tomatoes, and avocados) may falsely raise urinary 5HIAA. The tumour can be localized by ultrasound, CT, or MRI. As more than 80% of carcinoid tumours have somatostatin receptors, radio-labelled octreotide is used to scan for localization and spread of disease. Galium-68 PET scanning is also used in complex cases.

Surgery is the mainstay of treatment and is often curative in early detected localized disease, as well as having a role in debulking of more advanced disease. Liver embolization or radioablation may also provide a means of debulking tumours. Surgery may precipitate an extreme carcinoid syndrome (carcinoid crisis) and so intravenous octreotide is given prophylactically. Octreotide treatment is also used for long-term treatment to manage symptoms but has not been shown to reduce tumour size. Tachyphylaxis may be seen. Alternative treatments are α-interferon and radioactive somatostatin analogues. Chemotherapy for advanced disease and radiotherapy for bone metastasis are also used.

Further Reading

Ramage J, Davies A, Ardill J, et al. (2012). Guidelines for the management of gastroenteropancreatic neuroendocrine (including carcinoid) tumours (NETs). *Gut* 61(1): 6–32.

59. B) Overnight dexamethasone suppression test

The symptoms and signs raise the possibility of Cushing's syndrome. The following tests can be used as an initial test to confirm Cushing's syndrome:

1) Overnight dexamethasone suppression test: 1 mg dexamethasone is given at midnight. A 9 am cortisol <50 nmol/L makes Cushing's very unlikely.

2) Low dose dexamethasone suppression test: 0.5 mg of dexamethasone is given six hourly for 48 hours. This should normally suppress cortisol level to <50 nmol/L in healthy individuals.

3) Elevated midnight sleeping serum cortisol (requires admission to the hospital). Late night salivary cortisol (available in some centres, at least two measurements). Loss of circadian rhythm of cortisol secretion is seen in Cushing's syndrome with cortisol >50 nmol/L around midnight.

4) A 24-hour urinary free cortisol test (at least three measurements): least recommended as low specificity. Reduced GFR (<30 ml/min) may lead to false negative results.

If two of the above are normal Cushing's is unlikely.

The following tests in screening or diagnosis are no longer recommended:

• Random serum cortisol or plasma ACTH levels
• Urinary 17-ketosteroids
• Insulin tolerance test
• Loperamide test

Tutorial

Excess cortisol secretion results in Cushing's syndrome (CS) whereas Cushing's disease is Cushing's syndrome secondary to a pituitary corticotroph adenoma (CA). The causes of CS are summarized in Figure 3.3. Whilst testing for CS should be carried out if there is any clinical suspicion after exogenous glucocorticoid use has been excluded, the most discriminating clinical features are proximal myopathy, easy bruising, striae, and facial plethora. Asymptomatic patients with an adrenal lesion should also be tested.

The cause of CS can be delineated by means of basal ACTH measurement, corticotrophin releasing hormone (CRH) test, and inferior petrosal sinus sampling (IPSS) as shown in Figure 3.3. The CRH test involves a 100 µg CRH infusion and assessment of cortisol and ACTH response. IPSS involves bilateral inferior petrosal sinus sampling of ACTH with simultaneous ACTH assessment in the peripheral blood. This is assessed at the basal level and after a CRH infusion. The high dose dexamethasone suppression test (2 mg instead of 0.5 mg every 6 hours for 48 hours) is no longer recommended if bilateral inferior petrosal sinus sampling is available. ACTH secretion by pituitary CA is most common (80–90%). If this is the case, ACTH is partially suppressed (>35% of basal value) and cortisol falls >50% of the basal value during high dose dexamethasone suppression test. Ectopic tumours are mostly resistant to this inhibitory feedback. However, 10% of ectopic tumours will suppress and 10% of pituitary tumours will not. A gadolinium enhanced MRI is used to localize pituitary tumours. MRI should not substitute the biochemical assays as an incidental pituitary tumour (present in 10% of healthy individuals) may not be the source of ACTH and an ectopic tumour is actually the source. Ectopic sources can be localized by multiple imaging modalities.

Pseudo-CS is believed to be due to central stimulation of CRH and is seen in alcohol abuse and also severe depression. Symptoms and signs of CS can be seen and biochemically a loss of circadian cortisol rhythm as well as lack of suppression with a low dose dexamethasone test. It is difficult to distinguish from other causes of CS but it usually resolves with abstinence from alcohol and to a lesser degree treatment of depression.

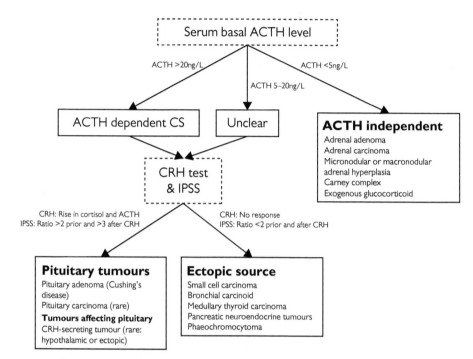

Figure 3.3 Differential diagnosis of Cushing's syndrome.

Further Reading

Nieman L, Biller B, Findling J, et al. (2008). The diagnosis of Cushing's syndrome: an endocrine clinical practice guideline. *Journal Clinical Endocrinology & Metabolism* 93: 1526–1540.

60. C) Increase carbimazole to 30 mg od and refer to the ophthalmologist urgently

The history suggests Graves' ophthalmopathy (GO). If there is any suspicion of optic neuropathy or corneal ulceration then urgent referral to the ophthalmology team should be made. Carbimazole dose should be increased, aiming for fT4 and fT3 in the normal range. Artificial tears or protective paraffin ointment should be prescribed as well. If diplopia is present and not resolving with steroid treatment an orthoptist review is recommended and glasses with prisms may be prescribed.

Tutorial

Patients with GO are not necessarily hyperthyroid. Up to 10% are euthyroid or hypothyroid. GO is present in half of patients with Graves' disease and can be sight-threatening in up to 5%. Therefore, it is vital they are referred to the ophalomologist promptly if there are any features as discussed above. Smoking may worsen GO and smokers are more likely to develop GO. The clinical features of GO are as follows:

- Eyelid retraction and a lid lag: sclera is visible above and below the limbi.
- Proptosis/exophthalmos: both terms mean forward displacement or protrusion of the eye. Proptosis can refer to any organ of the body that is displaced forward, exophthalmos is

restricted to the eye. Some class a protrusion less than 18 mm as proptosis and greater than 18 mm as exophthalmos. It can be documented using a Hertel exophthalmometer.

- Keratitis and corneal ulceration which can be confirmed with fluorescein or Rose Bengal stain.
- Periorbital oedema and chemosis as less efficient orbital drainage occurs.
- Optic atrophy: poor vision or documented decrease in visual acuity, poor colour vision, or an afferent pupillary defect.
- Ophthalmoplegia: diplopia can occur due to oedema or fibrotic effects on extraocular muscles.
- Papilloedema.

The active phase of GO is believed to be immune driven and therefore may respond to immunotherapy. Prednisolone or methylprednisolone has the most convincing evidence of efficacy. The active phase may last 1–2 years, after which stabilization and eventually remission usually occur. Lens sparing orbital radiotherapy may also be used in severe disease. Otherwise therapies include stopping smoking, controlling hyperthyroidism if present, artificial tears, botulinum toxin, and prisms.

Further Reading

Bartalena L, Tanda M (2009). Graves' ophthalmopathy. *New England Journal of Medicine* 360: 994–1001.

Wiersinga W, Perros P, Kahaly G, et al. (2006). Clinical assessment of patients with Graves' orbitopathy: the European Group on Graves' Orbitopathy recommendations to generalists, specialists and clinical researchers. *European Journal of Endocrinology* 155: 387–389.

61. D) Switch his antihypertensive to doxazosin, control hypokalaemia with supplementation and then perform an aldosterone/rennin assay

Given that many patients are asymptomatic, when should one screen for primary aldosteronism? Indications for screening include patients with hypertension not controlled on three or more agents; hypertension with hypokalaemia; hypertension before the age of 40; family history; and a lesion seen on adrenal imaging. Screening is carried out by measurement of aldosterone:renin ratio. Prior to this test, hypokalaemia should be controlled with supplementation and any medication that may interfere with the test should be stopped (see Box 3.7). Hypertension can be controlled in the interim with doxazosin. A high ratio is suggestive of primary hyperaldosteronism. The greater the ratio the more likely the diagnosis. It is also worth noting that chronic renal failure can lead to a false negative.

Box 3.7 Drugs interfering with aldosterone: renin measurement

False positives
Beta blockers
Methyldopa
Clonidine

False negatives
Calcium antagonists
ACE inhibitors
Diuretics

Tutorial

The adrenal cortex has three morphologically and functionally distinct regions. Aldosterone, the principal mineralocorticoid, is produced by the outer region (zona glomerulosa). The secretion of aldosterone is regulated by the rennin angiotensin system and by potassium ions. Aldosterone causes renal sodium retention and potassium loss, leading to expansion of body sodium content and volume expansion. The effect on the distal nephron is of sodium retention and loss of hydrogen and potassium ions leading to a hypokalaemic alkolosis (although serum potassium may be normal in up to 50% of cases). Aldosterone excess leads to an increased rate of cardiovascular events compared to patients with essential hypertension and similar risk profiles. This may be due to the aldosterone effect of inflammation, fibrosis, and necrosis in various target organs and endothelial dysfunction. The prevalence of hyperaldosteronism in unselected patients with hypertension is around 5%, and the causes and defining features are listed in Table 3.4.

The clinical features of primary aldosteronism are non-specific. Patients may be asymptomatic or experience symptoms related to hypertension (such as headache) and/or hypokalaemia (muscle cramps, polyuria/nocturia from hypokalaemic diabetes insipidus; occasionally profound weakness, tetany, and paraesthesia occur). Hypertension may be moderate or marked and often resistant to standard antihypertensives. Hypertension and symptoms often occur early in life. Rarely, primary aldosteronism is associated with phaeochromocytoma, primary hyperparathyroidism, or acromegaly.

Definitive biochemical diagnosis of aldosteronism can be made by inhibiting and stimulating aldosterone and renin secretion by physiologic manoeuvres of sodium loading and sodium depletion, respectively. Dietary sodium loading using either food with high sodium content or sodium chloride tablets will show failure to suppress urinary aldosterone secretion at the end of three days of loading in primary aldosteronism. In primary aldosteronism, aldosterone fails to suppress with a fludrocortisone test. It also fails to suppress after administration of 2 L of normal saline over four hours. This is followed up by seeing low renin levels under conditions of low sodium consumption or use of a diuretic captopril suppression test which has a lower specificity and sensitivity. Plasma renin and aldosterone can be used to distinguish between different causes; in practice these are not specific enough and imaging and/or adrenal vein sampling is needed to confirm the differential diagnosis.

Table 3.4 Causes of primary hyperaldosteronism

Causes	Pathology	Age	Blood pressure	Serum K+ level
Conn's syndrome (functional but benign adenoma).	Benign adenoma <2.5 cm diameter, yellow due to high cholesterol content	Middle aged, occasionally young.	Moderately high to very high but can occasionally be normotensive (in which case of uncertain clinical significance).	Greater degree of hypokalaemia than in idiopathic cause.
Adrenal carcinoma.	Tumour >4 cm may be evidence of invasion.	Middle aged, occasionally young.	Moderately high to very high.	Hypokalaemia often profound.
Primary adrenal hyperplasia (either unilateral or bilateral).	Macronodular or micronodular hyperplasia. No discrete tumour.	Usually older than in Conn's.	Moderately high to very high.	Lesser degree than in Conn's.
Glucocorticoid remedial aldosteronism (familial hyperaldosteronism type I).	Bilateral hyperplasia of zona glomerulosa. See below for biochemical defect.	Young: appears in childhood but often not diagnosed.	Slightly to moderately high.	Normokalaemia or low potassium.

Further Reading

Fogari R, Preti P, Zoppi A, et al. (2007). Prevalence of primary aldosteronism among unselected hypertensive patients: a prospective study based on the use of an aldosterone/renin ratio above 25 as a screening test. *Hypertension Research* 30(2): 111–117.

Ganguly A (1998). Primary aldosteronism. *Lancet* 339(25): 1828–1834.

Mulatero P, Bertello C, Verhovez A, et al. (2009). Differential diagnosis of primary aldosteronism subtypes. *Current Hypertension Reports* 11(3): 217–223.

62. D) Refer for psychiatric input

The patient's symptoms are classical for recurrent hypoglycaemia and the acute hypoglycaemic presentation with seizures supports that. In presence of hypoglycaemia, blood should be sent for venous glucose and serum sample for insulin and C-peptide. Once blood is taken, hypoglycaemia should be treated with intravenous 20% dextrose infusion. The inappropriate elevation of both insulin and C-peptide in the setting of hypoglycaemia confirms endogenous insulin production, therefore likelihood of insulinoma. Sulphonylurea abuse and exogenous insulin administration should be considered, especially when patients have access to these agents if they have relatives with diabetes. Sulphonylureas stimulate insulin secretion and will also elevate insulin and C-peptide, thus a urinary screen for sulphonylureas must also be sent and only if negative should an insulinoma be considered. In the above case, insulin is high in presence of hypoglycaemia and C-peptide is suppressed, which confirms administration of exogenous insulin. Thus, results should be explained to the patient and referral to the psychiatrist made. In case of insulinoma, imaging of the pancreas and calcium stimulation test help to localize a secreting pancreatic lesion. Mixed meal test helps with diagnosis of post-prandial hypoglycaemia, for example secondary to dumping syndrome. Diazoxide is a first-line medical treatment for hypoglycaemia in the case of insulinoma.

Tutorial

Abuse of insulin or oral anti-diabetic medications should always be excluded, when patient presents with recurrent hypoglycaemia. It is very important to take full family and occupational history. Hypoglycaemia could be caused by other anti-diabetic agents such as sulphonylureas, pioglitazone, or glinides, as well as salicylates or quinine. If substance misuse is confirmed, a psychiatrist/ psychologist should be involved.

An insulinoma is a rare neuroendocrine tumour of the endocrine pancreas that inappropriately oversecretes insulin. The majority are benign. It may occur sporadically (more likely to be unifocal) or as part of MEN-I (more likely to be multifocal; simultaneously or consecutively and develop earlier). The classical presentation was described by Whipple as 'Whipple's triad': (1) hypoglycaemia (glucose <2.2 mmol/L); (2) neuroglycopenic symptoms (visual disturbance, seizures, confusion, coma); and (3) symptoms that are corrected by the administration of carbohydrate. After excluding sulphonylurea and exogenous insulin, an initial screening test is performed with three separate glucose measurements each after a 15-hour fast. A glucose of <2.2 mmol/L should be found during symptoms, along with inappropriately high level of insulin and C-peptide. If these 15-hour fasts do not confirm the diagnosis, then carry out a 72-hour fast, with the same biochemical parameters. Both of these tests require close inpatient supervision and monitoring. Due to their small size no imaging modality is 100% sensitive for localizing insulinomas but an MRI with gadolinium +/– endoscopic ultrasound will provide the best imaging before surgical exploration of the whole pancreas. Surgical removal provides a high cure rate. Rarely, insulinomas may metastasize (especially to the liver) or a patient may not be a candidate for surgery. In those circumstances medical options should be employed, which involve the use of diazoxide, octreotide, and radiolabelled somatostatin analogues, often in combination. In case of metastatic disease, palliative surgery may temporarily relieve symptoms and chemotherapy can be considered.

Further Reading

Okabayashi T, Shima Y, Sumiyoshi T, et al. (2013). Diagnosis and management of insulinoma. *World Journal of Gastroenterology* 19(6): 829–837.

63. C) MRI of the pituitary gland

The blood results in this case are consistent with hypogonadotrophic hypogonadism and secondary hypothyroidism. The gynaecomastia is due to an increase in the ratio of oestrogen to androgen due to decreased testosterone. Therefore, MRI of the pituitary gland should be arranged to look for a pituitary lesion which is causing decrease in pituitary hormones. For completion, screening for impairment in the ACTH-cortisol and growth hormone axis should also be performed, as if the patient does have a mass but is for medical treatment, they may require additional hormone replacement. Doxazosin can rarely cause gynaecomastia, but the patient has been on the drug for many years and has only just developed gynaecomastia. Furthermore, there is a more likely alternate explanation here. Should the MRI head reveal no pituitary lesion and repeat hormone testing show a normal pituitary axis (i.e. the first test was spurious), stopping doxazosin may be worth trying. A testicular ultrasound would be indicated if a scrotal mass was found on examination and biochemistry confirms hypergonadotrophic hypogonadism. Mammography followed by biopsy should be carried out if a mass is suspected. A breast biopsy is not a routine investigation for bilateral gynaecomastia. An abdominal CT would not be helpful in the above case and chronic kidney and liver disease has been ruled out on biochemistry.

Tutorial

Increased male breast glandular tissue is due to an increase in the oestrogen:androgen ratio by either increased oestrogen or decreased testosterone levels. Sometimes both can occur simultaneously as increased luteinizing hormone (LH) or human chorionic gonadotrophin (hCG) will increase conversion of testosterone to oestrogen, as will testosterone replacement therapy. Additionally, in hyperthyroidism and chronic liver disease increased SHBG will affect the free testosterone as it will bind testosterone with greater affinity. Therefore, in clinical assessment of gynaecomastia, knowledge of oestrodiol, testosterone, LH, and hCG levels, along with a prolactin level will help identify the cause (Table 3.5). A large number of medications can cause gynaecomastia by different mechanisms and these are discussed in the tutorial to question 177. An increase in subareolar fat rather than an

Table 3.5 Diagnosis in gynaecomastia

Result	Diagnosis	Further investigation
↓LH ↓Testosterone	1) Prolactinoma—raised serum prolactin 2) Secondary hypogonadism—normal/low prolactin. NB: may be associated low levels of other pituitary hormones—panhypopituitarism.	MRI head and visual field testing.
↓Testosterone ↑LH	Primary hypogonadism	
↑LH ↑testosterone	Androgen insensitivity syndrome	
↑hCG/oestrodiol	1) Germ cell tumour. 2) Non-gonadal oestrodiol/hCG secreting tumours (large cell lung cancer, hepatoma, renal cell carcinoma).	1) Testicular examination including ultrasound. 2) CT of chest, abdomen and pelvis.
↑Oestrodiol and normal or ↓LH	1) Leydig or Sertoli tumour. 2) Adrenal tumour. 3) Increased testosterone to oestrogen conversion (e.g. liver disease, thyroid replacement therapy) or exogenous oestrogens.	1) Testicular examination including ultrasound. 2) CT of abdomen and pelvis.
All tests normal	Idiopathic gynaecomastia or rule out lipomastia.	

expansion of breast gland is termed lipomastia or pseudogynaecomastia. On examination, a ridge of glandular tissue can be felt when drawing a thumb from each side of the breast. However, this will not occur with lipomastia which also improves with weight loss. Systemic causes of gynaecomastia are chronic liver disease, chronic renal disease, HIV, and malnutrition.

Treatment of gynaecomastia predominantly involves treating the primary cause. Tamoxifen or clomiphene can be useful in the early stages to reduce swelling and pain but become less effective after a year, as a fibrotic process has usually then occurred. Danazol may also be used but has a greater degree of side effects, especially weight gain.

Further Reading

Johnson R, Murad M (2009). Gynaecomastia: pathophysiology, evaluation and management. *Mayo Clinic Proceedings* 84: 1010–1015.

64. B) He may have McCune-Albright syndrome

McCune-Albright syndrome is defined as the association of (a) polyostotic fibrous dysplasia; (b) irregular unilateral *café au lait* spots; and (c) endocrinopathies, including benign thyroid nodules, as seen in this case. A clinical diagnosis needs two out of these three associations. It is caused by a post-zygotic somatic mutation (not inherited) in GNAS1 gene. Mutational analysis of this gene is available in the UK. In neurofibromatosis type 1 (NF1) *café au lait* lesions have regular edge and are bilateral; multiple neurofibromas are present and associated endocrinopathies include phaeochromocytoma or gut neuroendocrine tumours. NF2 does not have association with endocrine conditions but bilateral acoustic neuromas and deafness are characteristic.

Tutorial

The clinical presentation of McCune-Albright is highly variable due to mosaicism, and the following features occur to different extents from patient to patient. These are summarized in Box 3.8.

Box 3.8 Clinical features of McCune-Albright syndrome

Polyostotic fibrous dysplasia (PFD)

- Multiple pathological fractures early in childhood with a predilection for one side of the body.
- Visible or palpable lesions or osteosarcoma, gait abnormalities may be the presentation, as well as symptoms and signs from nerve entrapment.
- The lesions do not resolve. They will either worsen or remain the same over time.
- Very difficult to treat.
- No evidence that bisphosphonates improve the underlying pathology, but may help in pain relief.
- Orthopaedic surgery for fractures may be complicated by bleeding and so traction management is preferred if possible.
- Radiotherapy has little effect.

Café au lait spots

- Usually strikingly unilateral (on the same side as PFD lesion) and stop abruptly at the midline if encroaching this area.
- They are prominent with irregular edges 'coast of Maine' variants (as opposed to the smaller, rounded and smooth edged 'coast of California' spots seen in neurofibromatosis type I).

Endocrinopathies

- Precocious puberty
- Thyroid anomalies (adenomas, goitrous colloid/hypertrophic nodules, rarely thyroid cancer)

- Acromegaly and prolactinomas
- Hypophosphataemic rickets
- Diabetes mellitus
- Cushing's syndrome

Other features
- Cardiomegaly
- Microencephalopathy
- Splenomegaly
- Pancreatitis, altered liver function tests secondary to cholestasis

Further Reading

Dumitrescu C, Collins M (2008). McCune-Albright syndrome. *Orphanet Journal of Rare Diseases* 19(3): 12.

65. D) The patient has Liddle's syndrome

The patient is most likely to have Liddle's syndrome. He has a low serum potassium and inappropriately high urinary potassium with a mild metabolic alkalosis. The suppressed rather than increased aldosterone is against Conn's syndrome (and Bartter's and Gitelman's syndrome). Mutation in SLC12A1 is found in Bartter's syndrome. Liddle's syndrome should not be treated with spironolactone as aldosterone is already suppressed in this condition. Table 3.6 is a guide to differentiate between the renal tubular abnormalities of Bartter's, Gitelman's, and Liddle's syndromes. Details of each are discussed below.

Table 3.6 Differential diagnosis of renal tubular abnormalities

	Bartter's	**Gitelman's**	**Liddle's**
Age (average) of presentation	Infancy	Early adulthood	Childhood
Blood pressure	Normal	Normal	Raised
Inheritance	AR	AR	AD
Serum K+	Low	Low	Low
Metabolic alkalosis	Yes	Yes	Yes
Serum magnesium	Normal or low	Low	Normal
Renin	Increased	Increased	Decreased
Aldosterone	Increased	Increased	Decreased
Urinary calcium	Increased or Normal	Decreased	Normal
Urinary prostaglandin-E2	Increased	Normal	Normal
Diuretic picture it is biochemically similar to	Loop diuretic	Thiazide diuretic	N/A

Tutorial

Liddle's syndrome

This is due to gain of function mutations in the epithelial sodium channel (ENaC) in the distal nephron, leading to increased sodium retention with lack of inhibition of the channel by high intracellular sodium levels. Hypertension with oedema is often seen. Hypokalaemia, metabolic alkalosis with decreased renin and aldosterone levels are present. It should be considered in a young hypertensive patient with mild hypokalaemia with a similar family history. Muscle weakness and cramps may result from the hypokalaemia. Treatment involves a low salt diet with amiloride or triamterene (K+ sparing diuretics that close the sodium channel directly). Spironolactone is of no use as it acts on the mineralocorticoid receptor and aldosterone is not causing the channel to be open.

Bartter's syndrome

A rare autosomal recessive disorder involving defects in the bumetanide-sensitive Na-K-2Cl channel or apical potassium channel or the basal chloride channel in the thick ascending limb of loop of Henle. It results in similar biochemical changes seen with loop diuretic use, salt wasting and volume depletion occur. The renin-angiotensin system is obviously activated, leading to secondary hyperaldosteronism and therefore a hypokalaemic metabolic alkalosis. However, there is no hypertension. The four identified mutations are listed in Table 3.7. It usually presents in childhood or adolescence with polyuria, polydipsia, cramps, muscle weakness, and may involve seizures and tetany. As well as the changes in sodium, potassium, and alkalosis, an increased urinary calcium (due to impaired calcium reabsorption leading to nephrocalcinosis) is seen. It is often also associated with other congenital defects such has growth retardation and, in the case of Bartter's type IV, sensorineural deafness. Treatment is lifelong and involves normalizing potassium with amiloride and oral potassium supplementation. NSAIDs (commonly indomethacin) can be effective by decreasing prostaglandins production.

Gitelman's syndrome

This is an autosomal recessive condition with loss of function mutations (SLC12A3 gene) to the thiazide sensitive Na-Cl co-transporter (NCCT) in the distal convoluted tubule, resulting in salt wasting, hypovolaemia, and metabolic alkalosis, along with secondary hyperaldosteronism and hypokalaemic metabolic alkalosis as seen in Bartter's syndrome. However, the differentiating feature when compared to Bartter's syndrome, is the increased calcium reabsorption and increased urinary magnesium and hypomagnesaemia. In this respect it is akin to thiazide diuretic use. It presents in adulthood with the biochemical features listed in Table 3.6 with a less severe clinical picture than Bartter's syndrome and usually with less volume depletion. These patients may be treated with potassium sparing diuretics (usually amiloride) and also require to varying degree potassium and magnesium replacement.

Table 3.7 Bartter syndrome subtypes

Syndrome and affected channel	Gene with mutation
Bartter syndrome type I (Na-K-2Cl transporter defect)	SLC12A1
Bartter syndrome type II (apical potassium channel defect)	ROMK 1
Bartter syndrome type III Bartter syndrome type IV (two defects associated with the basal chloride channel (ClC-K) in the thick ascending limb of Henle)	CLCNKB CLCNKA/BSND
Barter syndrome type V (activating mutation of calcium sensing receptor)	CASR

Further Reading

Mauricio B, Curtis J, Warnock D (1994). Liddle's syndrome revisited—a disorder of sodium reabsorption in the distal tubule. 1994. *New England Journal of Medicine* 330: 178–181.

Shaer A (2001). Inherited primary renal tubular hypokalemic alkalosis: a review of Gitelman and Bartter syndromes. *American Journal of Medical Science* 322(6): 316–332.

66. E) Testing of the HFE gene for mutations

The clinical suspicion is of haemochromatosis with cardiac, liver, pancreas, and skin involvement. There are no indications in the history or blood tests of a secondary cause of haemochromatosis, so hereditary haemochromatosis is likely. His diabetes is likely secondary to haemochromatosis and hypogonadotrophic hypogonadism secondary to iron deposits in the pituitary gland. Measuring serum iron has no value in diagnosis in hereditary haemochromatosis. Increased serum ferritin levels to >200 μg/L in premenopausal women and >300 μg/L in men and postmenopausal women indicate primary iron overload. This is supported by a plasma transferrin saturation of >60% in men and >50% in women. Transferrin saturation is influenced by inflammation and liver disease itself and therefore is not diagnostic, but is a good initial screening test. A large proportion of women below 30 years, who have haemochromatosis may have normal transferrin saturation. A histological diagnosis has been required for diagnosis (Perl's Prussian blue stain on liver biopsy showing iron accumulation in hepatocytes and biliary epithelial cells with relative sparing of Kupffer cells). This is in contrast to secondary causes of iron overload which occur predominantly in Kupffer cells. However, in many centres genetic testing demonstrating homozygosity for the Cys282Tyr mutation of the HFE gene is used. The raised alpha-fetoprotein also indicates a potential complication of hepatocellular carcinoma.

Tutorial

Hereditary haemochromatosis is an autosomal recessive disorder with high iron absorption resulting in progressive iron overload. It occurs in neonatal, juvenile, and adult forms. The adult form is usually due to a mutation on chromosome 6 within the HFE gene. Substitution of a cysteine for a tyrosine at amino acid position 282 of HFE is found in most cases. Excess iron is found in almost all tissues, leading to cell loss and fibrosis but the liver, heart, pancreas, spleen, pituitary, testes, and parathyroids are typically involved. Men are affected more than women and prevalence is 1 in 300, with most in northern Europe.

Although present from birth, iron accumulation with tissue damage takes years to develop in the adult form of the disease and commonly presents between 40 and 70 years of age. Early symptoms include lethargy, impotence, and arthralgia. Skin hyperpigmentation (or 'bronzing') occurs later, with the classic triad of diabetes, hepatomegaly/cirrhosis, and skin changes being the most common. Other features that may occur are hypogonadism, hypoparathyroidism, cardiomyopathy, conduction disturbances, arthropathy, hypothyroidism, and splenomegaly.

A normal life expectancy can be achieved if therapy aimed at removing iron is started before the development of cirrhosis. Treatment involves weekly venesection until iron depletion is demonstrated by normalization of serum ferritin and transferrin saturation. Thereafter venesection is usually carried out 2–3 monthly. In those with end stage liver disease, liver transplantation may be carried out, with a five-year survival of 42%. The liver disease seen can have a degree of reversibility with iron removal if caught in the early stages. Hepatocellular carcinoma is one of the most serious complications of haemochromatosis.

Secondary haemochromatosis involves the same pattern of tissue damage. Causes are listed in Box 3.9. Patients with secondary haemochromatosis often have anaemia and venesection is not appropriate for treatment. Chelators such as desferrioxamine, deferiprone, and deferasirox are an alternative treatment. They need to be given continuously rather than intermittently as only a small percentage of body iron is non-transferrin bound and accessible to chelators.

Box 3.9 Secondary causes of haemochromatosis

Hereditary causes

Thalassaemia
Sickle cell anaemia
Pyruvate kinase deficiency
Congenital dyserythropoietic anaemia
Hereditary spherocytosis
Sideroblastic anaemia (X-linked)
Diamond-Blackfan anaemia

Acquired causes

Myelofibrosis
Aplastic anaemia
Acquired sideroblastic anaemia
Myelodysplastic syndromes

Further Reading

Powell W, Seckington R, Deugnier Y (2016). Haemochromatosis. *Lancet* 388: 706–716.

67. D) Paget's disease

Whilst the initial presentation is with congestive cardiac failure, the raised ALP and radiological signs with normal calcium and phosphate indicate likely Paget's disease. One important complication of Paget's disease is high output cardiac failure, which precipitated this patient's admission. It is worth noting that the patient's ECG does show evidence of left ventricular hypertrophy which also supports this diagnosis. Another complication is osteogenic sarcoma. Whilst this complication is rare, any increase of pain in a patient with Paget's disease should arouse suspicion of sarcomatous degeneration and/or increase in disease activity. There are no auscultatory findings to suggest mitral valve prolapse. He has no chest pain or intrascapular pain and his BP is not significantly different between each arm. In severe vitamin D deficiency, patients complain of generalized not localized bony aches.

Tutorial

Paget's disease is due to an abnormal balance of excessive bone resorption (abnormal osteoclastic activity) with disordered bone formation (abnormal osteoblastic activity). The resultant bone is larger, less dense, and weaker as well as being more vascular. The exact aetiology is unclear. The greatest prevalence is seen in Europe (predominantly England, France, and Germany), Australia, and New Zealand. It is rare in those younger than 25 years and increases in frequency with age.

The majority are asymptomatic and the condition is picked up on incidental radiograph or blood tests. It may be monostotic or polyostotic, with new sites occurring after diagnosis. Bone pain is the most common symptom. Other symptoms are hearing loss, congestive cardiac failure, dysaesthesias, and weakness due to nerve root compression. Physical signs include bowing of the long bones, frontal bossing of the skull, and kyphosis. Due to the increased vascularity of the involved bone it may be warm over the affected bone, superficial temporal arteries may be prominent, and high output cardiac failure may develop. Nerve compression may lead to neuropathies at various locations but the most common is deafness due to compression of the VIIIth cranial nerve.

The alkaline phosphatase (ALP) is raised but serum calcium and phosphate are normal (with the exception of hypercalcaemia after a period of immobility). ALP measurements are also used to monitor response to treatment. However, in monostotic disease levels may not be raised and any liver isoforms seen in liver disease may mask changes. Increased urinary hydroxyproline indicates increased bone turnover. Diagnosis is predominantly made with radiology in which three patterns may be seen representing the three phases of the disease:

1. Predominantly lytic
   a) Radiolucency especially of the skull where it is called *osteoporosis circumscripta*
   b) V-shaped pattern demarcating healthy and Pagetic bone in the long bones ('cutting cone', 'blade of grass')
   c) 'Brim sign'—thickened ilio-pectineal line in the pelvis
2. Mixed lytic and sclerotic phase
   a) Loss of cortico-medullary differentiation
   b) Cortical thickening
   c) 'Framed vertebrae'
3. Predominantly sclerotic phase
   a) Increased bone size
   b) Thickening of long bones

Fractures may also be seen. The uptake of tracer with isotope bone scanning indicates disease activity and fracture risk.

Bisphosphonates licensed in the UK for the treatment of Paget's disease are etidronate, pamidronate, risedronate, tiludronic acid, and zoledronic acid. These agents decrease bone turnover by inhibiting osteoclastic activity and reducing pain. Deafness is irreversible and it is unclear if over the long term these drugs reduce any of the other complications of Paget's disease (Box 3.10). The more aggressive the initial regimen, the longer the remission as monitored by symptoms, ALP, and isotope scanning.

Box 3.10 Complications of Paget's disease

- Nerve entrapment: most commonly VIII cranial nerve
- Spinal cord compression (usually thoracic)
- Osteoarthritis
- Osteogenic sarcoma
- High output cardiac failure

Further Reading
Paul T (2017). Adult Paget's disease of bone: a review. *Rheumatology* (Oxford). 56(12): 2050–2059.

68. C) IV fluid resuscitation, 100 mg hydrocortisone IV stat and 6-hourly IM afterwards

Pituitary apoplexy refers to the haemorrhage or ischaemia of the pituitary gland and patient's post-partum presentation is likely to be secondary to Sheehan's syndrome, especially as her morning cortisol is low. Hydrocortisone is needed to prevent cardiovascular collapse due to cortisol deficiency because of insufficient ACTH. In this case, parenteral hydrocortisone administration should not be delayed, while fluid resuscitation is continued. An MRI of the head should be performed next to confirm if pituitary apoplexy has occurred. CT imaging has lower resolution and will detect only a big bleed/big pituitary lesion. It is used when MRI is contraindicated. Even if this patient may have secondary hypothyroidism, L-thyroxine replacement should be started only after glucocorticoids are adequately replaced, which usually takes place after 3–4 days. If given too early this may provoke Addisonian crisis.

Tutorial

The commonest cause of pituitary apoplexy is extensive infarction of a pituitary adenoma with haemorrhage. Other causes include radiation therapy, anticoagulant therapy, disseminated intravascular coagulopathy, reduction in intracranial pressure, and post-partum ischaemic infarction (Sheehan's syndrome; usually due to severe hypotension following post-partum haemorrhage). It often presents with associated cardiovascular collapse from cortisol deficiency, along with the classic features of raised intracranial pressure. Occasionally the onset is more insidious with symptoms of hypopituitarism. The causes of pituitary apoplexy are summarized in Table 3.8.

Hypopituitarism denotes deficiency of all or some of the pituitary hormones (anterior and/ or posterior). It may be due to destruction or compression of pituitary tissue, hypothalamic dysfunction or reduction in the blood supply of the hypothalamic-pituitary portal circulation. The causes of hypopituitarism are summarized in Table 3.8. The usual sequence in which hormone function is lost is: GH → LH & FSH → TSH → ACTH. Prolactin deficiency and ADH deficiency are rare. The clinical features of hypopituitarism are those of insufficiency of the target gland as summarized in Table 3.9.

If hypopituitarism is suspected, biochemical assessment of pituitary function, formal visual field assessment, and imaging of the pituitary fossa (MRI with contrast) are required. Measurement of pituitary hormones alone is not enough as target hormone levels may be low even with normal pituitary hormones (i.e. inappropriately normal). The following are usually assessed:

- LH and FSH, 9 am testosterone or oestradiol.
- TSH and thyroxine (serum free T4).
- A 9 am cortisol and short Synacthen test (note less than six weeks deficiency may lead to falsely normal results as the adrenal cortex may not have atrophied within that time).
- Prolactin (hyperprolactinaemia is more often seen than low prolactin in hypopituitarism from stalk compression by intrasellar mass or infiltration).
- IGF-1 and insulin tolerance test or glucagon test are used to assess GH and cortisol reserve.
- Plasma and urine osmolality and 24-hour urine volume to screen for diabetes insipidus. A water deprivation test to confirm (note ACTH deficiency reduces glomerular filtration rate, which may mask diabetes insipidus, so testing needs to be done after glucocorticoid replacement).

Treatment involves replacement of the target hormone or in the case of growth hormone deficiency, replacement of the pituitary hormone. If visual fields are significantly affected or cranial nerves palsy is present a surgical decompression is indicated. ACTH deficiency requires glucocorticoid replacement (mineralocorticoid replacement is not needed as this is under control of the renin-angiotensin system). For most patients 20 mg of hydrocortisone daily is sufficient in divided doses. It is important to avoid long-term over replacement due to side effects. A cortisol day curve is used to assess the adequacy of replacement. Prednisolone may also be used which has a longer half-life. Advice should be given on doubling the dose if the patient is acutely unwell. If the patient is unable to tolerate PO medication (e.g. vomiting and diarrhoea or severe illness/ surgery) then parenteral therapy is needed. Steroid equivalent dosing is important to remember (Box 3.11).

Thyroid replacement is as for primary hypothyroidism, although TSH is obviously of no use in monitoring treatment, and free thyroid hormone concentrations as well as clinical assessment are used. There are bone mineral density and quality of life benefits to adult growth hormone replacement and NICE have produced guidelines on its use in this situation. Both males and female require sex steroid replacement to prevent osteoporosis. If a patient is not keen for HRT/testosterone replacement or it is contraindicated, an alternative bone protection can be used, for example bisphosphonates.

Further Reading
Sibal L, Ball S, Connolly V, et al. (2004). Pituitary apoplexy: a review of clinical presentation, management and outcome in 45 cases. *Pituitary* 7(3): 157–163.

69. B) Osteomalacia

Looser's zones described in X-ray report are pathognomonic for osteomalacia. This diagnosis is supported further by mild hypocalcaemia and hypophosphataemia. In osteoporosis, bone density will be generally decreased but X-ray may look normal. In the case of Paget's disease, primary V-

Table 3.8 Causes of hypopituitarism

Cause	Examples
Tumours	Pituitary adenomas, craniopharyngiomas, gliomas, meningiomas, secondary malignancy (breast, lung)
Infiltration	Sarcoidosis, haemochromatosis, histiocytosis X
Infection	TB, syphilis, meningitis, pituitary abscess
Autoimmune	Lymphocytic hypophysitis
Congenital	Kallman syndrome, Pit1 and Prop1 gene mutations
Trauma	Trauma to the hypophysis
Empty sella syndrome	
Treatment related	Surgery (e.g. transsphenoidal adenomectomy), radiotherapy
Infarction/haemorrhage (apoplexy)	Sheehan's syndrome, apoplexy of pituitary adenoma, DIC, anticoagulant therapy,
Other	Russell viper snake bite

shaped lytic lesions can be seen, followed by cortical thickening and at later stage osteosclerosis.

Table 3.9 Clinical features of hypopituitarism

Hormone deficiency	Features
ACTH	Same as Addison's disease except no hyperpigmentation and K+ is normal
Growth hormone	Adult: poor exercise capacity, psychological effects, reduced lean body mass
LH/FSH	Reduced libido, infertility, and loss of secondary sexual characteristics Dysmenorrhoea, erectile dysfunction, testicular atrophy
TSH	Features of hypothyroidism
Prolactin	Lack of lactation
ADH	Polyuria, polydipsia (diabetes insipidus)

Box 3.11 Steroid equivalents

- Prednisolone 5 mg
- Hydrocortisone 20 mg
- Dexamethasone 750 µg
- Methylprednisolone 4 mg

In sarcoma, X-ray will identify bone deformity. Whilst myeloma must be considered in this clinical presentation it is unlikely with a normal Hb, low calcium, and phosphate.

Tutorial

Inadequate mineralization of the bone in the adult leads to osteomalacia. In childhood (before fusion of the epiphyseal plates) it leads to rickets, where non-mineralized osteoid occurs at the growth plates. Causes can be classified into vitamin D deficiencies, hypophosphataemic causes, defective bone matrix, and defective mineralization as described in Table 3.10.

Presentation may be vague and insidious with generalized aches and pains to more specific bone

Table 3.10 Causes of osteomalacia/rickets

Vitamin D deficiency	Decreased production	● Poor sunlight exposure ● Poor dietary intake ● Malabsorption
	Decreased 1-hydroxylation	● Renal failure ● VDDR type I
	Decreased clearance	● For example, enzyme inducers such as phenytoin
	Decreased action	● VDDR type II
Hypophosphataemia	Increased renal losses	● Hyperparathyroidism ● Fanconi syndrome ● X-linked hypophosphataemia ● Oncogenic osteomalacia (FGF23 production leads to phosphaturia) ● Acidosis ● Corticosteroids ● Diabetes ● Alcoholism
	Decreased absorption	● Malabsorption ● Phosphate binders
	Movement into cells	● Insulin ● Sepsis ● Salicylates
Other		● Fibrogenesis imperfecta ossium ● Fluoride ● Bisphosphonates

VDDR = Vitamin D Dependent rickets.

pain, fracture, and deformity. Clinical features of hypocalcaemia may be present. A definitive diagnosis can only be made with bone biopsy. However, the clinical and biochemical picture with or without characteristic radiological features, usually gives a secure diagnosis:

- ↓or normal serum calcium
- ↓ or normal phosphate (may be raised with renal failure)
- ↑ ALP
- Low or normal vitamin D levels (except in vitamin D dependent rickets type II or associated secondary hyperparathyroidism when it can be raised)
- Looser's zones/pseudo-fractures: linear areas of decreased opacity on X-ray due to decreased mineralization
- Biconcave vertebrae and intervertebral disc ballooning (codfish vertebrae)
- Rickety rosary (enlarged costa-chondral junction)

Causes of vitamin D deficiency may be classified into decreased production, decreased 1-hydroxylation, decreased clearance, and decreased action as described in Table 3.10. Vitamin D supplementation with or without calcium supplementation (depending on calcium level and intake in diet) is needed. Ergocalciferol (vitamin D2) or cholecalciferol (D3) is the preferred form of replacement, while 1-alpha-calcidol is used with impaired 1-alpha hydroxylation (renal failure).

Renal failure leads to failure of 1α-hydroxylase (phosphate is often raised in this situation). Vitamin D dependent rickets type I (VDDR type I) is due to a congenital absence of 1α-hydroxylase whereas VDDR type II is due to a defective vitamin D receptor and hence there is raised vitamin D. It may be associated with alopecia (VDDR type IIa, type IIb without alopecia).

There are many causes of hypophosphataemia, including Fanconi syndrome and X-linked hypophosphataemia. In Fanconi syndrome generalized renal tubular dysfunction leads to phosphaturia, aminoaciduria, glycosuria, renal tubular acidosis, proteinuria, hypercalciuria, and sodium and potassium loss.

Further Reading

Nair R, Maseeh A (2012). Vitamin D: the 'sunshine' vitamin. *Journal of Pharmacology and Pharmacotherapy* 3(2): 118–126.

70. B) CT scan chest and neck followed by USS guided FNA (fine needle aspiration) of the right thyroid nodule

This lady has a cold nodule in the right lobe of her thyroid, which is compressing her trachea and causing stridor. She has no symptoms of hyper- or hypothyroidism and TFTs are normal. The most likely diagnosis is a neoplastic lesion of her thyroid. A CT scan will reveal the extent of compression, identify secondary lesions, and provide structural detail of the lesion. An FNA of the nodule will provide histology to confirm the nature of the lesion. Flow volume loops will provide information on the level of tracheal encroachment, but CT will give more information. Serum calcitonin is used to monitor medullary carcinoma of the thyroid which usually presents in younger patients. Thyroglobulin is used to detect early recurrence of follicular/papillary carcinoma of the thyroid following total thyroidectomy and radioiodine ablation. Thyroid specific antibodies will not be helpful in diagnosis of thyroid cancer, though anti-thyroglobulin Ab should be checked before thyroglobulin level is interpreted.

Tutorial

Goitre may be diffuse or nodular as listed in Table 3.11. Presentation may be asymptomatic or associated with symptoms of hypo-/hyperthyroidism or due to local pressure symptoms (difficulty swallowing or difficulty breathing with stridor). The presence of associated lymphadenopathy, a firm non-tender fixed nodule, is more indicative of malignancy, which is seen in less than 5%. *Pemberton's sign* (jugular venous distension and facial erythema on raising the arms is a sign of superior vena cava obstruction caused by a substernal mass) may be seen.

Investigations for goitre involve the following:

- Thyroid function tests (TSH, T4, and T3):
  - To check for hypo/hyperthyroidism.
  - Subclinical hyperthyroidism (suppressed TSH, normal T4 and T3) is common in patients with goitre.
- Thyroid antibodies for autoimmune disease:
  - Anti-TPO suggestive of Hashimoto's thyroiditis.
  - TSH receptor antibody pointing towards Graves' disease.
- Calcitonin: the pentagastrin test:
  - If medullary thyroid carcinoma is suspected, for example MEN-II.

- Thyroglobulin:
  - This is used as a follow-up marker after treatment of thyroid carcinoma rather than a screening test.
- Plain X-rays/CT/respiratory flow loops:
  - Imaging of the thoracic inlet may demonstrate retrosternal extension of a goitre and compression of adjacent structures.
  - Respiratory flow loops will support this, giving information on tracheal encroachment, but rarely used now.
- US:
  - Provides information on thyroid size.
  - Useful to distinguish cystic from solid nodules.
  - Cannot differentiate between benign and malignant lesions.
  - Monitoring of lesion size over time.
- Scintigraphy:
  - Not routinely used.
  - Accumulation of radioiodine (^{123}Iodine) or technetium scan (^{99m}TC) gives a guide as to increased or decreased function within the thyroid. 'Hot'/toxic and 'cold'/suspicious of malignancy, but could be caused by cyst.
  - Identifies retrosternal goitre and ectopic thyroid tissue.
- Fine needle aspiration or cytology (FNA, FNAC):
  - This is the most accurate diagnostic test and the first-line test if the nodule is technically feasible to biopsy.

Table 3.11 Cause of goitre

Diffuse goitre	Physiological	Pregnancy
		Puberty
	Thyroiditis	Subacute (de Quervain's)
		Riedel's disease
	Autoimmune	Graves' disease
		Hashimoto's
	Iodine deficiency	
	Goitrogens	Antithyroid medication
		Lithium
		Iodine excess
Nodular goitre	Multi-nodular	Toxic
		Non-toxic
	Solitary nodule	Toxic adenoma
		Benign nodule
		Malignant nodule
		Lymphoma
		Metastasis
Infiltration		Tuberculosis
		Sarcoidosis

Treatment is then aimed at the underlying cause. For example,: thyroidectomy for malignant or suspicious nodules; T4 replacement for hypothyroidism in Hashimoto's goitre; or surgery (partial or total thyroidectomy) for benign non-toxic nodules causing significant local pressure effects. For a toxic multinodular goitre or nodule, the patient is rendered euthyroid first with medical management, for example carbimazole. However, due to the autonomous nature of the pathology, radioiodine treatment or surgery is needed for long-term control.

Further Reading

Mehanna H, Jain A, Morton R, Watkinson J, Shaha A (2009). Investigating the thyroid nodule. *British Medical Journal* 338: b733.

Song J, Dmytriw A, Yu E, et al. (2018). Investigation of thyroid nodules: a practical algorithm and review of guidelines. *Head Neck* 40(8):1861–1873.

71. C) Refer for radioactive iodine treatment

Subclinical hyperthyroidism is diagnosed when TSH is suppressed with normal levels of T4 and T3. This may occur with over replacement of levothyroxine in hypothyroidism or as a result of toxic nodule/multinodular goitre or early Graves' disease. If TFTs are consistent with subclinical hyperthyroidism, then they should be first repeated after eight weeks. If TSH is still suppressed to <0.1 mU/L or there is increased risk of osteoporosis/arrhythmias (this patient has both), treatment should be considered, especially if a thyroid uptake scan is suggestive of toxic nodule. In this case, radioiodine as treatment should be considered. Carbimazole could be an alternative if the patient is not keen for radioiodine or surgery. Subclinical hyperthyroidism may recur though, after stopping it.

Tutorial

Subclinical hyperthyroidism as defined above is usually asymptomatic or presents with mild symptoms. Whether or not this syndrome should be treated has been a matter of debate, but increasing evidence indicates subclinical hyperthyroidism is associated with increased incidence of AF and mortality and morbidity from cardiovascular disease and osteoporosis, especially in the elderly.

In the case of those on thyroxine treatment the dose of levothyroxine should be reduced. It should also be reduced if accelerated bone loss, new angina, cardiac failure, or atrial fibrillation occurs. Those not on levothyroxine generally should be offered treatment if TSH persistently below 0.1 mU/L. Treatment of patients with TSH levels between 0.1 and 0.4 mU/L should depend on other risk factors and patient age (treat if >70 years old). All patients with endogenous subclinical hyperthyroidism should first have investigations to exclude nodular thyroid disease (thyroid uptake scan) and Graves' disease (TSH receptor antibodies, uptake scan).

If thyroid uptake is diffusely increased, it suggests Graves' disease and anti-thyroid medications should be started. If uptake is consistent with solitary nodule/multi-nodular goitre, radioiodine is the first line of treatment. In frail elderly people small dose of anti-thyroid medication lifelong could be an option. Graves' disease (GD, 50–60%), toxic multinodular goitre (MNG, 15–20%), subacute thyroiditis (15–20%), and toxic adenoma (3–5%) make up 85–95% of causes of thyrotoxicosis (Table 3.12). Secondary hyperthyroidism is rare. TSH is suppressed in thyrotoxicosis except for a TSH producing pituitary tumour and T4 and/or T3 are raised.

Table 3.12 Causes of thyrotoxicosis

Primary	Graves' disease
	Toxic multinodular goitre or toxic solitary nodule
	Toxic adenoma
	Post-partum thyroiditis
	Drug induced (e.g. amiodarone, thyroxine)
	Subacute, silent, and post-partum thyroiditis
	Hashitoxicosis (hyperthyroid phase of Hashimoto's disease)
	Ectopic: for example struma ovarii
	Thyroid carcinoma
Secondary	Pituitary adenoma (TSH producing)
	Trophoblastic tumours

Further Reading

Bahn R, Burch H, Cooper D, et al. (2011). Hyperthyroidism and other causes of thyrotoxicosis: management guidelines of the American Thyroid Association and American Association of Clinical Endocrinologists. *Endocrine Practitioner* 17(3): 456–520.

Collet T, Gussekloo J, Bauer D, et al. (2012). Subclinical hyperthyroidism and the risk of coronary heart disease and mortality. *Archives Internal Medicine* 172(10): 799–809.

Cooper D (2007). Approach to the patient with subclinical hyperthyroidism. *Journal of Clinical Endocrinology & Metabolism* 92(1): 3–9.

72. C) Hydrocortisone

High TSH level in the setting of high dose of thyroxine treatment may simply be caused by lack of compliance, which must first be ruled out. If the patient takes thyroxine on the day of the test fT4 could be in normal range, but TSH will still be deranged. This patient is taking over 1.5 μg/kg/day of thyroxine with a persistently raised TSH which should alert to this. Other causes of TFTs suggestive of inadequate replacement in this situation are: malabsorption, including coeliac disease and *Helicobacter pylori* gastritis; drugs which interfere with levothyroxine absorption; or altered drug-induced liver metabolism. Drugs implicated include phenytoin, omeprazole, rifampicin, calcium carbonate, ferrous sulphate, sucralfate, and cholestyramine. Therefore, both of his medications may contribute to the above picture.

Tutorial

Hypothyroidism is a clinical syndrome that is due to deficiency in thyroid hormones T4 and T3. It may be primary or secondary as listed in Box 3.12. Traditionally the most common cause worldwide has been iodine deficiency but, in the UK, autoimmune thyroid disease and hypothyroidism after treatment for hyperthyroidism remain the most common causes. The presentation is usually gradual. Classical symptoms are cold intolerance, tiredness, weight gain, constipation, myalgia, and menstrual irregularities (usually heavy bleeding). Classical signs are dry skin, bradycardia, hair loss, slow relaxing reflexes, carpal tunnel syndrome, macroglossia, and hoarse voice with or without goitre. Congenital cases are usually picked up on routine neonatal screening.

Hypothyroidism results in accumulation of mucopolysaccharides with water in tissues which causes myxoedema. This can result in cardiomegaly, pericardial effusions, megacolon, and neuropathy. With increasing severity, cerebellar ataxia, hypothermia, encephalopathy, and coma can occur. Myxoedema crisis/coma is a rare but life-threatening presentation seen in severe untreated hypothyroidism and is often precipitated by an intercurrent illness or cold exposure.

TSH will be high with low fT4 and fT3 in primary hypothyroidism. The TSH will be low or inappropriately normal in secondary hypothyroidism. A full assessment of pituitary function should be carried out if secondary hypothyroidism is suspected. Thyroid peroxidase auto-antibodies are elevated in most of patients with Hashimoto's thyroiditis.

Treatment involves correcting any reversible cause, for example iodine deficiency and restoring metabolic rate by T4 (thyroxine) replacement. Treatment should be started at a low dose and gradually increased (particularly in the elderly or those with co-morbidities) as cardiac arrhythmias may be precipitated. The usual starting dose of thyroxine is 50–75 μg (25 μg in the elderly or with cardiac disease) and it is increased 4–8 weekly according to clinical symptoms and TSH (use fT4 in those with secondary hypothyroidism). Be aware that pregnancy increases thyroid binding globulin and so dose should be increased. Myxoedematous coma/crisis requires intensive support and slow rewarming. Intercurrent illness such as pneumonia should be treated and hyponatraemia and hypoglycaemia corrected with close monitoring. The best method of starting thyroxine in such a crisis is a matter of debate whether to use T4 or T3. Liothyronine (T3) has a more rapid onset of action and shorter half-life, though it is more likely to cause arrhythmias. Both can be given via NG and liothyronine is available in intravenous form.

Box 3.12 Causes of primary hypothyroidism

- Autoimmune thyroiditis (Hashimoto's)
- Burnt-out phase of Graves' disease
- Previous treatment for thyrotoxicosis (radioiodine, thyroidectomy)
- Iodine deficiency or excess (Wolff-Chaikoff effect)
- Drugs, for example amiodarone, lithium, radiation treatment
- Subacute thyroiditis
- Post-partum thyroiditis
- Infiltration, for example amyloidosis
- Congenital (thyroid agenesis, inborn errors of thyroid hormone synthesis, Pendred's syndrome)

Further Reading

Almandoz J, Gharib H (2012). Hypothyroidism: etiology, diagnosis, and management. *Medical Clinics of North America* 96(2): 203–221.

Chaker L, Bianco A, Jonklaas J, Peeters R (2017). Hypothyroidism. *Lancet* 390: 1550–1562.

73. C) She should be recommended lifestyle measures and alendronate

The Royal College of Physicians and the National Osteoporosis Guideline Group have published guidance on the prevention and treatment of glucocorticoid-induced osteoporosis (see Further Reading). As well as leading to loss of bone mineral density, glucocorticoids increase fracture risk at the hip and spine. Those aged over 65 years and those under 65 years but with a previous fragility fracture, are high risk and should be recommended to start bone protective therapy as well as lifestyle measures, even before bone mineral density is known. Those aged under 65 years without a previous fragility fracture should be assessed first with a DEXA scan of hip and spine. Bone protection therapy and lifestyle measures are recommended in those with a T-score of −1.5 or lower. Those with a T-score of 0 or above should be recommended lifestyle measures and only have a repeat DEXA scan if on high doses of glucocorticoids. Those with T-scores between −1.5 and 0 should be recommended lifestyle measures and have repeat DEXA scans every 1–3 years whilst on steroids. Secondary causes of osteoporosis should be investigated for those with previous fragility fractures and or a suggestive clinical history. HRT is not recommended as a first-line treatment for postmenopausal women with osteoporosis due to increased risk of stroke, breast cancer, coronary disease, and thrombosis. Those who are receiving HRT for management of menopausal symptoms will have the benefit of bone protection for the duration of treatment with HRT.

Tutorial

Bone mass peaks in the third decade of life, which is influenced by genetic factors, weight-bearing exercise, nutrition, and exposure to oestrogen. Osteoporosis involves loss of structural integrity of microarchitecture of the bone, usually with reduction in the amount of bony tissue, with increased risk of fracture. This may occur due to an earlier/greater rate than average loss of bone mass in adult life or failure to form sufficient bone during maturation. Diagnosis of osteoporosis is made by quantitative assessment of bone mineral density (BMD). This is carried out using dual energy X-ray absorptiometry (DEXA) with BMD at the femoral neck the reference point. The T-score is BMD compared with peak bone mass whereas the age-adjusted bone mass is known as the Z-score. T-scores are used for postmenopausal women and men aged 50 years or more. A BMD 2.5 standard deviations below the young adult (T-score $\leq$ −2.5) is classed as osteoporosis. The same score in the setting of a fragility fracture is classed as established (severe) osteoporosis. Osteopenia is a T-score between −1 and −2.5.

Any secondary causes of osteoporosis (as described in Table 3.13) should be identified and treated. After this, the risk of fracture should be calculated and then the best treatment instigated. The clinical risk factors for fracture are listed in Box 3.13. An algorithm, known as the FRAX® algorithm, calculates a ten-year probability of hip fracture from the information on clinical risk factors. Post-menopausal women with a previous fragility fracture should be treated without the need for a risk assessment. In the rest (men and women), the risk score is charted against age and those with a score below the lower assessment threshold can be reassured. Those above the upper assessment are treated and those in the intermediate grade are assessed with BMD. The BMD is then entered into a BMD adjusted FRAX® score and patients treated if above the intervention threshold.

Management involves lifestyle measures and pharmacological therapy. A well-balanced diet and adequate calcium and vitamin D intake should be ensured. Weight-bearing exercise should be encouraged and smoking and excess alcohol consumption discouraged. Pharmacological interventions include the bisphosphonates, denosumab, raloxifene, strontium, and parathyroid hormone (teriparatide). All these agents reduce the risk of vertebral fracture. Alendronate, risedronate, zoledronate, denosumab, and strontium reduce the risk of hip fracture and other non-vertebral fractures. Alendronate has the lowest cost and is recommended as first-line treatment.

Table 3.13 Secondary causes of osteoporosis

Gastrointestinal	Cirrhosis
	Inflammatory bowel disease
	Coeliac disease
	Malabsorption
Endocrine	Hyperthyroidism
	Diabetes mellitus
	Cushing's syndrome
	Hyperparathyroidism
	Hypopituitarism
	Acromegaly
	Hypogonadism
Drugs	Heparin, glucocorticoids, cyclosporin
Bone marrow-related disease/bone marrow infiltration	Myeloma, mastocytosis, amyloidosis,
Other	Anorexia nervosa, osteogenesis imperfecta, prolonged immobility

Box 3.13 Clinical risk factors for fracture in osteoporosis

Age
Sex
Low body mass index
Previous fragility fracture
Parental history of hip fracture
>3 months of glucocorticoid treatment
Smoking
>3 units of alcohol intake per day
Secondary causes of osteoporosis
Falls

Further Reading

Buckley L, Guyatt G, Fink H, et al. (2017). 2017 American College of Rheumatology Guideline for the prevention and treatment of glucocorticoid-induced osteoporosis. *Arthritis & Rheumatology* 69(8): 1521–1537.

Compston J, Cooper A, Cooper C, et al. (and the National Osteoporosis Guideline Group- NOGG) (2017). UK clinical guideline for the prevention and treatment of osteoporosis. *Archives of Osteoporosis* 12(1): 43.

FRAX® tool for calculating a 10-year probability of a hip-fracture. Available at: www.shef.ac.uk/FRAX

74. **A 61-year-old woman was referred to the gastroenterology clinic for investigation and management of chronic diarrhoea. She reported opening her bowels 4–5 times each day, and described the stools as watery but not bloody. She also experienced intermittent abdominal cramps. Her past medical history included osteoarthritis, for which she took regular paracetamol and naproxen. Colonic biopsies demonstrated a lymphocytic infiltrate with a 22 μm collagen band in the subepithelial layer.**

   What is the most likely diagnosis?

   A. Behçet's disease
   B. Crohn's disease
   C. Irritable bowel syndrome
   D. Microscopic colitis
   E. Ulcerative colitis

75. **A 24-year-old man was reviewed in the inflammatory bowel disease clinic. He had a 12-year history of ulcerative colitis, for which he took mesalazine. He reported an eight-month history of nausea and vomiting, non-bloody diarrhoea, and had lost 10 kg of weight over the preceding year. On examination, he had peripheral oedema to both knees and on percussion of the chest there was dullness bibasally, with diminished breath sound. His abdomen was also distended, with dullness in the flanks.**

```
Investigations:
  Hb                       108 g/L
  MCV                      81.2 fL
  WCC                      7.4 × 10⁹/L
  Plt                      210 × 10⁹/L
  Urea                     2.4 mmol/L
  Creatinine               42 µmol/L
  Na                       137 mmol/L
  K                        3.5 mmol/L
  Corrected calcium        2.05 mmol/L
  Phosphate                0.45 mmol/L
  Bilirubin                18 µmol/L
  ALT                      33 IU/L
  ALP                      95 IU/L
  Albumin                  12 g/dL
  INR                      1.45
  IgA                      0.5 g/L (0.8-3.0)
  IgG                      4.7 g/L (6.0-13.0)
  IgM                      0.2 g/L (0.4-2.5)
  Anti-TTG                 negative
  Urine dipstick           negative for protein
  Oesophagoduodenoscopy:   normal oesophagus, mild gastritis,
                           normal D2 appearances
  Colonoscopy:             mild proctitis, no evidence of
                           proximal inflammation
```

What is the most appropriate test to confirm the cause of his current symptoms?

A. ANA and liver biopsy
B. Anti-gliadin antibodies and trial of gluten free diet
C. Duodenal biopsy with PAS staining
D. Enteroscopy with jejunal biopsy
E. Urine 24-hour protein collection and urinary protein:creatinine ratio

76. **A 57-year-old woman was reviewed in the inflammatory bowel disease clinic. She reported increasing abdominal bloating and loose stools since undergoing a right hemicolectomy a year previously for terminal ileal Crohn's disease that was complicated by a fibrotic stricture. She described the diarrhoea as different to that associated with her active Crohn's disease, appearing loose and non-bloody, occasionally floating, and containing fat globules. She took mesalazine 2.4 g once daily. Her clinical examination was unremarkable.**

Investigations:

Hb	112 g/L
MCV	83.0 fL
WCC	6.1 × 10⁹/L
Plt	387 × 10⁹/L
Urea	4.6 mmol/L
Creatinine	68 µmol/L
Na	133 mmol/L
K	3.9 mmol/L
Corrected calcium	2.40 mmol/L
Phosphate	0.83 mmol/L
Bilirubin	15 µmol/L
ALT	42 IU/L
ALP	48 IU/L
Albumin	38 g/dL
INR	0.99
CRP	3.4 mg/L
ESR	7 mm/hr
Colonoscopy	Macroscopically normal mucosa.
Biopsy	No evidence of active inflammation.

What is the most appropriate next step to confirm the cause of her current symptoms?

A. Fasting serum gastrin levels

B. Meckel's scan

C. Octreotide scan

D. Serum VIP levels

E. Trial of bile acid sequestrant

77. **A 37-year-old man presented to A&E with a two-week history of bloody diarrhoea and lower abdominal pain. He had no past medical history or history of recent travel. On examination, he was thin, had palpable lymphadenopathy in the cervical, supraclavicular, and inguinal regions. On inspection of his mouth, oral candidiasis was seen.**

Investigations:

Hb	104 g/L
MCV	73.2 fL
WCC	4.3×10^9/L
Plt	67×10^9/L
Urea	4.3 mmol/L
Creatinine	62 µmol/L
Na	141 mmol/L
K	3.6 mmol/L
CD4 count	45 cells/mm^3
HIV serology	positive for HIV-1
HIV viral load	250,000 copies/mL
Flexible sigmoidoscopy	confluent inflammation and ulceration
Biopsy	lymphocytic infiltration with scattered inclusion bodies

What is the most likely diagnosis?

A. Cryptosporidiosis

B. Cytomegalovirus infection

C. Kaposi sarcoma

D. Lymphogranuloma venereum

E. *Mycobacterium avium-intracellulare* infection

78. A 45-year-old woman developed paraesthesia in her fingers and toes on a background of chronic fatigue and weight loss. Her past medical history included gastro-oesophageal reflux, for which she took regular omeprazole, and an appendicectomy. On examination, she had loss of pinprick sensation to the wrists and shins bilaterally.

```
Investigations:
   Hb                                  78 g/L
   MCV                                 120.0 fL
   WCC                                 5.1 × 10⁹/L
   Plt                                 110 × 10⁹/L
   Urea                                4.3 mmol/L
   Creatinine                          62 µmol/L
   Na                                  141 mmol/L
   K                                   3.6 mmol/L
   CRP                                 4 mg/L
   Ferritin                            164 µg/L
   Serum folate                        5.3 µg/L
   Serum B₁₂                           70 ng/L
   Anti-TTG                            negative
   Anti-intrinsic factor antibodies    negative
   Anti-parietal cell antibodies       negative
   OGD                                 normal gastric mucosa
                                       and D2

   MR small bowel                      no small bowel inflammation
                                       or thickening
```

Which of the following is true?

A. A diagnosis of Crohn's disease is probable

B. A diagnosis of pernicious anaemia is probable

C. A trial of tetracycline is indicated

D. Capsule endoscopy would be indicated

E. The patient does not have vitamin B_{12} malabsorption

79. **A 31-year-old female with extensive small bowel Crohn's disease was reviewed in clinic. She reported fatigue but no exertional dyspnoea, chest pain, or pre-syncope.**

```
Investigations:
  Hb                              83 g/L
  MCV                             73 fL
  WCC                             8.3 × 10⁹/L
  Plt                             515 × 10⁹/L
  Ferritin                        150 μmol/L
  Serum iron                      4 μmol/L
  Iron-binding saturation         8%
  Total iron binding capacity     110 μmol/L
  Blood film                      microcytic, hypochromic
                                  erythrocytes, target and
                                  pencil cells present
```

What is the most appropriate means of treatment for her anaemia?

A. Blood transfusion

B. Dietary advice

C. Intravenous iron dextran

D. Intravenous iron sucrose

E. Oral ferrous sulphate

80. **A 68-year-old man presented with a large volume of haematemesis from a suspected gastric ulcer. His past medical history included ischaemic heart disease with a myocardial infarction eight years previously, and a metallic mitral valve replacement. He took aspirin, simvastatin, ramipril, bisoprolol, and warfarin.**

```
Investigations:
  Hb                79 g/L
  MCV               78.0 fL
  WCC               9.1 × 10⁹/L
  Plt               510 × 10⁹/L
  Urea              14.8 mmol/L
  Creatinine        71 μmol/L
  Bilirubin         8 μmol/L
  ALT               35 IU/L
  ALP               42 IU/L
  Albumin           41 g/dL
  APTT              31s
  PTT               62s
  INR               5.2
  Fibrinogen        2.7 g/L
```

How should his coagulopathy be managed?

A. Cryoprecipitate

B. Fresh frozen plasma

C. Omit warfarin only

D. Prothrombin complex concentrate

E. Vitamin K

81. **An 18-year-old man presented with a three-day history of fever, vomiting, bloody diarrhoea, and abdominal cramp after returning from a holiday in India. A stool sample was sent for culture, which identified Gram negative rods.**

Which would be the most appropriate antimicrobial agent to initiate?

A. Azithromycin
B. Ciprofloxacin
C. Co-amoxiclav
D. Metronidazole
E. Tinidazole

82. **A 53-year-old woman with was referred with dysphagia to both solids and liquids, along with regurgitation of undigested food. Her symptoms were non-progressive. Physical examination revealed evidence of significant weight-loss but was otherwise unremarkable. Chest X-ray demonstrated mediastinal widening with an air-fluid level in the oesophagus. Oesophago-gastroduodenoscopy (OGD) did not demonstrate a stricture.**

Which investigation is most appropriate to establish the diagnosis?

A. Anti-centromere antibodies
B. Barium swallow
C. Computed tomography of the thorax
D. Oesophageal impedance monitoring
E. Oesophageal manometry

83. **A 78-year-old lady presented with a six-month history of severe diffuse abdominal pain, which was constant and colicky in nature. She also reported pain 15–20 minutes after eating which could last for over an hour. On further questioning, she mentioned she had early satiety, weight loss, and an altered bowel habit. On examination, the abdomen was mildly tender on palpation, but there was no rebound tenderness or guarding. Her past medical history included a recent myocardial infarction and poorly controlled type II diabetes. She was a lifelong smoker. There was no history of recent travel.**

What is the most useful next investigation?

A. Colonoscopy
B. CT abdomen
C. CT angiography
D. Faecal elastase
E. Ultrasound abdomen

84. **A 45-year-old woman was referred for investigation of painless jaundice and weight loss.**

Investigations:

Hb	104 g/L
MCV	99.0 fL
WCC	9.3 × 10^9/L
Plt	445 × 10^9/L
Urea	5.2 mmol/L
Creatinine	76 µmol/L
Na	141 mmol/L
K	4.3 mmol/L
Bilirubin	76 µmol/L
ALT	99 IU/L
ALP	359 IU/L
GGT	556 IU/L
Albumin	29 g/dL
INR	1.25
Amylase	710 IU/L
ESR	51 mm/hr
IgA	2.2 g/L (0.8–3 g/L)
IgG	32.6 g/L (6.0–13.0 g/L)
IgM	1.2 g/L (0.4–2.5 g/L)
ANA	positive at 1:40
ANCA	negative

Autoantibodies:

Anti-mitochondrial	negative
Anti-smooth muscle	negative
Anti-LKM-1	negative
CT abdomen	there is diffuse pancreatic enhancement and enlargement. The biliary tree appears normal. There is a large retroperitoneal inflammatory mass, and significant para-aortic adenopathy.

What is the most likely diagnosis?

A. Adenocarcinoma of the pancreas
B. Autoimmune hepatitis
C. Autoimmune pancreatitis
D. Primary biliary cirrhosis
E. Primary sclerosing cholangitis

85. **A 34-year-old man presented with abdominal pain and vomiting. He had a history of ileocolonic Crohn's disease and HIV infection. His medications included prednisolone, mesalazine, tenofovir, emtricitabine, ritonavir, ferrous sulphate, and folic acid. His investigations are as follows.**

```
Investigations:
  Hb                    99 g/L
  MCV                   80.5 fL
  WCC                   15.2 × 10⁹/L
  Plt                   550 × 10⁹/L
  Urea                  7.3 mmol/L
  Creatinine            90 µmol/L
  Na                    139 mmol/L
  K                     4.6 mmol/L
  Calcium               2.47 mmol/L
  CRP                   85 mg/L
  Bilirubin             9 µmol/L
  ALT                   38 IU/L
  ALP                   67 IU/L
  Albumin               28 g/dL
  INR                   0.98
  Amylase               1700 IU/L
  CD4 count             890 cells/mm³ (>500 cells/mm³)
  HIV viral load        undetectable
```

Which drug is likely to be responsible for the patient's symptoms?

A. Emtricitabine

B. Ferrous sulphate

C. Mesalazine

D. Prednisolone

E. Ritonavir

86. **A 55-year-old Cantonese woman visiting the UK presented with jaundice. She was a non-smoker and drank around 8–10 units of alcohol per week. On examination she was afebrile, icteric, and had mild epigastric tenderness with guarding but no rebound.**

```
Investigations:
    Hb                              129 g/L
    WCC                             11.1 × 10⁹/L
    Neutrophils                     8.2 × 10⁹/L
    Lymphocytes                     1.5 × 10⁹/L
    Eosinophils                     0.8 × 10⁹/L
    Plt                             355 × 10⁹/L
    Urea                            4.5 mmol/L
    Creatinine                      65 μmol/L
    Na                              141 mmol/L
    K                               4.7 mmol/L
    Bilirubin                       112 μmol/L
    ALT                             31 IU/L
    ALP                             320 IU/L
    INR                             1.05
    Amylase                         350 IU/L
    IgA                             1.7 g/L (0.8–3.0 g/L)
    IgG                             10.2 g/L (6.0–13.0 g/L)
    IgM                             1.8 g/L (0.4–2.5 g/L)
    Cholesterol                     5.1 mmol/L
    Triglycerides (non-fasting)     4.7 mmol/L
    LDL                             3.2 mmol/L
    Plain AXR                       normal
    US abdomen                      dilatated common bile duct to
                                    1.1 cm, with a normal gall
                                    bladder
```

What is the most likely diagnosis?

A. Ascariasis
B. Autoimmune pancreatitis
C. Gallstones
D. Primary sclerosing cholangitis
E. Strongyloides

87. A 17-year-old male was referred for investigation of persistent diarrhoea. He had symptoms for over a year. He had loose stools but reported no blood or mucus. He found that they were sometimes difficult to flush. He had also experienced intermittent bouts of abdominal pain. He had a past medical history of cystic fibrosis. On examination, he was thin and had clubbing of his fingers with coarse crackles bilaterally on auscultation of the chest. His abdomen was soft and non-tender, with no palpable masses or organomegaly.

```
Investigations:
   Hb                      98 g/L
   MCV                     98.8 fL
   WCC                     6.3 × 10⁹/L
   Plt                     380 × 10⁹/L
   Urea                    3.6 mmol/L
   Creatinine              48 µmol/L
   Na                      139 mmol/L
   K                       3.8 mmol/L
   Corrected calcium       2.10 mmol/L
   Phosphate               0.58 mmol/L
   CRP                     10 mg/L
   Bilirubin               9 µmol/L
   ALT                     32 IU/L
   ALP                     39 IU/L
   Albumin                 39 g/dL
   INR                     1.32
```

What is the most appropriate test to confirm the cause of his current symptoms?

A. Colonoscopy

B. Faecal elastase-1

C. Fasting gut hormone profile

D. SeHCAT scan

E. Xylose breath test

88. **A 37-year-old man presented with severe left hypochondrial pain radiating to his back, associated with nausea and vomiting. He had a past medical history of type II diabetes mellitus. He did not smoke and drank five units of alcohol each week. On examination, he was in marked discomfort, with diffuse abdominal tenderness and guarding.**

```
Investigations:
  Hb                       148 g/L
  WCC                      15.1 × 10⁹/L
  Plt                      358 × 10⁹/L
  Creatinine               unable to measure as sample was lipaemic
  Amylase                  unable to measure as sample was lipaemic
Urine dipstick analysis:
  Glucose                  +++
  Ketones                  ++
  Blood                    not detected
  Protein                  not detected
  Leucocytes               not detected
  Nitrites                 not detected
Venous blood gas:
  pH                       7.39
  Na                       118 mmol/L
  K                        4.9 mmol/L
  Glucose                  27 mmol/L
  Plain AXR                sentinel loop of bowel in the left upper
                           quadrant
```

What is the most appropriate test to confirm the cause of his current symptoms?

A. Abdominal ultrasound

B. Plasma ketones

C. Serum lipase

D. Serum troponin

E. Urinary amylase

89. **A 36-year-old woman was investigated for fatigue following a trip to the far-east three months previously. Routine blood tests were performed and abnormal liver function tests were noted.**

```
Investigations:
  Bilirubin                     28 µmol/L
  ALT                           72 IU/L
  ALP                           55 IU/L
Given the derangement, serology for hepatotropic viruses
  was sent.
  Hepatitis A IgM               negative
  Hepatitis A IgG               negative
  HBsAg                         not detected
  Anti-HBs IgG                  positive
  Anti-HBc IgG                  positive
  HBeAg                         negative
  Anti-HBe IgG                  positive
  Anti-Hepatitis C IgG          negative
```

Which of the following statements is correct?

A. Liver biopsy would be useful to stage and grade the disease

B. The patient has acute hepatitis B infection

C. The patient has resolved hepatitis B infection

D. The patient is highly infective

E. The results demonstrate previous vaccination against hepatitis B

90. **A 29-year-old woman was admitted to hospital with jaundice. She was 36 weeks pregnant with her first pregnancy and had previously been well. She had no personal or family history of liver disease. The pregnancy had been otherwise uncomplicated, apart from mild early morning sickness during the first trimester. Over the preceding two weeks, she had experienced increasing headache and fatigue, and now had a recurrence of nausea, vomiting, and abdominal discomfort. She noted that her urine had become darker and her stools paler. Her BP was elevated at 180/105 mmHg.**

```
Investigations:
   Hb                      109 g/L
   WCC                     12.2 × 10⁹/L
   Plt                     80 × 10⁹/L
   Urea                    8.7 mmol/L
   Creatinine              190 µmol/L
   Na                      141 mmol/L
   K                       3.4 mmol/L
   Bilirubin               140 µmol/L
   ALT                     600 IU/L
   ALP                     350 IU/L
   Albumin                 29 g/dL
   INR                     1.7
   Urate                   550 µmol/L
   Glucose                 3.5 mmol/L
   Blood film              neutrophilia, thrombocytopaenia,
                           normoblasts, target cells and giant
                           platelets present.
   Abdominal ultrasound    the echotexture of the liver is
                           bright, moderate ascites is present
   Urinalysis              protein ++
```

What is the most likely diagnosis?

A. Acute fatty liver of pregnancy

B. Budd-Chiari syndrome

C. HELLP syndrome

D. Hyperemesis gravidarum

E. Obstetric cholestasis

91. **A 37-year-old male presented with right hypochondrial pain, nausea, and vomiting. He had no past medical history. He had travelled to Spain and the USA in the previous year and worked as a farmer. On examination he was apyrexial, looked systemically well but was noted to have hepatomegaly.**

```
Investigations:
  Hb                 141 g/L
  WCC                6.6 × 10⁹/L
  Neutrophils        4.8 × 10⁹/L
  Eosinophils        0.3 × 10⁹/L
  Plt                370 × 10⁹/L
  Bilirubin          12 μmol/L
  ALT                41 IU/L
  ALP                11 IU/L
  Albumin            34 g/dL
  INR                1.05
  CRP                12 mg/L
  HIV serology       negative for HIV-1 and HIV-2
Amoebic serology:
  IFAT               positive
  CAP                negative
  CT liver           large, well-defined hypodense cyst involving
                     the postero-superior segment of the right
                     lobe. Three smaller 'daughter' cystic
                     lesions seen in both hepatic lobes.
```

What is the most appropriate course of treatment?

A. Biopsy and trans-arterial chemoembolization

B. Cefuroxime and metronidazole

C. Cyst aspiration and empirical TB treatment

D. Cyst aspiration and tinidazole

E. Cystectomy and albendazole

92. **A 68-year-old woman was admitted for investigation of increasing fatigue and jaundice. She had a past medical history of hypothyroidism treated with replacement levothyroxine. Physical examination revealed widespread excoriations and hepatosplenomegaly.**

```
Investigations:
   Hb                        100 g/L
   MCV                       114 fL
   Bilirubin                 20 µmol/L
   ALT                       65 IU/L
   ALP                       320 IU/L
   Albumin                   41 g/dL
   INR                       1.1
   Red cell folate           310 µg/L
   Vitamin B₁₂               60 ng/L
   IgA                       6.4 g/L (0.8-3.0)
   IgG                       8.4 g/L (6.0-13.0)
   IgM                       1.9 g/L (0.4-2.5)
```

Which of the following is most likely to be detected in the patient's serum?

A. Anti-centromere antibody

B. Anti-mitochondrial antibody

C. Anti-neutrophil cytoplasmic antibody (ANCA)

D. Anti-nuclear antibody (ANA)

E. Anti-smooth muscle antibody

93. **A 53-year-old woman presented with increased lethargy, dyspnoea, and confusion. She reported a chronic cough, with intermittent respiratory tract infections. She smoked five cigarettes per day and had a ten pack-year history. On examination, she had peripheral cyanosis, palmar erythema, and multiple spider naevi. Her chest was hyperexpanded and hyper-resonant with diffuse wheeze. Hepatosplenomegaly was also noted.**

```
Investigations:
  Hb                        172 g/L
  Bilirubin                 13 µmol/L
  ALT                       38 IU/L
  ALP                       261 IU/L
  INR                       1.2
Arterial blood gases:
  pH                        7.25
  P_aO_2                    6.8 kPa
  P_aCO_2                   7.2 kPa
  HCO_3                     30 mmol/L
She was treated with nebulizers, steroids, and antibiotics,
  with which she clinically improved. Spirometry was performed
  when she was back to baseline, which showed:
  FEV_1                     0.8 L (predicted 2.3L)
  FVC                       2.1 L (predicted 3.1L)
  FEV_1/FVC                 38%
  A liver biopsy was performed after imaging to investigate
    the cause of her hepatosplenomegaly. This showed numerous
    PAS-positive globules within hepatocytes, alongside
    periportal fibrosis and early cirrhosis.
```

Which of the following investigations is most likely to be abnormal?

A. *PiZZ* genotype

B. Serum α-galactosidase activity

C. Serum caeruloplasmin

D. Serum ferritin

E. Urinary copper

94. **A 45-year-old Indian female was investigated for weight loss. She denied any gastrointestinal or respiratory symptoms. She had never smoked. Her past medical history included previous miscarriages and vertebral fractures. There was no family history of gastrointestinal disease or malignancy.**

```
Investigations:
  Hb                       107 g/L
  WCC                      8.3 × 10⁹/L
  Plt                      149 × 10⁹/L
  MCV                      95.0 fl
  Corrected calcium        2.21 mmol/L
  AST                      25 iU/L
  ALT                      35 iU/L
  GGT                      40 iU/L
  ALP                      234 iU/L
  Bilirubin                13 µmol/L
  Albumin                  35 g/L
  Vitamin B₁₂              14 ng/L
  Ferritin                 3 µg/L
  Serum TTG                6 U/mL
  Serum IgA                0.2 g/L (0.8–3.0 g/L)
  Serum IgG                20.5 g/L (6.0–13.0 g/L)
  Serum IgM                1.63 g/L (0.4–2.5 g/L)
```

What is the most appropriate next investigation?

A. Colonoscopy

B. CT abdomen

C. Isotope bone scan

D. OGD and duodenal biopsy

E. Tuberculin skin test

95. **A 26-year-old pregnant lady was found to have positive serology for hepatitis B during antenatal screening. She was 28 weeks into her first pregnancy and was asymptomatic.**

```
Her liver enzymes and hepatitis B serology were as follows:
  Hepatitis B sAg          positive
  Hepatitis B eAg          positive
  Hepatitis B (DNA)        4.2 ×10⁶ copies/mL
  AST                      30 IU/ml
  ALT                      42 IU/ml
```

What treatment should be given to her and/or her newborn?

A. Hepatitis B immune globulin and vaccination to the newborn

B. Hepatitis B vaccination to the newborn

C. Lamivudine monotherapy to the mother

D. Lamivudine to the mother and the newborn at delivery

E. Lamivudine to the mother and vaccination to the newborn

96. **A 54-year-old man with NASH cirrhosis was admitted with haematemesis and melaena. At upper GI endoscopy (OGD), he was found to have oesophageal varices with evidence of recent bleeding, and was treated with endoscopic variceal ligation (EVL) as well as intravenous terlipressin and antibiotics. After 72 hours of observation, he was discharged home.**

Which of the following is the most appropriate treatment strategy following discharge?

A. Propanolol 40 mg bd

B. Propanolol 40 mg bd and omeprazole 40 mg od

C. Propanolol 40 mg bd and repeat OGD+/−EVL at two weeks following discharge

D. Repeat OGD+/−EVL at two weeks following discharge

E. Trans-jugular intrahepatic porto-systemic shunt (TIPSS) work-up

97. **A 55-year-old man presented with a four-month history of right upper quadrant pain. There was no history of nausea, vomiting, or steatorrhoea. His weight had been stable. His past medical history included osteoarthritis of the knees, type II diabetes, and hypertension, for which he took gliclazide and lisinopril. He also had a history of impotence, which has been attributed to past use of atenolol and thiazide which had been discontinued. He had been to Thailand six months previously, where he stayed for two weeks on a business trip. He consumed approximately 14 units of alcohol per week.**

On examination his BMI was 33. He was not jaundiced and there were no peripheral stigmata of chronic liver disease. There were no palpable lymph nodes. On examination of the abdomen, the liver edge was smooth, tender and palpable 5 cm below the costal margin. There was no palpable spleen. The flanks were dull to percussion, with no evidence of shift.

```
Investigations:
  Hb                     160 g/L
  WCC                    5 × 10⁹/L
  Platelets              175 × 10⁹/L
  Sodium                 136 mmol/L
  Potassium              4.5 mmol/L
  Urea                   5 mmol/L
  Creatinine             120 µmol/L
  AST                    65 iU/L
  ALT                    78 iU/L
  ALP                    150 iU/L
  Bilirubin              13 µmol/L
  Albumin                35 g/L
  Glucose                14 mmol/L
  HbA1c                  86 mmol/mol (20-42 mmol/mol)
  Ferritin               380 µg/L
  Total cholesterol      6.5 mmol/L
  Triglycerides          6.1 mmol/L
  Serum IgA              3.8 g/L (0.8-3.0 g/L)
  Serum IgG              19.2 g/L (6.0-13.0 g/L)
  Serum IgM              2.0 g/L (0.4-2.5 g/L)
  Hep B sAg              negative
  HCV IgG                negative
  ANA                    negative
  ANCA                   negative
  Anti-mitochondrial     negative
  Anti-smooth muscle     negative
  Anti-LKM-1             negative
```

What is the most likely diagnosis?

A. Alcoholic hepatitis

B. Auto-immune hepatitis

C. Haemochromatosis

D. Non-alcoholic steatohepatitis

E. Primary biliary cirrhosis

74. D) Microscopic colitis

This question tests the candidate's knowledge of the different subtypes of inflammatory bowel disease. Any of the conditions listed may present with non-bloody diarrhoea, although the presence of blood and mucus is more likely in colitis associated with Behçet's disease, Crohn's disease, and ulcerative colitis. NSAIDs, such as naproxen, can exacerbate any form of inflammatory colitis, but are also recognized to predispose to microscopic colitis.

Macroscopic inflammation is usually visible at the time of endoscopy in Behçet's disease, Crohn's disease (discrete skip lesions, aphthous ulceration, and a cobblestone appearance to the mucosa), and ulcerative colitis (continuous inflammation extending proximally from the rectum, with pseudo-polyp formation). Histologically, Behçet's is characterized by vasculitis; Crohn's disease by transmural inflammation, with non-caseating granulomas in at least 50%; and ulcerative colitis by inflammation confined to the mucosa, crypt distortion, and goblet cell depletion.

An absence of macroscopic inflammation would be compatible with either irritable bowel syndrome or microscopic colitis. The presence of inflammatory cells on biopsy excludes the former. The observation of lymphocytic inflammation with a collagen band >10 μm suggests a diagnosis of collagenous colitis, a subtype of microscopic colitis.

Tutorial

The term microscopic colitis encompasses two disease entities: collagenous colitis and lymphocytic colitis. Both present with watery diarrhoea, macroscopically normal mucosa on colonoscopy, but inflammatory infiltrates on histology. They are sometimes associated with cramping abdominal pain and weight loss. Stool samples are positive for leukocytes in 50%, but negative for blood.

Microscopic colitis has a prevalence of 1 in 1000. It is classically said to affect women more frequently than men (3–9:1 ratio). The peak age of onset is 50–70 years, although it can occur at any age. Associations include autoimmune disease (particularly coeliac disease, but also thyroiditis, rheumatoid arthritis, and type I diabetes mellitus) and certain medications (particularly NSAIDs, but also aspirin, proton pump inhibitors, and SSRIs).

Biopsies demonstrate increased CD8 T lymphocytes, plasma cells, and macrophages within the mucosa. In collagenous colitis there is also a thickened subepithelial band of collagen I and III. This appears to result from reduced collagenase activity rather than exaggerated deposition. It likely represents a secondary phenomenon, as opposed to directly causing diarrhoea, as disease severity correlates more with the intensity of the inflammation than with the extent of collagen formation. Several studies demonstrate that patients with microscopic colitis exhibit impaired absorption and increased secretion of electrolytes, and this is thought more relevant to symptom generation.

The treatment of choice is budesonide. Any predisposing drugs should be discontinued if possible. There is some evidence to support use of mesalazine for mild active disease or long-term maintenance of disease remission. Severe recalcitrant cases may require azathioprine or methotrexate. Anti-diarrhoeal agents such as loperamide help ameliorate symptoms.

Approximately 50% of patients enter complete remission, but in the remainder the course is chronic with frequent relapses.

Further Reading

Chetty R, Govender D (2012). Lymphocytic and collagenous colitis: an overview of so-called microscopic colitis. *Nature Reviews Gastroenterology and Hepatology* 21(4): 209–218.

Pardi D, Kelly C (2011). Microscopic colitis. *Gastroenterology* 140: 1155–1165.

Stewart M, Seow C, Storr M (2011). Prednisolone and budesonide for short- and long-term treatment of microscopic colitis: systematic review and meta-analysis. *Clinical Gastroenterology and Hepatology* 9: 881–890.

75. D) Enteroscopy with jejunal biopsy

This question tests the candidate's knowledge of the causes of hypoalbuminaemia. The patient presents with a combination of gastrointestinal symptoms, and generalized oedema (the clinical examination highlighting signs consistent with bilateral pleural effusions and ascites, as well as the elevated JVP and peripheral oedema). The latter relates to his low plasma oncotic pressure, caused by severe hypoalbuminaemia.

Hypoalbuminaemia can result from insufficient dietary protein intake, impaired hepatic synthesis, or excess loss from the body (either in the urine as part of a nephrotic syndrome, or from the gastrointestinal tract due to a protein-losing enteropathy). Of note, the renal function (when accounting for probable loss of muscle mass) and urine dipstick are normal, as are the bilirubin and serum aminotransferases. The calcium and phosphate are low (a picture consistent with vitamin D insufficiency), and the elevated INR may indicate vitamin K deficiency. Together, they imply potential malabsorption of fat-soluble vitamins. Given the patient's relatively normal colonoscopy, it is important to realize that their symptoms are not due to ulcerative colitis and that they have a protein-losing enteropathy.

The most likely diagnosis is intestinal lymphangiectasia which is best diagnosed by enteroscopy and jejunal biopsy. This investigation may also allow further tissue sample for histological assessment of other intestinal pathologies that the OGD and colonoscopy have otherwise missed (e.g. intestinal TB, Whipple's disease, Crohn's disease, lymphoma).

A duodenal biopsy with PAS staining is the test for Whipple's disease, which can cause a protein-losing enteropathy, but this is very rare (incidence of 1 in 1,000,000) and often presents with other non-GI symptoms. In any case, PAS staining could also be done on the jejunal biopsy obtained during enteroscopy. The patient does have malabsorption of fats which can sometimes be due to cholestasis secondary to liver disease. Many candidates will think first of the connection of ulcerative colitis and primary sclerosing cholangitis. However, this patient does not have any evidence of liver dysfunction or cholestasis. Furthermore, a biopsy without imaging of the liver and biliary tract would not be done in clinical practice.

Coeliac disease is probably the commonest cause of protein-losing enteropathy. However, anti-TTG (tissue transglutaminase) is a more sensitive antibody than anti-gliadin, and thus the latter would not add anything in this case. The patient does have a low IgA, but this is a global picture due to their protein-losing enteropathy, which goes against a false negative antibody test result. Given normal macroscopic morphology of the duodenum and negative anti-TTG, coeliac disease is very unlikely. A trial of a gluten-free diet is only going to delay further investigation in this patient. Exclusion of nephrotic syndrome would normally be indicated here but given the negative urine dipstick there is likely to be very little proteinuria. More commonly, nephrologists now use protein:creatinine ratios instead of, as opposed to in conjunction with, 24-hour urine collection test as it is a lot easier to arrange.

Tutorial

Protein-losing enteropathies are rare syndromes characterized by loss of serum proteins into the gastrointestinal tract. In healthy individuals, approximately 1–2% of serum protein is lost through the enteric system; this can rise to up to 60% in protein-losing enteropathy. Blood tests show profound hypoalbuminaemia, and there may be deficiencies of fat-soluble vitamins. Complications secondary to decreased plasma oncotic pressure include peripheral oedema, ascites, and pleural and pericardial effusions. Causes of protein-losing enteropathy include:

- Inflammatory bowel disease
- Coeliac disease
- Tropical sprue
- NSAID enteropathy
- Whipple's disease
- Ménétrier's disease
- Intestinal lymphoma
- Intestinal sarcoidosis
- Amyloidosis
- Mesenteric vein thrombosis
- Intestinal lymphangiectasia
- Sclerosing mesenteritis
- Graft-versus-host disease
- Right heart failure (through lymphatic obstruction related to increased central venous pressure)
- Fontan procedures (for a single cardiac ventricle)

The initial step in evaluation is to exclude other aetiologies of hypoproteinaemia, including malnutrition, chronic liver disease, and nephrotic syndrome. Historically, the next step would involve confirming a protein-losing enteropathy by comparing blood and 24-hour stool samples for quantities of α1-antitrypsin, but due to the technically difficult nature of this test as well poor sensitivity it is no longer done. Nuclear scintigraphy using ^{99m}Tc-labelled albumin may also be used to quantify enteric protein excretion, but this again does not help with identifying the cause of the enteropathy. Further gastrointestinal imaging looking for obstruction and tissue sampling now remain the mainstay of diagnosis and are likely to give the highest diagnostic yield.

There is no specific therapy for protein-losing enteropathy. Treatment is directed at the underlying cause, with careful monitoring of nutrition and correction of micronutrient deficiencies. A high protein diet is recommended, and there is anecdotal evidence to suggest that octreotide can decrease protein exudation from the bowel. Long-term use of intravenous albumin infusions is generally unrewarding. Surgery may be required for refractory cases.

Further Reading

Umar S, DiBaise J (2010). Protein-losing enteropathy: case illustrations and clinical review. *American Journal of Gastroenterology* 105: 43–49.

76. E) Trial of bile acid sequestrant

This question tests the candidate's knowledge of some of the rarer causes of chronic diarrhoea. In this patient, although the development of loose stools could indicate recurrence of Crohn's disease, this is essentially excluded by the normal blood tests, and endoscopic and histological findings. The description is consistent with intermittent fat malabsorption and steatorrhoea. The most likely cause in this patient is bile acid malabsorption, often caused by disruption of the terminal ileum and consequently of bile acid enterohepatic recirculation. In this case, the patient has two predisposing factors: ileocaecal Crohn's disease and surgical removal of the terminal ileum by the preceding right hemicolectomy. The diagnosis may be confirmed by selenium homocholic acid taurine (SeHCAT) study (see tutorial), but in practice NICE guidelines suggest empirical treatment should be tried first as the scan is not cost effective.

Meckel's diverticula arise from a persistent vitelline duct. They are found in 2% of the population and are usually asymptomatic. When they do present, the most common manifestations are painless lower gastrointestinal bleeding in children, and obstruction in adults, rather than diarrhoea. Diverticulitis and emergent carcinoma are rare complications. Diagnosis may be achieved using scintigraphy with technetium pertechnetate (the 'Meckel's scan'), a tracer which is taken up by heterotopic gastric mucosa.

Gastrinomas cause chronic diarrhoea in up to 70% of patients, sometimes with associated steatorrhoea. They are associated with fasting serum gastrin concentration of >1000 pg/ml. A key feature, present in >75% of patients, is epigastric pain related to peptic ulceration, driven by hypergastrinaemia as part of the Zollinger-Ellison syndrome. VIPomas are characterized by profound watery diarrhoea, with secondary dehydration, hypokalaemia, and hypochloraemia. Octreotide scans are useful in the diagnosis and monitoring of most neuroendocrine tumours, most commonly carcinoids producing vasoactive hormones such as serotonin and histamine. Most patients are asymptomatic, although the carcinoid syndrome can include diarrhoea and abdominal cramps. These are, however, usually also associated with cutaneous flushing and wheeze.

Tutorial

Bile acids are synthesized in the liver, then excreted into the hepatic duct in water-soluble form conjugated to cholic or chenodeoxycholic acid. Intraluminal bacteria then deconjugate these into insoluble deoxycholic and lithocholic acids. This permits their enterohepatic recirculation, with uptake of >95% in the terminal ileum, and return to the liver via the portal vein. This process can be interrupted by exclusion of the terminal ileum following its surgical removal, due to inflammatory diseases (such as Crohn's disease or radiation enteritis) or, rarely, due to congenital deficiencies in the sodium-bile acid co-transporter.

Patients with bile acid malabsorption present with bloating, abdominal discomfort, diarrhoea (due to increased delivery of deconjugated bile acids to the colon, which inhibit carbohydrate transporters, reduce intraluminal pH, and directly damage enterocytes), steatorrhoea (fat malabsorption occurs secondary to reduced bile acids in the small bowel for solubilization of lipids and micelle formation), gallstones, and renal oxalate stones. The prevalence of undiagnosed bile acid malabsorption may be as high as 30% in patients meeting criteria for diarrhoea-predominant irritable bowel syndrome.

The most common diagnostic test employed is the SeHCAT study. Selenium-labelled bile acid is administered orally and total body retention measured using a γ-camera after seven days. A retention value <10% is abnormal and indicative of malabsorption. Novel techniques involve measuring levels of the bile acid precursor 7α-hydroxy-4-cholesten-3-one (C4), which has a high negative predictive value if normal. Its positive predictive value is, however, only 74%, limiting this test's utility to exclusion of the disorder.

Treatment is with bile acid sequestrants, such as cholestyramine or colesevelam. Patients should maintain adequate oral fluid intake to minimize risk of urinary oxalate calculi.

Further Reading

Borghede M, Schlütter J, Agnholt J, et al. (2011). Bile acid malabsorption investigated by selenium-75-homocholic acid taurine ((75) SeHCAT) scans: causes and treatment responses to cholestyramine in 298 patients with chronic watery diarrhoea. *European Journal of Internal Medicine* 22: e137–140.

Gracie D, Kane J, Mumtaz S, et al. (2012). Prevalence of, and predictors of, bile acid malabsorption in outpatients with chronic diarrhea. *Neurogastroenterology and Motility* 24: 983–e538.

77. B) Cytomegalovirus infection

This question tests the candidate's knowledge of the causes of diarrhoea in severely immunocompromised patients. The patient presents with advanced HIV disease (evidenced by the profound reduction in circulating CD4 T lymphocytes) and clinical findings of severe colitis. All the conditions listed as possible answers typically arise in the context of severe immunocompromise. In HIV-infected individuals, they are rare when the CD4 count exceeds 200/mm^3. The presence of inclusion bodies is highly suggestive of cytomegalovirus (CMV) infection, which can be confirmed by immunohistochemical analysis.

Tutorial

Cytomegalovirus is a herpes virus, for which there is serological evidence of acquisition in 60–100% of individuals in adult populations. Primary infection is typically mild, and either asymptomatic or presents as an undifferentiated viral syndrome or mononucleosis-like illness. Although this is self-limiting, CMV remains latent within mononuclear cells, with potential to reactivate in later life. CMV disease occurs in up to 10% of patients with AIDS. In addition to reactivation of latent infection, the virus can also be sexually transmitted. Ileocolitis presents with pain, diarrhoea, and bleeding. CMV is also recognized to exacerbate inflammatory bowel disease in HIV-uninfected patients.

Diagnosis is achieved by demonstrating mucosal ulceration with characteristic intracytoplasmic and intranuclear inclusion bodies on biopsy. This can be supported by detection of CMV antigen by immunohistochemistry or PCR. The latter two are important, as the sensitivity of routine histological staining is only 27–63%. Viral cultures require over two weeks' incubation, and are prone to contamination. Treatment is with intravenous ganciclovir, or oral valganciclovir. Foscarnet is used for resistant disease.

The differential diagnosis of diarrhoea in HIV-infected individuals is broad, and includes:

- Protozoa: *Cryptosporidium* is a protozoal infection acquired from ingesting contaminated water. Individuals are most susceptible with CD4 counts <50/mm^3. It predominantly infects the small bowel, and presents with high-volume non-bloody diarrhoea, nausea, vomiting, and abdominal cramps. The diagnosis is confirmed on stool microscopy using a modified acid-fast stain or immunofluorescence. Treatment is primarily supportive, until anti-retrovirals re-establish immune competence. Other protozoa that may present in a similar fashion are *Microsporidia* (diagnosed by electron microscopy of stool, or Giemsa or modified trichrome stain of mucosal biopsies), and *Cyclospora* and *Isospora belli* (both diagnosed on stool microscopy for oocysts, or on PCR).

- Tuberculosis: HIV significantly increases the risk of latent *Mycobacterium tuberculosis* reactivation. This can present at any stage of HIV disease, although it is more common as immunodeficiency progresses. It most frequently affects the ileocaecal region, and diagnosis usually requires colonoscopy or laparoscopy, as immunocompromise reduces the sensitivity of tuberculin skin testing and interferon-γ release assays.

- Non-tuberculous mycobacteria: *Mycobacterium avium-intracellulare* is now rare following the widespread use of anti-retrovirals, and typically only presents when the CD4 count falls under 100/mm^3. The most common manifestation is as a systemic disseminated illness with fever and severe anaemia. Gastrointestinal tract involvement occurs in up to 80%, with diarrhoea, malabsorption, and abdominal pain. Characteristic 1–3 mm white nodules are seen on endoscopy, with chronic inflammation on microscopy, typically without granuloma formation. The diagnosis is confirmed by demonstrating organism in tissue samples, peripheral blood cultures, or bone marrow; stool culture is not helpful as it does not differentiate colonization from tissue invasion.

- Lymphogranuloma venereum: chlamydial infection, causing a proctocolitis. It should be considered in any HIV-infected homosexual man presenting with acute bloody diarrhoea. Diagnosis is made by PCR of viral swabs, and treatment is with doxycycline. Herpes simplex virus and gonorrhoea may also cause severe relapsing proctocolitis; characteristic vesicles are seen on endoscopy with the former.

- Neoplasia: causes of diarrhoea in HIV-infected individuals include Kaposi's sarcoma and lymphoma. Kaposi's sarcoma is more common in the proximal intestine than the large bowel, and typically presents with haemorrhage. Oral involvement predicts endoluminal tumours elsewhere. It is diagnosed endoscopically, where appearances can be varied but are most frequently violaceous nodules. Histologically, the tumour arises from cells of the lymphatic endothelium and contains characteristic spindle cells. The underlying cause is infection with human herpes virus-8.

- Non-infective: other causes of diarrhoea in HIV-infected individuals may arise even when the CD4 count is preserved. Diarrhoea as a side effect of anti-retroviral therapy is common, particularly with nelfinavir and ritonavir. Infections with *Salmonella, Shigella*, and *Campylobacter* are more common, although the incubation period is short (up to 72 hours), and rates of *C. difficile* are increasing. Giardiasis is frequently observed in men who have sex with men, as cycles of acquisition and reacquisition are established with oro-anal intercourse.

Further Reading

Mentec H, Leport C, Leport J, et al. (1994). Cytomegalovirus colitis in HIV-1-infected patients: a prospective research in 55 patients *AIDS* 8: 461–467.

Nelson M, Dockrell D, Edwards S, on behalf of the BHIVA Guidelines (2011). British HIV Association and British Infection Association guidelines for the treatment of opportunistic infection in HIV-seropositive individuals 2011. *HIV Medicine* 12(2): 1–140.

Sanchez T, Brooks J, Sullivan P, et al. (2005). Bacterial diarrhoea in persons with HIV infection, United States, 1992–2002. *Clinical Infectious Diseases* 41: 1621–1627.

78. C) A trial of tetracycline is indicated

This question tests the candidate's knowledge of the causes and investigation of vitamin B_{12} deficiency. The patient presents with macrocytic anaemia and sensory polyneuropathy in a glove-and-stocking distribution, which blood tests demonstrate are due to vitamin B_{12} deficiency. Given the history of previous GI surgery and omeprazole use, she is at high risk of small bowel overgrowth. Negative anti-intrinsic factor and anti-parietal cell antibodies make the diagnosis of pernicious anaemia unlikely. Given the lack of inflammatory response and a negative MR small bowel, Crohn's disease is also unlikely. A capsule endoscopy can be diagnostic for small bowel overgrowth. However, given that she has had a previous operation and is likely to have strictures, it would be unsafe to do this without first doing a 'patency test' to see if the capsule might get stuck. This involves swallowing a dummy pill made of chalk. If it is not passed, it can be seen radiographically (e.g. on CT scanning or an external radio scanner) to identify the site of the obstructed pill, likely to represent an adhesion or some other cause of blockage. The advantage is that the pill, which is made of lactulose and barium, will dissolve in the gut by 72 hours, thus will itself not cause obstruction.

A Schilling test which was previously done for B_{12} malabsorption is no longer routinely performed. This is not corrected by addition of exogenous intrinsic factor (excluding a diagnosis of pernicious anaemia), nor pancreatic enzyme supplementation with Creon®. A normal small-bowel follow through with this degree of vitamin B_{12} deficiency similarly makes the diagnosis of Crohn's disease unlikely.

A diagnostic, and potentially therapeutic, trial of antibiotic therapy with tetracycline is indicated to determine whether the cause is malabsorption secondary to small bowel bacterial overgrowth. Faecal elastase which hasn't been listed as an option would also be a prudent test to look for possible pancreatic insufficiency if empirical antibiotic treatment had failed.

Tutorial

Vitamin B$_{12}$ (cobalamin) is found in animal-derived dietary products. It is a co-factor for two enzymes: methionine synthase and L-methyl-malonyl-coenzyme A mutase. Deficient function of these enzymes leads to defective maturation of erythrocytes resulting in megaloblastic anaemia, and demyelination of peripheral nerves of the dorsal and lateral columns of the spinal cord. Patients may also develop glossitis. Laboratory assays for the direct measurement of vitamin B$_{12}$ are neither 100% sensitive or specific, and where there is clinical doubt, measurement of serum methylmalonic acid is helpful, being elevated in >98% of patients with clinical vitamin B$_{12}$ deficiency.

Vitamin B$_{12}$ absorption in the gastrointestinal tract requires two proteins: intrinsic factor (produced by gastric parietal cells) and R binder protein. Most vitamin B$_{12}$ initially binds to R binder in the stomach. The complex is subsequently cleaved by pancreatic trypsin, and free cobalamin then binds to intrinsic factor. The intrinsic factor-cobalamin complex binds to the cubilin receptor in the ileum, which mediates its endocytosis. Finally, vitamin B$_{12}$ is transported to tissues bound to transcobalamin II.

Vitamin B$_{12}$ deficiency can result from inadequate dietary intake, inadequate release of food-bound cobalamin, loss of active intrinsic factor, proximal small bowel disease, pancreatic disease, disease of the terminal ileum, or drug therapy. Causes include:

- Vegan diet
- Alcohol misuse
- Achlorhydria (may be secondary to proton pump inhibitor use)
- Autoimmune pernicious anaemia
- Gastrectomy
- Congenital lack of intrinsic factor
- Pancreatic exocrine insufficiency
- Small bowel bacterial overgrowth
- Crohn's disease
- Ileocaecal tuberculosis or lymphoma
- Terminal ileal resection
- R binder deficiency
- Metformin or colchicine use

The first-line investigation in non-vegan patients is to measure parietal cell and intrinsic factor auto-antibodies, to exclude pernicious anaemia which is B$_{12}$ deficiency due to absence of intrinsic factor. Previously, Schilling tests were performed, which measured absorption of radio-labelled cobalamin following ingestion by measuring urine concentrations. The test occurs in multiple stages, each occurring only if the previous was abnormal. It involves giving the patient nothing, giving intrinsic factor, giving antibiotics, and finally giving pancreatic extract. Whilst it has a high specificity, given its complexity and the availability of cheaper, quicker, and easier tests which look for the specific causes of B$_{12}$ deficiency, it is no longer offered in the majority of centres.

Small bowel bacterial overgrowth refers to an increase in the normally low bacterial colonization of the proximal gastrointestinal tract. It can cause vitamin malabsorption, malnutrition, and weight loss. Predisposing factors include reduced host defences (hypogammaglobulinaemia, immunodeficiency, old age, and hypochlorhydria) and delayed small bowel clearance (jejunal disease and autonomic neuropathy). Microbiological culture is the gold standard for diagnosis, with $>10^5$ colonies/ml identified on duodenal aspirate. Hydrogen breath test two hours after glucose or lactulose ingestion are less invasive. Treatment is with antimicrobial therapy with activity against aerobic and anaerobic bacteria; tetracycline is most frequently used, although co-amoxiclav, co-trimoxazole, or ciprofloxacin are alternatives. A single one-week course is often effective, but sometimes continuous rotating antibiotics are necessary. The efficacy of probiotics remains unproven.

Treatment of vitamin B_{12} deficiency itself is classically achieved using intramuscular hydroxycobalamin, 1 mg three times weekly for two weeks, then 1 mg every three months. High dose daily oral cobalamin is, however, equally effective. In the case of combined deficiency, vitamin B_{12} should be corrected prior to folate supplementation, to avoid precipitating subacute combined degeneration of the spinal cord.

Further Reading

Bures J, Cyrany J, Kohoutova D, et al. (2010). Small intestinal bacterial overgrowth syndrome. *World Journal of Gastroenterology* 16: 2978–2990.

Stabler S (2013). Vitamin B_{12} deficiency. *New England Journal of Medicine* 368: 149–160.

Toh B, van Driel I, Gleeson P (1997). Pernicious anemia. *New England Journal of Medicine* 337: 1441–1448.

79. C) Intravenous iron dextran

This question tests the candidate's knowledge of the methods of iron supplementation and correction of iron deficiency anaemia. The patient has iron deficiency anaemia secondary to diffuse small bowel Crohn's disease. The blood film demonstrates a microcytosis with hypochromasia, with target and pencil cells, indicative of severe disease. Ferritin is usually low in iron deficiency anaemia, reflecting depletion of body stores. In this case, however, it is elevated due to the presence of active inflammation, where it rises as an acute phase protein. Ferritin can also be raised in anaemias of chronic disease. Whilst this may well co-exist with iron deficiency in patients with Crohn's disease, this patient's main problem is iron deficiency as seen by the indices of reduced total serum iron and iron-binding saturations, and elevated total iron binding capacity. This is discussed further in the tutorial.

The standard approach to correction of iron deficiency anaemia is oral supplementation of iron. Where this has failed (either due to lack of efficacy or tolerance of oral iron preparations), or there is a likelihood of insufficient absorption of enteral iron (in this case due to extensive small bowel Crohn's disease), parenteral iron should be used. It is worth noting that there have been promising trials of a new oral supplement: ferric maltol which has been shown to be better tolerated and has an increased rise of haemoglobin in patients with inflammatory bowel disease compared with conventional oral iron supplements. It is expected to be recommended by NICE in the near future. Currently iron dextran is the choice of parenteral supplementation and has largely replaced iron sucrose in clinical practice as it is possible to infuse larger doses more quickly. Blood transfusion is reserved only for patients with haemodynamic compromise, ongoing high-volume bleeding, or severe symptoms.

Tutorial

The commonest causes of iron deficiency anaemia are menstrual and gastrointestinal blood losses (especially peptic ulceration, colonic neoplasia and, worldwide, hookworm infection). Approximately 4% of men and post-menopausal women, and 20% of pre-menopausal women, have iron deficiency. Normally, 1–2 mg of iron is absorbed each day, equivalent to 3–5 ml of whole blood. Consequently, persistent loss of >5 ml blood per day leads to deficiency.

Haematinics (iron studies, vitamin B$_{12}$, and folate) and ferritin should be measured in any patient found to be anaemic, or to have a red cell microcytosis. The MCV is typically 70–80 fL, in contrast to thalassaemia trait where it is often substantially lower. Interpretation of iron studies is highlighted in Table 4.1.

Table 4.1 Interpretation of iron studies. Note the iron indices in anaemia of chronic disease, which is frequently misdiagnosed as iron deficiency anaemia

Condition	Iron	TIBC	Iron binding saturation	Ferritin
Iron deficiency	↓	↑	↓	↓
Anaemia of chronic disease	↓	↓	↓	↔/↑
Haemolysis	↑	↔/↓	↑	↑
Sideroblastic anaemia	↔/↑	↔/↓	↑	↑

There are two principles in the treatment of iron deficiency: prevent ongoing losses and replace iron. In general, iron replacement should commence with an oral iron supplement (such as ferrous sulphate or ferrous gluconate), taken on an empty stomach. Concomitant antacids or milk should be avoided, whereas use of vitamin C increases absorption. Iron supplementation should be provided for six weeks to correct anaemia, and three months to replenish stores. An increase in haemoglobin of 2–4 g/dL after three weeks should be seen. Reasons for failing to achieve this include poor compliance, malabsorption or ongoing iron loss, co-existent anaemia of chronic disease, or erythropoietin deficiency secondary to chronic kidney disease. If treatment fails because the first oral supplement is not tolerated, a different preparation with lower elemental iron should be trialled.

Intravenous iron therapy should be considered if multiple oral treatments are not tolerated or effective; in inflammatory bowel disease (where extensive small bowel involvement can limit absorption, or oral therapy may precipitate a flare); and in dialysis patients. These formulations allow increments in haemoglobin of up to 5 g/dL, at a rate of 1 g/dL per week, after 1–3 doses depending on the preparation used.

Further Reading

Gomollón F, Gisbert J (2013). Intravenous iron in inflammatory bowel disease. *Current Opinion in Gastroenterology* 29: 201–207.

Richards T (2012). Anaemia in hospital practice. *British Journal of Hospital Medicine* (London) 73: 571–575.

Weiss G, Goodnough L (2005). Anemia of chronic disease. *New England Journal of Medicine* 352: 1011–1023.

80. D) Prothrombin complex concentrate

This question tests the candidate's knowledge of the correction of coagulopathy, including warfarin reversal. The patient has had a significant upper gastrointestinal haemorrhage, as evidenced by the volume of haematemesis, drop in haemoglobin, and disproportionate rise in urea. The clotting tests are consistent with over-anticoagulation with warfarin, which elevates the prothrombin time and INR, but does not affect the APTT or plasma fibrinogen. The normal liver function tests imply that impaired hepatic synthetic function is an unlikely cause of these results. Nonetheless, the indication for warfarin therapy is robust, as stroke risk with a metallic mitral valve is high (up to 6.5% per patient-year), and hence prolonged reversal is undesirable.

All the options provided would correct the INR, but at different rates. Omission of warfarin, whilst part of the overall management plan, would result in correction only after 2–3 days if used as the sole measure. Similarly, vitamin K would only begin working after approximately six hours, due to the time required to synthesize new clotting factors. Neither of these is appropriate for the severe and ongoing bleed described in the scenario.

Fresh frozen plasma refers to the non-cellular fraction of blood, frozen and preserved subsequent to blood donation. It contains all clotting factors, although lacks fibrinogen in high concentrations. It produces suboptimal warfarin reversal and should only be used if prothrombin complex concentrate is not available. Risks include potential for transmission of infection, anaphylactoid reactions, alloimmunization, and high-volume transfusion (10–15 ml/kg body weight).

Cryoprecipitate refers to the proteins that precipitate when fresh frozen plasma is slowly thawed, then refrozen within one hour. It contains fibrinogen, von Willebrand factor, and factors VIII and XIII. It is the only product that contains therapeutic amounts of fibrinogen replacement when the latter is depleted from plasma, and should therefore be reserved for patients with a consumptive coagulopathy and hypofibrinogenaemia.

Prothrombin complex concentrates are pooled plasma-derived products that contain the vitamin K-dependent clotting factors II, VII, IX, and X. They correct clotting factor deficiencies more rapidly and completely than fresh frozen plasma, and reduce the risks of infection, anaphylaxis, and fluid overload. They are the agents of choice for rapid warfarin reversal.

Tutorial

The need for, and rapidity and permanence of, reversal of warfarin depend on the clinical scenario and indication for its use. In ongoing significant gastrointestinal haemorrhage, anticoagulation should be reversed rapidly. The modality of choice for warfarin is prothrombin complex concentrate, used alongside intravenous vitamin K if a degree of longer lasting reduction in the INR is desirable. Fresh frozen plasma is inferior to prothrombin complex concentrate for this purpose but can be used if the latter is unavailable. Anticoagulation reversal for non-major bleeding should be achieved with intravenous vitamin K alone. Patients who are not bleeding with an INR of 5–8 should have 1–2 doses of warfarin withheld and their maintenance dose reduced; those with an INR >8 should receive 1–5 mg oral vitamin K.

Antiplatelet drugs, such as aspirin and clopidogrel, are often prescribed for patients at high risk of arterial thrombosis. The decision to discontinue or reverse the antiplatelet effect needs to be balanced against the risk to the patient of suboptimal treatment of coronary artery or cerebrovascular disease. Most antiplatelet drugs have short plasma half-lives, but prolonged biological effects because of irreversible platelet inhibition. There are no specific reversal agents, although platelet transfusion can be considered as an emergency measure in life-threatening haemorrhage.

Increasing numbers of patients are now being treated with direct oral thrombin inhibitors (such as dabigatran), or factor Xa inhibitors (such as rivaroxaban). There are no specific reversal agents for these drugs. Managing haemorrhage in these patients is discussed in more detail in the tutorial of question 190.

Further Reading

Makris M, Van Veen J, Tait C, Mumford A, Laffan M, and British Committee for Standards in Haematology (2012). Guideline on the management of bleeding in patients on antithrombotic agents. *British Journal of Haematology* 160: 35–46.

Samama C (2008). Prothrombin complex concentrates: a brief review. *European Journal of Anaesthesiology* 25: 784–789.

81. A) Azithromycin

This question tests the candidate's knowledge of the microbiological causes of gastroenteritis and their antimicrobial sensitivities. The Gram stain on the stool culture identifies the causative organism in this case as *Campylobacter*, a Gram-negative microaerophilic spiral bacteria. In most cases of acute bacterial gastroenteritis (including those caused by *E. coli*, *Salmonella*, and *Shigella*), a fluoroquinolone such as ciprofloxacin is the most appropriate initial antibiotic choice. However, in the Indian sub-continent and Southeast Asia resistance to ciprofloxacin is now quite high and widespread. Hence macrolides such as azithromycin are now the recommended first-line therapies. For confirmed cases of *Campylobacter*, the health protection agency of England and Wales recommends clarithromycin.

In terms of the other antimicrobial drugs listed, metronidazole is the appropriate first-line treatment of *C. difficile* infection, with oral vancomycin second-line and fidaxomicin for recalcitrant disease. Tinidazole is highly effective for giardiasis.

Tutorial

Acute diarrhoea and vomiting are most frequently infectious in origin. The majority (up to 70%) of cases are viral, with most of the remainder being bacterial. They can be subdivided into those in which vomiting is the predominant feature (often due to ingestion of a pre-formed toxin or spores), and those causing bloody or non-bloody diarrhoea respectively. Small bowel involvement is suggested by high volume, watery stools and mid-abdominal pain. Large bowel involvement manifests with lower abdominal pain, and mucoid or bloody diarrhoea. Causative organisms are highlighted in Box 4.1.

Box 4.1 Causative organisms responsible for gastroenteritis

Vomiting pre-dominant
- *Staphylococcus aureus* (toxin mediated)
- *Bacillus cereus*
- *Clostridium perfringens*

Non-bloody diarrhoea
- Viral gastroenteritis (rotavirus, norovirus, and adenovirus)
- *Salmonella* species
- Enteropathogenic or enterotoxigenic *E. coli*
- *Campylobacter* species
- *Vibrio* species
- *C. difficile*
- *Giardia lamblia*
- *Strongyloides stercoralis*

Bloody diarrhoea
- *Campylobacter* species
- *Shigella* species
- *Salmonella* species
- Enterohaemorrhagic or entero-invasive *E. coli*
- *Yersinia enterocolitica*
- *Entamoeba histolytica*
- *Trichuris trichiura*
- *Schistosoma* species

The diagnostic yield of stool cultures ranges from 1.5–5.6%, with significant associated costs. Consequently, initial clinical evaluation should focus on assessment of illness severity, need for rehydration, and identification of likely microbiological cause, based on history and examination. Most diarrhoeal illnesses are self-limiting or viral, and approximately half are of less than 24 hours' duration. Microbiological investigation is therefore usually unnecessary, unless patients are dehydrated, febrile, have blood or pus in the stool, or present with a protracted illness.

Campylobacter is usually acquired from ingestion of contaminated meat, most frequently undercooked chicken. Horizontal transmission between people is also common. Two principal subspecies cause human disease: *C. jejuni* and *C. coli*. The incubation period is 48–96 hours; patients present with nausea and vomiting, severe abdominal cramps, and diarrhoea that is frequently bloody. Guillain-Barré syndrome is a recognized post-infective complication.

The mainstay of treatment is replacement of fluid and electrolyte losses. This is most effectively provided with oral rehydration salts. Antibiotics are indicated for cases of febrile diarrhoea where the patient is believed to have moderate or severe invasive disease (passage of >4 stools/day for >3 days and at least one of: abdominal pain; fever; rectal bleeding; vomiting; myalgia; or severe headache); confirmed *Shigella*, enteropathogenic *E. coli*, or *C. difficile* infection; travellers' diarrhoea; or proven parasitic infection. These are most effective if initiated within four days of symptom onset.

Further Reading

Giddings S, Stevens A, Leung D (2016). Traveller's diarrhea. *Medical Clinics in North America* 100(2): 317–330.

82. E) Oesophageal manometry

This question tests the candidate's knowledge of the investigation of oesophageal obstruction and dysmotility. The history of non-progressive dysphagia to both solids and liquids, with regurgitation of undigested food and an air-fluid level on the chest X-ray, is highly suggestive of achalasia. The gold standard investigation for assessment and diagnosis of oesophageal motility disorders is manometry, which characterizes peristaltic performance, contraction wave configuration, and lower oesophageal sphincter pressures and relaxation.

Barium swallow is a less invasive alternative to manometry and can identify both physical obstructing lesions and dysmotility. Its limitations include the subjective nature of its evaluation, the study of only a small number of swallows, lack of standardization, and non-quantitative assessment. Upper gastrointestinal endoscopy should be performed in all patients to exclude a mucosal lesion, but is usually normal in achalasia (although subtle changes can be detected by an experienced endoscopist).

Oesophageal impedance monitoring is used to detect the flow of liquids through a hollow viscus, by measuring changes in electrical resistance when a bolus traverses an electrode pair. It is helpful in non-obstructive dysphagia, and acid and alkaline reflux disorders, but less suitable for the evaluation of achalasia. Ambulatory 24-hour pH monitoring is the other investigation frequently employed to investigate oesophageal disease, but is particularly helpful in cases of potential gastro-oesophageal reflux. A pH probe is positioned 5 cm above the lower oesophageal sphincter, following which the patient proceeds with daily life, recording their symptoms, meals, and sleep in a diary. It is not necessary in most patients with typical reflux symptoms, but can be helpful in those with refractory or atypical features. Finally, anti-Scl70 antibodies would be a good test to do if there was a suspicion of limited cutaneous form of systemic sclerosis (sometimes called CREST syndrome) which can cause oesophageal dysmotility. However, there are no other features of this condition present in this case. Even if it was the underlying diagnosis, manometry would still be needed to diagnose oesophageal dysmotility.

Tutorial

Achalasia is an oesophageal motility disorder characterized by failure of relaxation of the lower oesophageal sphincter leading to functional obstruction at the distal oesophagus, food stasis, and oesophageal dilatation. The cause is unknown, but reduced numbers of ganglion cells can be demonstrated in the myenteric nerve plexus. The age of onset is most commonly 30–50 years, and clinically achalasia presents with dysphagia to both solids and liquids, regurgitation, weight loss, and chest discomfort. Differential diagnoses include oesophageal spasm, trypanosomiasis (Chagas disease), and pseudo-achalasia (oesophageal dilatation and dysphagia, usually due to malignant obstruction). There is an increased risk of oesophageal squamous cell carcinoma.

The diagnosis is established on the basis of history, radiologic, and manometric findings. Chest radiography may demonstrate an air–fluid level, and barium swallow a dilated oesophagus with reduced peristalsis. Endoscopy is essential in all patients to exclude mucosal pathology. Oesophageal manometry is diagnostic, and shows raised lower oesophageal sphincter pressures and incomplete or absent sphincter relaxation.

The treatment goal is reduction of the pressure gradient across the lower oesophageal sphincter. Drug therapies, including nitrates and calcium channel blockers, can be useful but are short-acting. Local botulinum toxin injection provides more durable relief of symptoms, but needs to be repeated at 6–12 monthly intervals. Endoscopic dilatation is effective in 60–70%, but often requires multiple procedures; complications include perforation and reflux. Surgical myotomy is effective in 90%, but as it causes reflux in 10% an anti-reflux procedure is often performed concurrently.

Further Reading

Fisichella P, Carter S, Robles L (2012). Presentation, diagnosis, and treatment of oesophageal motility disorders. *Digestive and Liver Disease* 44: 1–7.

Rohof W, Boeckxstaens G (2012). Treatment of the patient with achalasia. *Current Opinion in Gastroenterology* 28: 389–394.

83. C) CT angiography

This question tests the candidate's knowledge of the differential diagnosis of abdominal pain. In this case, the differentials include mesenteric ischaemia, gastroduodenal ulceration, chronic pancreatitis, biliary disease, or a functional disorder. The early satiety and weight loss are 'red flags' that make a functional disorder unlikely.

Postprandial pain is more common with gastroduodenal disease, chronic pancreatitis, biliary disease, and mesenteric ischaemia. However, the diffuse nature of the pain favours mesenteric ischaemia, particularly of the midgut region (supplied by the superior mesenteric artery). By contrast, gastroduodenal disease and pancreatic disease would localize to the epigastric region, and biliary disease to the right upper quadrant.

Early satiety is an important red flag symptom for upper GI malignancy, and would merit an upper GI endoscopy, which would typically be requested in addition to the CT angiography listed above.

Therefore, to discriminate the options listed, a specific imaging protocol is required to image the mesenteric arterial vessels—this could be CT or MRI angiography. Ultrasound would be a useful initial evaluation for biliary disease, and a standard CT abdomen would be a useful initial screening test for chronic pancreatitis, along with the faecal elastase. Colonoscopy is not usually helpful for investigating abdominal pain, but may be required for the change in bowel habit if other first-line investigations are negative. Consequently, the correct answer is CT angiography.

Tutorial

Chronic mesenteric ischaemia is typically caused by long-standing atherosclerotic disease of the mesenteric vessels, and therefore has the same risk factors as peripheral vascular disease, including smoking, hypertension, dyslipidaemia, and diabetes mellitus. It usually presents with moderate to severe postprandial pain, which is poorly localized in nature. Patients may describe a fear of eating due to the postprandial pain. There is also usually a history of weight loss, nausea or vomiting, and a change in bowel habit. On examination, the abdomen may be soft and non-tender, or there may be some mild tenderness which is disproportionate to the severity of the pain. It is important to listen for an abdominal bruit and look for signs of cardiovascular or peripheral vascular disease.

Management includes full dose anticoagulation, and revascularization either by interventional radiology or surgery.

Rare causes of mesenteric ischaemia include large vessel vasculitis, such as Takayasu's arteritis, or external compression of mesenteric vessels such as coeliac artery compression syndrome where the coeliac trunk is compressed by the median arcuate ligament or the coeliac ganglion.

Further Reading

Mastoraki A, Mastoraki S, Tziava E, et al. (2016). Mesenteric ischemia: pathogenesis and challenging diagnostic and therapeutic modalities. *World Journal of Gastrointestology and Pathophysiology* 7(1): 125–130.

84. C) Autoimmune pancreatitis

This question tests the candidate's knowledge of autoimmune diseases of the pancreatobiliary system. The patient presents with painless jaundice, which the liver function tests characterize as obstructive in nature (elevated ALP and γGT). The amylase is moderately elevated, and associated with pancreatic abnormalities on CT scanning. The principal concern initially in this case should be of a cancer in the head of the pancreas, causing extrinsic compression and obstruction of the biliary tree. This possibility is less likely, however, as pancreatic imaging shows global enlargement as opposed to a focal mass, and the diagnosis would not explain the diffuse biliary tree stricturing.

Autoimmune hepatitis, primary biliary cirrhosis, and primary sclerosing cholangitis can all cause painless jaundice. Although this patient has a positive ANA, this is at low titre and of unlikely clinical significance (>1:80 typically of relevance). Although type III autoimmune hepatitis is classically autoantibody negative, a hepatitic picture of liver function tests would be expected (ALT elevated in excess of ALP and γGT). Primary biliary cirrhosis is associated with elevated IgM and anti-mitochondrial antibodies, which are normal in this case. Primary sclerosing cholangitis would be consistent with the LFT results, and although p-ANCA is elevated in 65–85% it need not be detectable. However, this diagnosis would not explain the pancreatic or retroperitoneal abnormalities. Whilst endoscopic visualization and MRCP remain the modality of choice for PSC, a CT demonstrating a normal biliary tree also goes against this diagnosis.

Autoimmune pancreatitis (AIP) can be subdivided into types I and II. Type I AIP is part of the spectrum of conditions known collectively as IgG4-related systemic disease. It most commonly presents as obstructive jaundice, and can mimic cancer of the head of the pancreas (which is the principal differential diagnosis to be excluded). It is frequently associated with elevated serum IgG. Extra-pancreatic involvement is common, particularly mediastinal or upper abdominal lymphadenopathy (80%), interstitial nephritis (45%), secondary Sjögren's syndrome affecting the salivary and lacrimal glands (up to 40%), and retroperitoneal fibrosis (10%). Lung, liver, pituitary, thyroid, and prostatic lesions have also been reported. Co-existent biliary disease occurs frequently, and although the principal cause of jaundice in this disorder remains obstruction of the common bile duct by an inflammatory pancreatic mass, stricturing in the remainder of the biliary tree is increasingly recognized. Retroperitoneal inflammatory masses are important, as they can rapid progress and involve the ureters leading to obstructive uropathy. The disease is exquisitely sensitive to steroid therapy.

Tutorial

The autoimmune pancreatitides are rare chronic diseases, affecting 0.82 per 100,000 of the population, and accounting for up to 6% of chronic pancreatitis. The typical presentation is with obstructive jaundice; manifestation as acute pancreatitis is unusual. Diabetes mellitus or impaired fasting glucose are complications in up to 70%. Type I AIP is the more common. It has peak incidence between the ages of 50–60 years, affects men twice as frequently as women, and is the pancreatic manifestation of a systemic fibro-inflammatory disorder called IgG4-associated systemic disease. Type II is associated with inflammatory bowel disease, affects a younger cohort, does not demonstrate a gender difference, and is not associated with other organ involvement.

Type I AIP can mimic most other pancreatic diseases in its presentation, and often needs to be differentiated from pancreatic cancer. Diagnosis uses the HISORt criteria:

- **H**istology: presence of periductal lymphoplasmocytic infiltrates with obliterative phlebitis and storiform fibrosis, and/or lymphoplasmocytic infiltrates with >10 IgG4+ plasma cells/high power field.
- **I**maging: typically shows diffuse gland enlargement with a diffusely attenuated pancreatic duct. Other appearances include focal masses or strictures, atrophy, calcification, or active pancreatitis.
- **S**erology: elevated serum IgG4 (in 70%).
- **O**ther organs: hilar/intrahepatic strictures, biliary strictures, parotid and lacrimal gland, mediastinal lymphadenopathy, and/or retroperitoneal fibrosis.
- **R**esponse to steroid **t**reatment.

Pancreatic imaging is key to diagnosis, either with CT or MRI. The characteristic appearance is of a low bile duct stricture in association with either diffuse pancreatic enlargement (a 'sausage pancreas') or a focal mass. ERCP for brush cytology, and endoscopic ultrasound with core biopsy (fine needle aspiration is rarely sufficient), are required to exclude malignancy and formalize the diagnosis. Serum IgG4 is elevated in approximately 70%, and is 90% specific.

AIP type I responds well to corticosteroids, although up to 40% of patients relapse after the initial course. There is an evolving role for CT-PET scanning in the monitoring of remission and detection of relapse.

Further Reading

Kalaitzakis E, Webster G (2011). Review article: autoimmune pancreatitis—management of an emerging disease. *Alimentary Pharmacology and Therapeutics* 33: 291–303.

Sugumar A, Chari S (2011). Autoimmune pancreatitis. *Journal of Gastroenterology and Hepatology* 26: 1368–1373.

85. E) Ritonavir

This question tests the candidate's knowledge of the causes of drug-induced pancreatitis. The patient presents with abdominal pain and vomiting, and the accompanying elevation in serum amylase is essentially diagnostic of acute pancreatitis. The normal LFTs exclude alternative diagnoses of acute hepatitis or gallstone disease.

Over 500 drugs have been identified to date that are either proven or suspected to cause pancreatitis. Those employed in the management of inflammatory bowel disease are relatively common culprits, in particular the 5-aminosalicylates (pancreatitis constitutes approximately 10% of reported drug reactions), azathioprine and its derivative 6-mercaptopurine (3–5%), and corticosteroids. Infliximab, and other anti-TNF agents, are not, however, currently recognized as causes.

Anti-retroviral drugs used in the treatment of HIV infection have also historically been frequently identified precipitants. The most frequent offenders were didanosine and stavudine; these are now rarely encountered in the UK but are still often used in Eastern Europe and sub-Saharan Africa and hence need to be considered in patients recently arriving from these locations. Acute pancreatitis may also arise secondary to hyperlipidaemia induced by protease inhibitors.

The management involves drug withdrawal and subsequent avoidance, alongside supportive measures. Drug-induced pancreatitis is almost never chronic.

Tutorial

The majority (approximately 80%) of cases of acute pancreatitis are caused by gallstones or alcohol misuse. Of the remainder, drug therapies are recognized to be responsible for a minority (estimated at 1%). Mechanisms vary from idiosyncratic (type B) reactions (azathioprine, 6-mercaptopurine, metronidazole, and salicylates) to direct toxic effects (diuretics, glucocorticoids, and sulphonamides). Drug agents recognized to cause acute pancreatitis are listed in Box 4.2.

Box 4.2 Drugs known to cause pancreatitis

- Antibiotics: macrolides, isoniazid, metronidazole, nitrofurantoin, trimethoprim-sulphamethoxazole, pentamidine, rifampicin, tetracyclines
- Antivirals: ribavirin, lamivudine, interferon.
- Antiretrovirals: didanosine, stavudine, nelfinavir
- Corticosteroids
- NSAIDs
- Immunomodulators: 5-aminosalicylates (sulphasalazine, mesalazine), azathioprine, 6-mercaptopurine, tacrolimus
- Cardiac drugs: ACE inhibitors, furosemide, hydrochlorothiazide, amiodarone, procainamide
- Cytotoxic chemotherapy: cytosine arabinoside, ifosfamide, paclitaxel
- Neuropsychiatric drugs: valproic acid, clozapine, carbamazepine, risperidone, sertraline

---

The diagnosis is often challenging to establish, and typically involves a combination of an appropriate clinical presentation, temporally associated with drug introduction or dose escalation, with remission on drug withdrawal. There is generally no role for re-challenge.

Further Reading

Ksiądzyna D (2011). Drug-induced acute pancreatitis related to medications commonly used in gastroenterology. *European Journal of Internal Medicine* 22: 20–25.

Nitsche C, Maertin S, Scheiber J, et al. (2012). Drug-induced pancreatitis. *Current Gastroenterology Reports* 14: 131–138.

86. C) Gallstones

This question tests the candidate's clinical reasoning of common causes of a raised bilirubin due to biliary tree obstruction. The absence of visible gallstones on ultrasound is non-confirmatory but does not exclude the diagnosis of gallstones which remains the most likely cause of any patient presenting with obstructive jaundice. An MRCP would be the most sensitive test to confirm or refute this diagnosis.

The patient's ethnic origin, alongside the peripheral blood eosinophilia, raises the possibility of helminthic infection. A variety of parasites can access the bile ducts via the duodenum, and of them the roundworm *Ascaris lumbricoides* is the most common globally and given its size, can cause obstruction of the biliary tree. Given their relatively small size (less than 3 mm), *Strongyloides* is extremely unlikely to cause obstruction of the biliary tree, but there do exist case reports of the parasite causing papillary stenosis. Given her mild eosinophilia, she may well have a parasitic infection but it still is not the most likely cause of her obstructive jaundice.

AIP typically presents as a chronic disease and one would expect a degree of abdominal pain and a more profoundly raised amylase. This is discussed in more detail in the tutorial to question 84. Primary sclerosing cholangitis (PSC) is not the correct answer either for a number of reasons. First, PSC has far slower presentation, with pruritus being a key feature due to cholestasis. Second, the disease causes stenosis of the bile duct causing intra-hepatic duct dilation, not common bile duct dilation. Third, though ALP is indeed significantly raised, you would also expect a rise in transaminases. Lastly, there is no history of inflammatory bowel disease in this patient which is associated in 70–90% of cases.

Tutorial

It is worth familiarizing yourself with the causes of intra and extra-hepatic biliary obstruction. These are listed in Box 4.3 and 4.4 respectively.

Box 4.3 Causes of intraductal biliary obstruction

- Gallstones (*most* common).
- Strictures—majority are due to previous surgical trauma, for example during ERCP. Others may be due to recurrent stone disease, abdominal or pancreatic trauma, and malignancy.
- Malignancies—cholangiocarcinoma, ampullary carcinomas, and gall bladder carcinomas.
- Primary sclerosing cholangitis.
- Parasitic infections (discussed in more detail in the tutorial).
- AIDS related cholangiopathy.
- Biliary tuberculosis (rare).

Box 4.4 Causes of extra-ductal biliary obstruction

- Pancreatitis.
- Pancreatic malignancy occurring in the head of the pancreas.
- Metastatic tumours (usually gastrointestinal or breast).
- Mirrizzi's syndrome—gall bladder inflammation and distension due to obstructed stone in cystic duct or neck of gall bladder.

Among the infective causes, parasitic infections are more common in patients from the tropics. The majority of infections are asymptomatic, although the acute phase can manifest with a febrile illness and peripheral blood eosinophilia. A number of helminths acquired orally can migrate from the duodenum into the pancreatobiliary tree, which can subsequently become obstructed resulting in biliary colic, cholangitis, and/or pancreatitis. ERCP is indicated in these scenarios, at which time worms can be mechanically extracted.

Ascaris lumbricoides, the commonest helminthic infection in humans, has a widespread geographic distribution, but is most prevalent in the rural tropics. Its life cycle is not discussed here but it inhabits the small intestine where it can cause abdominal distension, pain, and malabsorption. In children, they have a tendency to aggregate in the terminal ileum where they cause partial obstruction, precipitating intussusceptions and volvulus. Occasionally, they can end up in the pancreatobiliary tree and cause obstruction here. The diagnosis is established by visualization of either eggs in stool samples, or of the worm itself expelled orally, per rectum or at endoscopy. Treatment is of the acute complication through standard means, and of the helminth with albendazole or piperazine.

Other hepatobiliary flukes that can obstruct the biliary system include *Clonorchis sinensis*, *Opisthorchis*, and *Fasciola hepatica*. *Clonorchis* is most frequently acquired in China and Southeast Asia, and *Opisthorchis* in Thailand, Laos, Cambodia, and Vietnam, both from eating infected fish. Cysts are digested in the duodenum, from which larvae are released and may enter the pancreatobiliary tree where they mature into adult worms. The treatment of both is with praziquantel. Chronic infection with *Clonorchis* is a risk factor for cholangiocarcinoma. *Fasciola hepatica* is principally acquired in the Americas (mainly Peru and Bolivia), Europe, and Oceania. The main source is consumption of raw vegetables contaminated with metacercariae from irrigation water. An acute phase of illness may occur related to parasite migration, causing eosinophilia and hepatomegaly, with track-like lesions on CT. The chronic phase is associated with biliary tree obstruction and cirrhosis. Treatment is with triclabendazole.

Further Reading

Bethony J, Brooker S, Albonico M, et al. (2006). Soil-transmitted helminth infections: ascariasis, trichuriasis, and hookworm. *Lancet* (2006). 367: 1521–1532.

Marcos L, Terashima A, Gotuzzo E (2008). Update on hepatobiliary flukes: fascioliasis, opisthorchiasis and clonorchiasis. *Current Opinions in Infectious Diseases* 21: 523–530.

87. B) Faecal elastase-1

This question tests the candidate's knowledge of the differential diagnosis of malabsorption and the investigation of possible pancreatic exocrine insufficiency. The patient presents with chronic diarrhoea, which is non-bloody, and the observation that the stools are difficult to flush suggests that he is describing steatorrhoea. Review of the blood tests show low serum calcium and phosphate concentrations (consistent with vitamin D insufficiency), and a mildly raised INR (potentially caused by lack of vitamin K). Taken together, they suggest a possible lack of fat-soluble vitamins.

The patient's past medical history is significant for cystic fibrosis. This causes blockage of the pancreatic duct through accumulation of dehydrated protein-rich secretions, as well as chronic pancreatitis (potentially responsible for his episodic abdominal pain). The pancreas has both endocrine and exocrine functions, the latter mediated through secretion of enzymes such as amylase, trypsin, and elastase. Lipase production is key for the digestion of dietary fats, and subsequently absorption of the fat-soluble vitamins A, D, E, and K. The overall clinical picture therefore is of pancreatic enzyme insufficiency, most appropriately diagnosed through measurement of faecal elastase-1 concentrations.

Of the other investigations listed, a colonoscopy would be of value if a mucosal lesion such as Crohn's disease was suspected. The fasting gut hormone profile is used in the diagnosis of neuroendocrine tumours, many of which present with chronic diarrhoea but less so with malabsorption, and other positive features to suggest these diagnoses are absent. The SeHCAT scan tests for bile acid malabsorption, principally present in patients with terminal ileal pathology. The $[^{14}C]$-D-xylose breath test is helpful in the diagnosis of small bowel bacterial overgrowth, in which 85% of patients exhale elevated $^{14}CO_2$ concentrations. This could account for the clinical features in this case but is a less likely diagnosis in view of the history of cystic fibrosis.

Tutorial

Pancreatic exocrine dysfunction manifests with features of malabsorption, which typically only occur when >90% of exocrine pancreatic function is lost. Causes include chronic pancreatitis, pancreatic resection, and cystic fibrosis. Clinical features include chronic diarrhoea with steatorrhoea, weight loss, and abdominal bloating. Malabsorption of fat-soluble vitamins (A, D, E, and K) may give rise to a range of clinical syndromes, including metabolic bone disease and coagulopathy. Management includes treatment of the underlying cause, pancreatic enzyme supplements (e.g. Creon®), prevention or treatment of osteoporosis, and replacement of fat-soluble vitamins.

A number of functional tests are available to assess pancreatic exocrine function. The gold standard involves direct sampling of pancreatic secretions at endoscopy after administration of a secretagogue (such as secretin). Duodenal aspirates are then assayed for volume, and bicarbonate and enzyme concentrations. Given the invasive nature of this test, it is rarely used in clinical practice. Several indirect tests have been developed, which rely on measurement of pancreatic enzymes in stool, or of metabolites of pancreatic enzyme breakdown. These are listed in Box 4.5.

Box 4.5 Biochemical tests to assess pancreatic exocrine function

- *Three-day faecal fat test*—normally <7% of ingested fat appears in the stool; any more than this implies malabsorption. This test is, however, relatively insensitive, and therefore rarely performed. Qualitative microscopic examination for oil on a single stool sample is nearly as sensitive.
- *Measurement of faecal elastase-1*—this is increasingly used as it is simple, non-invasive, and has sensitivity and specificity in excess of 90%. A faecal elastase-1 concentration <50 µg/g stool is highly specific for pancreatic exocrine insufficiency. The assay is not affected by concomitant use of pancreatic enzyme supplements.
- *Pancreolauryl test*—this test uses fluorescein dilaurate, which is split into fluorescein and lauric acid by pancreatic enzymes. The free fluorescein can then be absorbed in the intestine, following which it is conjugated in the liver and excreted in urine. The test runs over two days: on one day fluorescein dilaurate is used, and on the other just free fluorescein. The ratio between the two is then calculated, and a value <20% is abnormal. The para-aminobenzoic (PABA) test employs similar principles. However, in practice, these require greater resources and time to organize, and are largely superseded by faecal elastase-1 measurement.

Further Reading

Domínguez-Muñoz J (2011). Pancreatic exocrine insufficiency: diagnosis and treatment. *Journal of Gastroenterology and Hepatology* 26(2): 12–16.

Leeds J, Oppong K, Sanders D (2011). The role of fecal elastase-1 in detecting exocrine pancreatic disease. *Nature Reviews Gastroenterology and Hepatology* 8: 405–415.

Walkowiak J, Lisowska A, Blaszczyński M (2008). The changing face of the exocrine pancreas in cystic fibrosis: pancreatic sufficiency, pancreatitis and genotype. *European Journal of Gastroenterology and Hepatology* 20: 157–160.

88. E) Urinary amylase

This question tests the candidate's knowledge of the causes and investigation of acute pancreatitis. The patient presents with clinical features strongly suggestive of this diagnosis, but inability to measure the serum amylase. The principal abnormalities demonstrated on the available blood tests are a leukocytosis, apparent hyponatraemia, and hyperglycaemia. Urinalysis reveals glycosuria and ketonuria, in a patient known to have type II diabetes mellitus. The patient is not, however, acidotic, and hence this is ketosis-prone hyperglycaemia (likely related to vomiting) rather than diabetic ketoacidosis.

The patient's blood sample is lipaemic. Hypertriglyceridaemia is a risk factor for acute pancreatitis, and the probable aetiological factor here. The presence of lipaemic serum interferes with a number of biochemical assays. Elevated serum lipids, as well as hyperglycaemia, can cause an apparent reduction in the measured plasma sodium concentration; this is artefactual and will normalize on correction of these parameters. When serum lipids are very high, it is also sometimes not possible to measure other blood biochemical tests (including renal and liver function, and amylase), thus confounding the diagnosis of acute pancreatitis. Serum lipase is similarly affected and therefore not a viable substitute in this scenario. Surface ultrasound is a poor modality for imaging the pancreas, which is retroperitoneal and largely obscured by overlying bowel gas, and hence unlikely to provide useful information with the exception of excluding biliary tree pathology. Amylase is, however, renally excreted; this is unaffected by serum lipids. The diagnosis of acute pancreatitis can therefore be established by measuring the urinary amylase.

Tutorial

Measurement of serum amylase is helpful in the diagnostic work-up of possible acute pancreatitis. A rise >3× the upper limit of normal, in the absence of renal failure, is usually diagnostic. Levels do not correlate well with disease severity, and it may be normal in acute-on-chronic pancreatitis due to pancreatic tissue loss. A rise <3× the upper limit of normal may be consistent with acute pancreatitis, but is not diagnostic as there are other causes of hyperamylasaemia which are listed in Box 4.6.

Box 4.6 Differential diagnosis of a raised amylase

- Renal insufficiency.
- Macroamylasaemia: a benign condition characterized by an unusually large serum amylase molecule, most commonly resulting from the formation of immune complexes between amylase and immunoglobulins. The clearance of this larger molecule by the kidneys is reduced, and hence assays detect high levels in blood in the absence of disease.
- Biliary tract disease.
- Intestinal obstruction, ischaemia, or perforation.
- Acute appendicitis.
- Ovarian cyst rupture, ectopic pregnancy.
- Parotitis, salivary gland disease.
- Diabetic ketoacidosis.
- Lung carcinoma.

If the cause of raised amylase is unclear, it is helpful to measure the serum lipase, which will be disproportionately normal with extra-pancreatic sources of amylase. Lipase also remains elevated for a longer duration than amylase, which can be useful in patients who present late. Amylase isoenzymes can be measured to identify a salivary source, although this is rarely done in practice.

Plain abdominal radiographs are generally not helpful in the diagnosis of acute pancreatitis, but may show a sentinel bowel loop or ileus due to local peritonism. Ultrasound is of value in looking for gallstone disease, though imaging of the pancreas is poor. Computed tomography performed with both oral and intravenous contrast is useful in confirming the diagnosis, but should be delayed beyond 72 hours after presentation as earlier scans may underestimate the extent of any fluid collections or pancreatic necrosis. It is not required if the diagnosis is otherwise robust and disease mild. MRI with gadolinium is as accurate as CT, but more difficult to perform in critically unwell patients. It helps further delineate pancreatic duct involvement.

Hypertriglyceridaemia is common, and defined as fasting serum triglycerides >2.3 mmol/L. Severe hypertriglyceridaemia (>20 mmol/L) is rare, and often occurs in the context of inherited disorders of lipid metabolism. Genetic disorders leading to hypertriglyceridaemia include:

- Type IV hyperlipidaemia (familial hypertriglyceridaemia).
- Type I hyperlipidaemias (lipoprotein lipase and apolipoprotein CII deficiencies).
- Type IIb hyperlipidaemia (familial combined hyperlipidaemia).
- Type III hyperlipidaemia (remnant removal disease).

Secondary contributors to hypertriglyceridaemia include poorly controlled diabetes mellitus, obesity, a high fat diet, excess alcohol consumption, hypothyroidism, and certain medications (particularly thiazide diuretics and antiretrovirals).

Classic clinical findings in patients with severe chronic hypertriglyceridaemia include eruptive or palmar xanthomas, and lipaemia retinalis on fundoscopy. Acute myocardial infarction, stroke, and pancreatitis are the most significant clinical complications. The first-line treatment (apart from dietary change) is monotherapy with a fibrate drug (such as bezafibrate). These are efficacious and typically lower triglyceride levels very rapidly. Second-line agents include statins and nicotinic acid. In extremis, for rapid control in the context of severe or life-threatening acute pancreatitis, there are case reports of therapeutic benefit using continuous insulin or heparin infusions, or plasmapheresis.

Further Reading

Frossard J, Steer M, Pastor C (2008). Acute pancreatitis. *Lancet* 371: 143–152.

Lindkvist B, Appelros S, Regnér S, Manjer J (2012). A prospective cohort study on risk of acute pancreatitis related to serum triglycerides, cholesterol and fasting glucose. *Pancreatology* 12: 317–324.

Lippi G, Valentino M, Cervellin G (2012). Laboratory diagnosis of acute pancreatitis: in search of the Holy Grail. *Critical Reviews in Clinical Laboratory Sciences* 49: 18–31.

89. C) The patient has resolved hepatitis B infection

This question tests the candidate's understanding of the interpretation of hepatitis B serology. The patient presents with a non-specific symptom (fatigue). Screening blood tests are performed, which demonstrate a mild rise in bilirubin and ALT. The most likely explanation for the deranged liver functions tests are a viral illness. The patient may even have Gilbert's syndrome, a benign condition in which reduced activity of hepatic bilirubin uridine diphosphate glucuronosyltransferase-1 causes a transient unconjugated hyperbilirubinaemia, particularly during periods of fasting or intercurrent illness.

Nonetheless, hepatotropic virus serology is requested, which is abnormal. The HBsAg should be positive in patients with acute or active ongoing infection. Its absence, in the context of a positive anti-HBs antibody, could be explained either by previous hepatitis B infection that has now resolved, or immunization. The positive anti-HBc antibody clarifies that it results from the former, as immunization should produce a positive anti-HBs alone out of the test results listed in the question. The envelope 'e' antigen and antibody are indicative of viral load and the risk of transmitting infection. Detectable HBeAg implies high viral replication and infectivity; an anti-HBe antibody is the reciprocal and suggests low infectivity. Liver biopsy is only required to guide the need for antiviral therapy in active chronic disease, and therefore not indicated in this scenario. For a useful algorithm on how to appraise hepatitis B serology, please see the tutorial to question number 115.

Tutorial

Hepatitis B is common worldwide, and endemic in Southeast Asia. The most frequent mode of transmission is vertical from mother to baby at birth, although blood inoculation (transfusion, needle sharing for recreational intravenous drug use, and tattooing or piercing) and sexual transmission are also important.

The hepatitis B surface antigen (HBsAg) appears in serum 1–10 weeks after exposure, and prior to symptom onset or serum aminotransferase derangement. Most infections are silent, with fewer than 50% presenting with jaundice. As HBsAg disappears, the corresponding antibody (anti-HBs) titres rise, although there may be a window period when both are negative. Detection of IgM antibody against the hepatitis B core antigen (anti-HBc) is usually regarded as an indication of acute infection, and hence it is helpful to clarify this window period, although it may remain detectable for up to two years and reappear during exacerbations of chronic disease. Anti-HBc IgG takes longer to develop and simply indicates prior exposure to the virus.

In patients who recover, HBsAg becomes undetectable within six months. Persistence beyond this time is defined as chronic infection. This occurs in <5% of adult-acquired infections, but >90% of vertical transmissions. The presence of the hepatitis B envelope antigen (HBeAg) is indicative of a high circulating viral load and implies a highly infective patient. The presence of the antibody (anti-HBe) is the reciprocal of this, suggesting low infectivity.

Hepatitis B DNA should be measured on a six-monthly basis in HBsAg$^+$/HBeAg$^-$ patients to assess for ongoing viral replication, and in HBeAg$^+$ patients to determine risk of progression and hence stratify need for antiviral therapy. Viral genotyping is available; at present this does not influence treatment strategy but is likely to do so within the next five years. Liver biopsy is rarely needed in the acute phase, but is helpful in chronic disease if active therapy is being considered. Non-invasive markers of liver fibrosis (ultrasound and blood tests) are being increasingly validated in clinical practice. All patients should be tested for co-infection with hepatitis C, delta virus (hepatitis D), and HIV.

Patients with acute hepatitis B do not generally require antiviral therapy, although there is a role in those with severe disease, acute liver failure (occurs in <2%, but treatment reduces the likelihood of re-infection following liver transplantation), a protracted course (jaundice for >4 weeks), immunocompromise (including old age), concomitant hepatitis C, or delta virus infection, or pre-existing liver disease.

Current guidelines suggest considering antiviral therapy in chronic hepatitis B infection in all patients with liver inflammation on biopsy and a circulating viral DNA level in excess of >2000 copies/mL. Antiviral therapy in viral hepatitis is a fast-moving field and varies according to local policies and funding. Currently available agents are listed in Box 4.7.

Box 4.7 Currently available treatments for hepatitis B

- Pegylated interferon-α. Advantages included a limited treatment course (48 weeks) and no risk of viral resistance as it works through immune modulation. Disadvantages include its subcutaneous route of administration and significant side-effect profile (flu-like symptoms, autoimmune reactions, myelosuppression, and depression). It is contraindicated in decompensated liver disease.
- Lamivudine: oral nucleoside analogue, which has minimal side effects. Resistance emergences in 25% after one year of treatment, and in 50% within three years.
- Tenofovir: oral nucleotide analogue, which currently demonstrates high rates of viral control and minimal resistance. It is appropriate for first-line monotherapy.
- Other recently approved agents include entecavir, adefovir, emtricitabine, and telbivudine.

Although the majority of adults exposed to hepatitis B will clear the virus, complications in chronically infected patients can be severe, and include:

- Cirrhosis: usually develops 30–40 years post-infection, but highly variable.
- Hepatocellular carcinoma: there is a 100-fold risk in comparison to the healthy population. Incidence is 0.5%/year in non-cirrhotic patients, and 2–6%/year in those with established cirrhosis. Patients should be screened every six months using serum α-fetoprotein and liver ultrasound.
- Membranous glomerulonephropathy.
- Polyarteritis nodosa.
- Mortality: five-year survival in chronically infected patients is 80%, which falls to 35% after an episode of decompensation.

Further Reading

Dienstag J (2008). Hepatitis B virus infection. *New England Journal of Medicine* 359: 1486–1500.

European Association for the Study of the Liver (2012). EASL clinical practice guidelines: management of chronic hepatitis B virus infection. *Journal of Hepatology* 57: 167–185.

Strassburg C (2010). Hyperbilirubinemia syndromes (Gilbert-Meulengracht, Crigler-Najjar, Dubin-Johnson, and Rotor syndrome). *Best Practice and Research: Clinical Gastroenterology* 24: 555–571.

90. A) Acute fatty liver of pregnancy

This question tests the candidate's knowledge of the causes of liver disease in pregnancy. Several disorders are unique to, or more likely to occur in, pregnant women. These should be considered alongside the causes of liver disease that occur in non-pregnant patients. Transient mild derangements in liver function tests are common and rarely require additional assessment beyond repeat monitoring to ensure normalization. Alkaline phosphate is normally elevated, as it is also produced by the placenta.

The patient has a mild anaemia (normal for this stage of pregnancy due to haemodilution), leukocytosis, thrombocytopaenia, and renal impairment. There is significant biochemical jaundice, associated with a raised ALT and INR; the ALP and albumin are within the normal ranges for this stage of pregnancy. The serum uric acid is elevated, and the patient has borderline hypoglycaemia. Furthermore, the patient has systemic hypertension and proteinuria, suggestive of pre-eclampsia. These features, alongside the timing and rate of progression of symptoms, are indicative of acute fatty liver of pregnancy. This is supported by the appearances on ultrasonography. Up to 40% of patients with this disorder also have associated pre-eclampsia or HELLP syndrome.

In terms of the differential diagnoses listed, Budd-Chiari syndrome refers to the consequences of hepatic vein thrombosis, which is more common in high oestrogen states, including pregnancy. The classical presentation is with painful hepatomegaly (due to acute liver capsular stretch) and ascites. Hepatic venous thrombosis can be confirmed by Doppler ultrasonography or triple-phase CT. Treatment is with anticoagulation, or in severe cases hepatic venous balloon dilatation or TIPS.

Hyperemesis gravidarum describes severe vomiting during the first trimester causing dehydration and ketosis; it typically resolves by 18 weeks' gestation. A reversible increase in serum aminotransferases occurs in 50%, with minor elevation in ALP and bilirubin in 10%. These are of no clinical significance.

The principal manifestation of obstetric cholestasis is with severe pruritus. It typically occurs in the second and third trimester. Jaundice is uncommon, although pale stools, dark urine, subclinical steatorrhoea, and fat and fat-soluble vitamin malabsorption may be detectable. LFTs may show mild elevation in bilirubin, and moderate elevation in aminotransferases and ALP, although only marginally raised γGT. Treatment is with ursodeoxycholic acid.

HELLP syndrome consists of a microangiopathic haemolytic anaemia, consumptive thrombocytopaenia (platelets aggregate into clots in the microvasculature) and elevated LFTs. To establish the diagnosis, there should be evidence on the blood film of mechanical intravascular haemolysis, with schistocytes and/or echinocytes and spherostomatocytes. The serum haptoglobin should be depleted, and LDH raised. There is also an overlap in this condition with pre-eclampsia.

Tutorial

Acute fatty liver of pregnancy is a microvesicular steatosis caused by mitochondrial dysfunction. It occurs in 1 in 14,000 pregnancies, predominantly in the third trimester (especially between weeks 34–37). Symptoms include headache, fatigue, nausea, vomiting, and abdominal pain. Jaundice may be severe. Urine is bile-stained, and stools pale. Progression can be rapid, and in fulminant cases cause acute liver failure, encephalopathy, and death within days. Serum aminotransferases are usually <750 IU/L. Hypoglycaemia and DIC are common. Hyperuricaemia is present in 80%. CT is sensitive for the detection of steatosis. The Swansea diagnostic criteria require six or more of: vomiting, abdominal pain, polydipsia/polyuria, encephalopathy, jaundice, hypoglycaemia, urate >340 μmol/L, white cell count >11 × 10^9 cells/L, elevated serum aminotransferase, hyperammonaemia, creatinine >150 μmol/L, coagulopathy, ascites or bright liver on ultrasound, and microvesicular steatosis on liver biopsy. Definitive management involves early delivery and supportive measures such as correction and prevention of hypoglycaemia. Without specialist care, foetal and maternal mortality is 10–20%. Although most cases are idiopathic, acute fatty liver of pregnancy is more common among heterozygous mothers carrying foetuses with long-chain 3-hydroxyacyl-CoA dehydrogenase (LCHAD) deficiency. These infants may develop non-ketotic hypoglycaemia, Reye's syndrome, or sudden infant death, and hence diagnostic testing for the *G1528C* mutation is recommended in all mothers with this condition.

Obstetric cholestasis is an intrahepatic process that accounts for 20% of cases of jaundice in pregnancy. It affects 0.5–1% of all pregnancies. The cause is unknown but may relate to impaired bile salt conjugation secondary to the high oestrogen state. It is relatively benign for the mother, but associated with increased risk for foetal prematurity, distress, and stillbirth. Serum bile acids are markedly elevated and foetal complications correlate with their concentrations. Ultrasound is necessary to exclude gallstone disease and MRCP is helpful if there is diagnostic uncertainty; liver biopsy is not required. Treatment is symptomatic with ursodeoxycholic acid for the duration of the pregnancy. Elective delivery is recommended by 38 weeks to minimize foetal complications.

HELLP syndrome is a thrombotic microangiopathy characterized by intravascular mechanical haemolysis, elevated liver enzymes, and thrombocytopaenia. It affects 0.2% of pregnancies, rising to 20% in patients with severe pre-eclampsia. Symptoms typically begin between weeks 28–36, but the condition can occur post-partum. Malaise and fatigue are followed by headache, abdominal pain, nausea, and vomiting. Massive LFT derangement or right shoulder tip pain are ominous as they indicate liver infarction or impending rupture. Maternal complications occur in 50%, and up to 25% develop DIC (D-dimer predicts severity). Urgent delivery is indicated.

Further Reading

Joshi D, James A, Quaglia A, Westbrook R, Heneghan M (2010). Liver disease in pregnancy. *Lancet* 375: 594–605.

Moore M, Nelson-Piercy C (2011). Pregnancy and the liver. *British Journal of Hospital Medicine (London)* 72: M170–173.

91. E) Cystectomy and albendazole

This question tests the candidate's knowledge of the diagnosis, investigation, and management of cystic liver lesions.

This patient has hydatid disease, caused by the tapeworm *Echinococcus granulosus*. This is common in Europe, particularly in rural communities. Hydatid cysts may be asymptomatic, but can cause pain from mass effects in the liver, or complications from rupture (anaphylaxis or secondary infection). The full blood count and LFTs may be normal, and eosinophilia is unusual unless the cyst is leaking. Serology is 90% sensitive, and CT is the gold standard imaging modality, with 95% accuracy for demonstrating characteristic 'daughter' cysts. Definitive treatment involves cystectomy or partial hepatectomy, with peri-operative albendazole cover.

Cefuroxime and metronidazole would be an appropriate treatment for bacterial pyogenic abscesses. These would usually present with high fevers (characteristically 'swinging' pyrexia), and a markedly elevated CRP. Rifampicin, isoniazid, pyrazinamide, and ethambutol is the drug combination used in treatment of tuberculosis. When this infects the liver it usually does so in a miliary pattern or as a diffuse granulomatous hepatitis, although isolated tuberculomas can occur. The presentation in this case would be extremely unusual given the history and demographic, particularly in the absent of immunocompromise. Similarly, the history and radiological appearances would be atypical for hepatic malignancy: with hepatocellular carcinoma a background of cirrhosis is typical, and with neuroendocrine tumours the carcinoid syndrome might be expected. These can be treated by a variety of therapies, of which transarterial chemoembolization constitutes one.

Tinidazole is a therapy for amoebic liver abscess, caused by *Entamoeba histolytica*. Abscesses are usually solitary. Blood tests typically show a normochromic normocytic anaemia, with neutrophilia and raised CRP. Liver function tests are usually normal, although albumin is often very low. Serology is >95% sensitive and specific. Two tests are available: the immunofluorescent antibody test (IFAT) and cellulose acetate precipitin (CAP). A positive IFAT is specific, but remains positive following previous, resolved infections; CAP is only detectable during active disease. Diagnostic aspiration is rarely required, but when performed the classic description is of a pink-brown 'anchovy sauce' aspirate).

Tutorial

Several processes can cause isolated liver lesions; these are principally infective or neoplastic in origin. The infective category fall into three main subgroups: pyogenic (bacterial) liver abscess, amoebic liver abscess, and hydatid disease.

Pyogenic abscesses may arise from systemic infection or local portal phlebitis. They are more common in the elderly, and associated with obstructive biliary disease, intra-abdominal infection (particularly diverticulitis and appendicitis), systemic infection (including endocarditis), and trauma. Infections are usually polymicrobial, with gut-derived anaerobes as well as Gram-negative and Gram-positive organisms. The presentation is often acute with right upper quadrant pain and fever. Ultrasound is 80–90% sensitive, and when there is doubt CT shows classic ring-enhancing lesions. Broad-spectrum antibiotic cover should be provided, and large abscesses drained percutaneously.

Amoebic liver abscesses are common in the Indian subcontinent, South America, West Africa, and Southeast Asia. Cysts of *Entamoeba histolytica* are ingested, from which trophozoites emerge and colonize the large bowel. Tissue invasion subsequently occurs, and organisms reach the liver via the portal vein. Liver lesions can arise in the absence of an overt preceding dysenteric illness. Antimicrobial therapy is with tinidazole or metronidazole; this should be accompanied by diloxanide to eliminate luminal bowel infection even in the absence of gastrointestinal symptoms. Aspiration or surgery is reserved for very large abscesses for which rupture is imminent or has occurred, or in those in whom antimicrobial therapy has failed. Treatment is successful in 85%.

Hydatid disease is common in rural communities, and farmers are at particular risk due to contact with the definitive host (dogs) and intermediate hosts (sheep, goats, and pigs). Eggs are shed from canines and contaminate soil, from which they can be ingested. They hatch in the small intestine and disseminate haematogenously and through lymphatics to generate cysts in the liver, lung and (rarely) bone, kidney, and spleen. The incubation period may be years. Treatment generally requires a combined medical and surgical approach, as only 30% are cured by medical therapy alone. During the operation, sterilization of the cyst with hypertonic saline and prevention of spillage by prior evacuation of its contents are essential, as accidental release of scolices into the peritoneum causes anaphylaxis and secondary peritoneal hydatidosis. For patients in whom surgery is unsuitable, percutaneous aspiration, injection, and re-aspiration (PAIR) can be attempted. Cysts are punctured under ultrasound guidance and contents withdrawn. Hypertonic saline is injected, left for 15 minutes, then re-aspirated. Peri-procedural albendazole cover is necessary. Recurrence occurs in up to 30%.

Further Reading

Bonder A, Afdhal N (2012). Evaluation of liver lesions. *Clinical Liver Disease* 16: 271–283.

Johannsen E, Sifri C, Madoff L (2000). Pyogenic liver abscesses. *Infectious Disease Clinics in North America* 14: 547–563.

McManus D, Zhang W, Li J, Bartley P (2003). Echinococcosis. *Lancet* 362: 1295–1304.

Stanley S (2003). Amoebiasis. *Lancet* 361: 1025–1034.

92. B) Anti-mitochondrial antibody

This question tests the candidate's knowledge of the serological investigation of patients with autoimmune hepatobiliary disease. The patient presents with jaundice alongside a cholestatic picture of LFT derangement and macrocytic anaemia. Testing of haematinics discloses vitamin B_{12} deficiency, and of immunoglobulins a raised serum IgM. The clinical picture (lethargy, jaundice, and marked pruritus as evidenced by widespread excoriation marks), elevated ALP in marked excess of ALT, and elevated IgM suggest a diagnosis of primary biliary cirrhosis. This is associated with anti-mitochondrial antibodies. A significant proportion of these cases have other concurrent autoimmune diseases, including hypothyroidism and pernicious anaemia.

Auto-immune hepatitis present with a hepatic picture (ALT/AST>ALP). Type I (80% of cases) is also associated with anti-smooth muscle antibodies and anti-nuclear antibodies (ANA), and IgG is raised in 97% of patients; it responds very well to immunosuppression unless cirrhosis has already developed. Type II is usually diagnosed in childhood, and associated with anti-LKM1 and anti-LC1 antibodies; ANA and anti-smooth muscle antibodies are usually negative. It is rapidly progressive and often refractory to medical therapy. Type III presents clinically in a similar fashion to type I, but classic autoantibodies are negative. Liver biopsy shows a periportal or lobular hepatitis, although there are no pathognomonic features.

Primary sclerosing cholangitis presents with progressive jaundice (although often with a fluctuating bilirubin level), and cholestatic LFTs. It is associated with inflammatory bowel disease in 3–10%, principally ulcerative colitis, where the risk of colorectal cancer is raised 50-fold. The p-ANCA is positive in 65–85%, and serum IgG4 is elevated in 6–12%. ERCP is the gold standard for diagnosis, although MRCP is usually sufficient, showing multifocal intrahepatic and extrahepatic strictures. Treatment is with ursodeoxycholic acid. It is controversial whether this actually improves symptoms or prognosis of liver disease, but there is increasing evidence that it provides chemoprevention against colorectal cancer in patients with concomitant colitis. Liver transplantation provides 80–90% five-year survival, but there is recurrence in 20% at five years.

Anti-centromere antibodies are found in systemic sclerosis; these patients are more predisposed to primary biliary cirrhosis.

Tutorial

Primary biliary cirrhosis is a chronic, progressive cholestatic disorder. It predominantly affects middle-aged women. The classic presenting features are pruritus and lethargy, although now up to 50% are identified in the early asymptomatic phase. Associated autoimmune diseases (sicca syndrome, thyroiditis, Raynaud's disease, pernicious anaemia, and systemic sclerosis) are common. Clinical signs include xanthelasma, excoriations, clubbing, and evidence of chronic liver disease. Investigations show markedly elevated ALP and γGT, with only mildly raised aminotransferases. Jaundice occurs late. Serum IgM is increased. Anti-mitochondrial M2 antibodies against the pyruvate dehydrogenase complex are found in >90%. Liver biopsy is not mandatory where the diagnosis is clear, but allows staging and grading.

Initial treatment is with ursodeoxycholic acid, which ameliorates symptoms, and reduces the likelihood of requiring transplantation as well as mortality. Colestyramine is an alternative useful adjunct for pruritus. Screen for fat-soluble vitamin deficiency and for osteoporosis, and treat accordingly. For end-stage disease, liver transplantation is highly effective (>80% five-year survival). Median survival overall is 10–16 years from presentation for asymptomatic patients, and 7–10 years for symptomatic patients.

Further Reading

Carey E, Ali A, Lindor K (2015). Primary biliary cirrhosis. *Lancet* 386: 1565–1575.

Karlsen T, Boberg K (2013). Update on primary sclerosing cholangitis. 2013. *Journal of Hepatology* 59(3): 571–582.

Lindor K (2007). Ursodeoxycholic acid for the treatment of primary biliary cirrhosis. *New England Journal of Medicine* 357: 1524–1529.

93. A) PiZZ genotype

This question tests the candidate's knowledge of metabolic liver diseases. The patient presents with an exacerbation of previously undiagnosed chronic obstructive airways disease. On the original admission, she is narcosed due to type II respiratory failure. Spirometry performed when well confirms an obstructive pattern. Clinical examination also reveals evidence suggestive of chronic liver disease. This is supported by the findings of abnormal LFTs on blood testing, and of anomalies on liver biopsy. The patient has α1-antitrypsin deficiency, which causes premature panlobular emphysema. Those individuals with the *PiZZ* genotype also develop chronic liver failure, characterized by accumulation of periodic acid Schiff (PAS) positive inclusions in periportal hepatocytes.

Elevated serum ferritin would be expected in haemochromatosis, or as an acute phase reactant. Low serum caeruloplasmin and elevated urinary copper excretion are seen in Wilson's disease. α-galactosidase deficiency causes Fabry's disease, a lysosomal storage disorder associated with cardiomyopathy, chronic kidney injury, and cutaneous angiokeratomas; hepatic involvement is not characteristic.

Tutorial

α1-antitrypsin deficiency is an autosomal recessive disorder, occurring in 1 in 1800 people of European descent. The normal protein functions as a proteolytic enzyme inhibitor, including of neutrophil elastase. Impaired cellular transport of α1-antitrypsin also leads to its intrahepatic accumulation, resulting in hepatocyte injury. Over 90 allelic variants in the α1-antitrypsin gene have been described, and annotated according to the Pi (protease inhibitor) nomenclature.

Point mutations are inherited in a Mendelian fashion. The normal genotype is designated *PiMM*, heterozygotes *PiMZ* or *PiMS*, and homozygotes *PiZZ*. Compound heterozygosity for the *S* and *Z* alleles leads to an intermediate phenotype.

The disease presents with premature emphysema, thought to be related to increased protease activity in the lung causing parenchymal injury. This is substantially accelerated by concurrent cigarette smoking. Pulmonary function tests show a reduced FEV1/FVC ratio, air trapping, and a low transfer factor. Inhaled α1-antitrypsin has been used therapeutically to limit progression of respiratory disease.

Liver disease presents in adulthood in 10% of *PiZZ* homozygotes. LFTs show raised cholestatic enzymes and transaminases. High rates of portal hypertension and hepatocellular carcinoma are reported. The diagnosis is established by finding serum α1-antitrypsin levels <75% of the lower limit of normal (<80 mg/dL), reduced α1-globulin on serum protein electrophoresis, the *PiZZ* genotype, and PAS-positive inclusions in peri-portal hepatocytes on liver biopsy. Management involves avoidance of additional hepatic insults, such as alcohol. Liver transplantation is the only recognized treatment for advanced disease, with an 80% five-year survival.

Haemochromatosis is caused by iron overload and may be primary (genetic) or secondary (usually due to repeated blood transfusions). Normal total body iron stores are 3–4 g; in genetic haemochromatosis these may be in excess of 20 g. Over 90% of primary cases are due to the *C282Y* polymorphism in the *HFE* gene on chromosome 6. Inheritance is autosomal recessive, with 10% of northern Europeans heterozygous and 1% homozygous. The polymorphism is, however, of low penetrance, partly due to menstrual iron losses in women. Clinical features include:

- Hepatosplenomegaly, cirrhosis, and hepatocellular carcinoma.
- Cardiomyopathy (usually dilated, but can be restrictive).
- Hypogonadotrophic hypogonadism (panhypopituitarism, testicular atrophy).
- Diabetes mellitus.
- Skin pigmentation ('bronze diabetes').
- Pseudogout.

A serum ferritin >1000 μg/L with transferrin saturation >45% strongly suggest iron overload. Liver biopsy remains the gold standard for diagnosis using Perl's haemosiderin stain and allows measurement of hepatic iron index, but is not required if the ferritin is >1000 μg/L and the patient *C282Y* homozygous. Genetic analysis is useful, but incomplete penetrance and the existence of other polymorphisms still necessitate full biochemical testing. MRI has high sensitivity and specificity for detecting liver iron overload. Treatment is with venesection, or iron chelation with desferrioxamine.

Wilson's disease is an autosomal recessive disorder affecting 1 in 30,000 people. Mutations in the *ATP7A* gene, encoding Wilson's disease protein, cause copper retention in the liver and failure of its incorporation into plasma caeruloplasmin. It most commonly presents between childhood and the age of 40, though can be first diagnosed in older individuals. Liver disease is the most common childhood presentation, compared to neuropsychiatric manifestations in adulthood. Other complications include parkinsonism and Coombs-negative haemolytic anaemia. Kayser-Fleischer rings may be seen on ocular slit lamp examination. The LFTs are usually non-specifically raised. Diagnosis can be achieved by identifying a low plasma caeruloplasmin (<200 mg/L), serum copper <11 μmol/L, and 24-hour urinary copper >3 μmol. Liver biopsy shows hepatic copper >250 μg/ g dry weight, and features of chronic hepatitis or necrosis. Genetic analysis is available, although the three most common mutations account for less than one-third of cases. Treatment is with chelation with D-penicillamine.

Further Reading

Fink S, Schilsky M (2007). Inherited metabolic disease of the liver. *Current Opinions in Gastroenterology* 23: 237–243.

Siddique A, Kowdley K (2012). Review article: the iron overload syndromes. *Alimentary Pharmacology Therapy* 35: 876–893.

Silverman E, Sandhaus R (2009). Clinical practice. Alpha1-antitrypsin deficiency. *New England Journal of Medicine*. 360: 2749–2757.

94. D) OGD and duodenal biopsy

This question tests the candidate's knowledge of the diagnosis of coeliac disease. This lady has no symptoms of diarrhoea, but presents with vertebral fractures and weight loss. The differential diagnosis includes malabsorption, malignancy, thyrotoxicosis, or tuberculosis. Primary metabolic bone disease must also be considered, but would not account for the weight loss. The blood tests demonstrate a normocytic anaemia. However, the biochemistry confirms iron and B_{12} deficiency; hence the patient is likely to have a *dimorphic* blood film despite the normal mean corpuscular volume. The elevated alkaline phosphatase represents osteomalacia due to vitamin D deficiency, since the normal gamma glutamyl transpeptidase makes hepatobiliary disease unlikely. The findings of weight loss and multiple nutrient deficiencies make malabsorption the most likely diagnosis. The sensitivity of the anti-TTG antibodies for coeliac disease is 95%. However, selective IgA deficiency is a cause of false negative antibodies, and hence duodenal biopsy is required for diagnosis (see below). Duodenal biopsy may also reveal other causes of enteropathy and malabsorption, such as giardiasis or vasculitis. The other investigations would be appropriate if features in the history suggested tuberculosis, such as fevers, or malignancy, such as a family history of GI cancer. Recurrent miscarriage may suggest the anti-phospholipid syndrome. However, in this context it is a feature of coeliac disease.

Tutorial

Coeliac disease is a disorder of the proximal small intestine that can involve the entire small intestine in some individuals. This proximal location in the small intestine often results in malabsorption of iron, folic acid, calcium, and fat-soluble vitamins, with resultant nutrient deficiencies and reduced bone density.

Coeliac disease predominantly affects white Europeans, primarily of Celtic ancestry. The advent of serological testing has shown the worldwide prevalence to be 1 in 266. However, coeliac disease can also affect non-European populations if they have an appropriate genetic background. Punjabi and Gujarati migrants living in England develop the disorder 2.7 times more commonly than Europeans when on a gluten-rich diet.

Coeliac disease is diagnosed in the presence of mucosal inflammation, crypt hyperplasia, and villous atrophy on a small intestinal biopsy sample, and improvements in clinical symptoms or histology after 4–6 months on a gluten-free diet. Positive serological tests lend support to the diagnosis, but are not essential.

Duodenal biopsy should be considered in several circumstances:

- Gastrointestinal symptoms including chronic diarrhoea, malabsorption, weight loss, and abdominal distension
- Iron-deficiency anaemia
- Osteopenia
- Short stature
- Delayed puberty

- Elevation of serum transaminases
- Recurrent foetal loss and infertility
- Peripheral neuropathy and cerebellar ataxia

The detection of IgA antibodies against TTG antibodies has a sensitivity of 95% and specificity of 96% for the diagnosis of coeliac disease. However, this should not replace small intestinal histology, which is required both to confirm the diagnosis, and as a baseline from which to monitor improvement.

Selective IgA deficiency occurs in 2.6% of patients with coeliac disease, ten-fold higher than that in the general population. Thus, individuals with selective IgA deficiency and coeliac disease will not have anti-TTG antibodies. These patients will, nevertheless, have a raised total IgG concentration. The diagnosis therefore rests upon measuring the serum IgA, and specific anti-endomysial and anti-TTG IgG antibody tests. The combination of IgA deficiency and a positive IgG test should prompt a biopsy.

This patient is likely to have coeliac disease and selective IgA deficiency, and therefore requires duodenal biopsy for diagnosis. Further investigations for malignancy or tuberculosis would only be indicated once coeliac disease has been excluded, particularly in the absence of fevers, colonic symptoms, or a family history of colon cancer.

Further Reading

Husby S, Murray J (2014). Diagnosing coeliac disease and the potential for serological markers. *Nature Reviews Gastroenterology and Hepatology* 11(11): 655–656.

Lundin K, Sollid L (2014). Advances in coeliac disease. *Current Opinions Gastroenterology* 30(2): 154–162.

Mehta G, Taslaq S, Littleford S, et al. (2008). The inchanging face of coeliac disease. *British Journal of Hospital Medicine* 69(2): 84–87.

95. A) Hepatitis B immune globulin and vaccination to the newborn

This question tests the candidate's knowledge of the management of hepatitis B in pregnancy. The correct answer involves the use of hepatitis B vaccination *and* immune globulin because the mother has a high viral load and hepatitis B eAg (see below). There is little evidence for the routine administration of lamivudine for the prevention of perinatal transmission of hepatitis B. Lamivudine and interferon are treatments for chronic hepatitis B infection. However, treatment is not typically initiated unless the ALT is greater than 2× the upper limit of normal, or if there is significant inflammation and fibrosis on liver biopsy. Correct management of mother and baby requires correct interpretation of hepatitis B serology.

Tutorial

Vertical transmission of hepatitis B may occur if the mother has chronic hepatitis B, or acute hepatitis B near the time of delivery. Most newborns with vertical transmission of hepatitis B are asymptomatic. The rate of transmission is greater than 90% to infants born to women who are both hepatitis B sAg and eAg positive. Almost all of these infected infants become chronic hepatitis B sAg carriers. By contrast, fewer than 10% of infants born to eAg negative mothers develop chronic infection. Infants with chronic hepatitis B infection are at increased risk of developing chronic liver disease or hepatocellular carcinoma. The Department of Health guidelines advise that all pregnant women should be offered antenatal screening for hepatitis B, and all babies born to infected mothers receive a complete course of immunization starting at birth.

Prevention of perinatal transmission of hepatitis B involves passive-active immunization. All infants born to mothers with hepatitis B sAg, or in whom the hepatitis B status is unknown, should receive the schedule of hepatitis B vaccination. The first dose should be administered within 24 hours, with further doses at one and two months of age. A booster dose is administered at one year of age, at the same time as follow-up testing.

Infants born to mothers with hepatitis B eAg should receive passive immunization with hepatitis B immune globulin within 24 hours of birth, due to the markedly increased risk of vertical transmission. With appropriate immunoprophylaxis, breast-feeding provides no additional risk for the transmission of hepatitis B.

Further Reading

Department of Health—Immunisation Branch (2011). Hepatitis B antenatal screening and newborn immunisation programme: best practice guidance. Available at: https://www.gov.uk/government/collections/hepatitis-b-guidance-data-and-analysis

96. C) Propanolol 40 mg bd and repeat OGD+/−EVL at two weeks following discharge

This patient has presented with his first variceal haemorrhage on the background of cirrhosis, and requires secondary prophylaxis. For primary prophylaxis, both non-selective beta blockers (NSBB) such as propranolol, and EVL, are equally effective in preventing the first variceal bleed. However, for secondary prophylaxis, there is an additional benefit in combining NSBB and EVL. Typically, EVL is performed by repeating the OGD at two-weekly intervals with repeat EVL until the varices appear obliterated.

Omeprazole is not indicated unless there is a concomitant mucosal lesion such as gastritis or ulceration. In fact, there is some evidence that PPIs can increase complications such as spontaneous bacterial peritonitis in cirrhosis. TIPSS is usually reserved as a salvage therapy for variceal bleeding that is refractory to endoscopic treatments.

Tutorial

Variceal bleeding is a serious complication of cirrhosis and portal hypertension. Although mortality rates have improved over recent years, largely due to better endoscopy and interventional radiology treatments, acute variceal bleeding remains a medical emergency. The detailed management of acute variceal bleeding is beyond the scope of this tutorial, but includes airway management, appropriate resuscitation using intravenous fluids or blood products, administration of splanchnic vasoconstrictors such as terlipressin, broad-spectrum antibiotics, correction of clotting abnormalities, and usually prompt endoscopic management of bleeding. Interventional radiology procedures, such as TIPSS, should be considered in specialist centres if the bleeding is refractory to endoscopic management, with balloon tamponade being used as a holding measure until this is arranged.

Since variceal bleeding is a significant complication, most patients with a diagnosis of cirrhosis should be regularly screened for varices by upper GI endoscopy. Newer guidelines (Baveno VI) use transient elastography (FibroScan), which measures liver stiffness, to risk stratify for variceal surveillance. These guidelines state that cirrhotic patients with a FibroScan <20 kPa and a platelet count >150,000 can safely avoid screening endoscopy, and have repeat FibroScan and blood count after one year. However, in instances where FibroScan is not available, all patients should have an endoscopy following diagnosis of cirrhosis, and if no varices are found this should be repeated every 2–3 years.

Primary prophylaxis should be considered once varices are detected. Since NSBB and EVL are equally effective, patient choice plays a key role in determining the strategy. NSBB have common side effects such as lethargy and sexual dysfunction, although no further endoscopy is required once these drugs are started unless bleeding occurs. By contrast, EVL requires repeat endoscopy every two weeks following variceal obliteration, followed by annual surveillance checks. There is also a small risk of bleeding from banding-related ulcers (up to 8%).

Following the first variceal haemorrhage, secondary prophylaxis is typically with NSBB and EVL. These patients should also be considered for liver transplantation, depending on their liver function tests and complications of cirrhosis.

Further Reading

Mehta G, Abraldes J, Bosch J (2010). Developments and controversies in the management of oesophageal and gastric varices. *Gut* 59(6): 701–705.

Tripathi D, Stanley A, Hayes P, et al. (2015). UK guidelines on the management of variceal haemorrhage in cirrhotic patients. *Gut* 64(11): 1680–1704.

97. D) Non-alcoholic steatohepatitis

This gentleman is obese and has diabetes, hypertension, and dyslipidaemia with hypertriglyceridaemia. All these features are associated with insulin resistance or, 'metabolic syndrome'. This has a common association with fatty liver disease. He presents with right upper quadrant pain and a transaminitis. With the given data, the most likely diagnosis from the above is non-alcoholic steatohepatitis (NASH). A history of diabetes, arthritis, and impotence, coupled with deranged liver function tests and raised ferritin might suggest a diagnosis of haemochromatosis; however, this is far less common than NASH. The absence of excess alcohol use makes alcoholic hepatitis less likely, although a history of alcohol misuse may be withheld on presentation, hence one must maintain a high index of suspicion for this diagnosis. Moreover, alcoholic hepatitis is associated with AST:ALT >2, whereas it is often <1 in NASH. Primary biliary cirrhosis is associated with a predominant cholestatic picture with positive anti-mitochondrial antibodies. The negative autoimmune serology and the absence of hypergammaglobulinaemia make autoimmune hepatitis unlikely.

Tutorial

Fatty liver disease can range from fatty liver alone (steatosis) to fatty liver associated with inflammation (steatohepatitis). Steatohepatitis can occur in the absence or presence of alcohol abuse. If steatohepatitis is present without a history of alcohol abuse, the condition is termed NASH. NASH results from excessive lipid accumulation within the hepatocytes. Simple fatty liver is benign, but it can progress to cirrhosis, fibrosis, and hepatocellular carcinoma. The most common association is the metabolic syndrome, and the main risk factors are obesity, diabetes, and hypertriglyceridaemia. Other causes of fatty liver disease are listed in Box 4.8. This condition occurs most commonly in females. Most patients are asymptomatic, but if questioned, 50% of patients report persistent fatigue, malaise, and right upper quadrant discomfort. Hepatomegaly is common, and splenomegaly and stigmata of portal hypertension may occur in patients with cirrhosis.

Both AST and ALT are elevated with AST:ALT <1. Sometimes, the AST and ALT may be normal in NASH. The ALP can be elevated, but often less than 2–3 times the ULN. Hyperbilirubinaemia is rare. Serum ferritin and iron may be elevated as in other chronic liver disorders including alcoholic hepatitis. Although, iron overload occurs in a small proportion of patients with NASH, these patients often have severe disease. An ultrasound scan demonstrates a bright hyperechogenic liver (steatosis is detected only when the fatty change is more than 30%). Liver biopsy is the gold standard for establishing the diagnosis. The diagnosis should be considered in patients with features of the metabolic syndrome and unexplained elevations in serum aminotransferases, negative viral, and autoimmune serology in the absence of alcohol abuse. Coeliac disease may also cause unexplained elevations of liver enzymes, and should be excluded.

There is no specific treatment. The optimal strategy is modification of metabolic risk factors through weight loss, improved diet, and glycaemic control. Insulin sensitizing drugs, specifically thiazolidinediones and metformin have shown some biochemical and histological improvement; however, long-term data is lacking.

Box 4.8 Causes of fatty liver disease

- **Diabetes**
- **Obesity**
- **Hyperlipidaemia**
- **Alcohol**
- **Drugs**
  Amiodarone
  Tamoxifen
  Methotrexate
  Valproate
  Tetracyclines
- **Metabolic diseases**
  Galactosaemia
  Glycogen storage diseases
  Homocystinuria
  Tyrosinaemia
- **Nutritional disorders**
  Severe malnutrition
  Over-nutrition
  Total parenteral nutrition
  Starvation diets

Further Reading

Machado M, Diehl A (2016). Pathogenesis of nonalcoholic steatohepatitis. *Gastroenterology* 150(8): 1769–1777.

Oseini A, Sanyal A (2017). Therapies in non-alcoholic steatohepatitis (NASH). *Liver International* 37(1): 97–103.

98. A 22-year-old man presented with a non-tender lump on the left side of his neck. He had noticed it for approximately four weeks. He denied any infective symptoms, weight loss, or night sweats, but on interrogation, he admitted to pain in the centre of his chest and his neck when drinking at the weekends. A core biopsy of the node showed Reed-Sternberg cells. A bone marrow aspirate/trephine was reported as normal, but a CT scan showed involvement of nodes in the left cervical, mediastinum, para-aortic, and internal iliac regions. There was also mild splenic enlargement with several lesions within the spleen.

The correct diagnosis is:

A. Stage IIIA Hodgkin's lymphoma
B. Stage IIIB Hodgkin's lymphoma
C. Stage IVA diffuse large B-cell lymphoma
D. Stage IVB diffuse large B-cell lymphoma
E. Stage IVA Hodgkin's lymphoma

99. **A 19-year-old student was referred after she presented to A&E with shortness of breath and chest pain. A CTPA showed a large pulmonary embolus. Her previous medical history included a DVT, diagnosed three months previously , soon after starting the combined oral contraceptive pill. This was stopped and she was commenced on warfarin. She subsequently presented several times to A&E complaining of severe abdominal pain and was referred to gynaecology for investigation of suspected endometriosis. The A&E staff suspected her of drug-seeking behaviour, as she repeatedly requested opioid analgesia. Student Health had recently treated her for a possible urinary tract infection with ciprofloxacin. Under direct questioning, she admitted binge drinking at weekends but denied other drug use. There was no family history of thrombotic events.**

On examination, she was thin and appeared anxious. Her oxygen saturations were 99% on 2 L/min O$_2$, heart rate of 99/min and BP of 130/70 mmHg. Examination was otherwise unremarkable.

```
Investigations:
  Hb                     90 g/L
  Platelets              447 × 10⁹/L
  WCC                    11.1 × 10⁹/L
  Neutrophils            7.0 × 10⁹/L
  INR                    2.3
  D-Dimer                2450 ng/ml (normal <500 ng/ml)
  Urinary                β-hcG negative
She was admitted and commenced on therapeutic tinzaparin but
24 hours later had an episode of abdominal pain and dropped
her Hb to 83. A full thrombophilia screen was sent.
```

Which of the following tests is *least* useful?

A. ANA (antinuclear antibody)

B. Haptoglobins

C. Serum bilirubin level

D. Urine sample for haemoglobinuria

E. USS abdomen

100. **A 44-year-old woman presented with prolonged bleeding following dental extraction. She had had previous dental work in her teens without bleeding complications, and denied menorrhagia. She had noticed several bruises over the preceding few weeks, but attributed these to helping her friend move to a new house.**

Her history was significant for previous IV drug use, although she had not used drugs for almost two years. She worked in a massage parlour when using drugs to fund her habit, but at the time of presentation worked for a rehabilitation charity. She drank spirits most nights and smoked 30 g tobacco per week.

On examination, she had several bruises on her arms and thighs, and a number of petechiae under her watchstrap.

```
Investigations:
   Hb                          101 g/L
   Platelets                   7 × 10⁹/L
   WCC                         10.9 × 10⁹/L
   Neutrophils                 8.5 × 10⁹/L
```

Which of these tests would be *least* helpful in determining the cause of her thrombocytopaenia?

A. dsDNA levels

B. Hepatitis A

C. Hepatitis C

D. HIV testing

E. Quinine antibodies

101. **A 24-year-old Filipino nurse presented with lethargy. She had been in the UK for nine months, and had never travelled elsewhere. She had become a vegan six months previously after she joined an animal rights group. She had previously had problematic menorrhagia, but this improved significantly after starting the combined oral contraceptive pill. She was on no other medications.**

```
Investigations:
   Hb                      80 g/L
   Hct                     0.27
   MCV                     61 fl/cell
   MCH                     18.2 pg/cell
   Platelets               363 × 10⁹/L
   WCC                     5.1 × 10⁹/L
   CRP                     3 mg/L
   Reticulocyte            1%
   INR                     1.0
   B₁₂                     450 ng/L
   Folate                  7.6 µg/L
   Ferritin                410 µg/L
   HbA2                    1.3% (<2.5%)
   HbF                     0.35% (0.3-4.4%)
```

Which is the most likely diagnosis?

A. Alpha-thalassaemia carrier

B. Alpha-thalassaemia trait

C. Beta-thalassaemia trait

D. HbH disease

E. Iron-deficiency anaemia

102. A 70-year-old woman was referred for investigation of anaemia. She reported increasing lethargy and shortness of breath on exertion over the preceding few months that interfered with her ability to complete a round of golf. She denied any overt blood loss, and her GP performed faecal occult blood sampling, which was negative. She was an ex-smoker but otherwise well. She had previously been on low dose aspirin, but had stopped this two months previously on the advice of her GP, when she was first noted to have anaemia.

```
Investigations:
  Hb                        84 g/L
  MCV                       87 fL
  Platelets                 201 × 10⁹/L
  WCC                       5.3 × 10⁹/L
  Neutrophils               3.1 × 10⁹/L
  Sodium                    133 mmol/L
  Potassium                 3.7 mmol/L
  Urea                      6.1 mmol/L
  Creatinine                123 µmol/L
  Corrected calcium         2.8 mmol/L
  LDH                       198 iU/L
  CRP                       3 mg/L
  Urine dip                 no abnormalities
  Serum electrophoresis     no paraprotein band detected
  Immunoglobulins           IgA 1.1 g/L (0.8–3.0 g/L)
                            IgG 7.1 g/L (6.0–13.0 g/L)
                            IgM 1.3 g/L (0.4–2.5 g/L)
  Chest X-ray               no lung lesions, but lytic lesions
                            in T7 and T10
```

Which of the following tests is most likely to be diagnostic?

A. Biopsy of thoracic bony lesion
B. Bone marrow biopsy
C. Parathyroid-related peptide levels
D. Serum erythropoietin levels
E. Urine cytology

103. **A 79-year-old man presented with malaise, weight loss, and a 'lumpy neck' which he first noticed when he began to have difficulty shaving. He had increasingly frequent episodes of chest pain and dyspnoea on exertion. He denied melaena, haematemesis, haematuria, haemoptysis, or any other symptoms of blood loss. On examination, he had bilateral non-tender cervical, supraclavicular, and axillary lymphadenopathy, ranging between 1 and 3 cm. His heart sounds were dual, with an ejection systolic murmur which did not radiate. His lung fields were clear, and there were no palpable masses in the abdomen.**

```
Investigations:
  Hb                       83 g/L
  Platelets                224 × 10⁹/L
  WCC                      18.9 × 10⁹/L
  Neutrophils              2.1 × 10⁹/L
  Lymphocytes              16.1 × 10⁹/L
  Reticulocytes            6%
  Haptoglobin              0.4 gL (0.13-1.63 g/L)
  Sodium                   134 mmol/L
  Potassium                4.1 mmol/L
  Urea                     5.1 mmol/L
  Creatinine               87 µmol/L
  GGT                      34 iU/L
  Troponin                 0.2 ng/ml (<0.3 ng/ml)
  CRP                      23 mg/L
  PT                       13 s
  APTT                     28 s
```

The most likely cause of his low haemoglobin is:

A. Autoimmune haemolytic anaemia

B. Gastric ulceration from NSAID use

C. Gastrointestinal losses related to valvular heart disease

D. Myelofibrosis

E. Red cell aplasia

104. **A 26-year-old woman was referred for advice in pregnancy after a thrombophilia screen showed the results below. The screen was performed because her mother had developed a deep vein thrombosis (DVT) and pulmonary embolus (PE) following a recent hysterectomy. The woman was 17 weeks pregnant with her first child, and so far there had been no problems during pregnancy other than moderate pregnancy-induced emesis for six weeks. She had no history of previous clots, and was on no regular medications, nor had she been in the past.**

```
Investigations:
  Lupus anticoagulant                  negative
  Anti-thrombin III                    85 iU/dL (80-110 iU/dL)
  Factor V Leiden                      heterozygous
  Protein C                            120 iU/dL (80-135 iU/dL)
  Protein S                            105 iU/dL (80-120 iU/dL)
  Prothrombin gene (G20210A)           negative
  mutation
  APTT                                 24 seconds
  INR                                  1.0
  Platelets                            204 × 10⁹
```

What advice would you give this woman?

A. She does not require any anticoagulation treatment

B. She has a very high risk of miscarriage with these results

C. She should begin treatment dose low-molecular-weight heparin (LMWH) immediately and there is no need to monitor anti-Xa levels

D. She should begin treatment dose LMWH immediately with weekly anti-Xa level monitoring

E. She should commence treatment dose unfractionated daily subcutaneous heparin

105. **A 77-year-old man was diagnosed with microcytic anaemia, and was undergoing investigation. He had a haemoglobin of 84 g/L, which exacerbated his angina. A blood transfusion was arranged for symptomatic relief. Twenty-six years previously, following a cholecystectomy, he required a blood transfusion and suffered a profound reaction, although he could not remember what had happened exactly. He was anxious that the same would occur this time.**

His cross-match showed A-positive blood type with no other antibodies detected. It was explained that advances such as leucodepletion had been made with transfusions since he had last required one.

Which of the following types of transfusion reactions is this man *least* likely to get with leucodepleted red blood cells?

A. ABO incompatibility reaction

B. Delayed haemolytic transfusion reaction

C. Febrile non-haemolytic transfusion reaction

D. Graft-versus-host disease

E. Transfusion-related acute lung injury

106. **A 56-year-old man presented over the course of three months with two large haematomas. Ultrasound on each occasion was consistent with bleeding into the muscle. He denied any trauma preceding these events.**

He was otherwise fit and well. He had had a laparoscopic cholecystectomy ten years previously with no complications, and was on no regular prescription drugs, although he took Omega 3 and glucosamine from his local pharmacy.

```
Investigations:
  Hb                     1 39 g/L
  Platelets              378 × 10⁹/L
  WCC                    8.8. × 10⁹/L
  Neutrophils            5.9 × 10⁹/L
  APTT                   96 seconds
  Corrected APTT         32 seconds
  2 hour corrected       88 seconds
  D-Dimer                1050 ng/ml (normal <500 ng/ml)
  Fibrinogen             3.6 g/L
```

Which of the following is the most likely diagnosis?

A. Acquired factor VIII inhibitor

B. Anti-thrombin III deficiency

C. Haemophilia A

D. Idiopathic thrombocytopaenic purpura

E. von Willebrand disease

107. An 81-year-old woman was referred with a one-year history of anaemia. She had had a normal gastroscopy and colonoscopy. Chest and abdominal X-rays were normal, although an abdominal ultrasound suggested a mildly enlarged spleen. She denied any symptoms other than fatigue.

She took aspirin 75 mg od, simvastatin 20 mg od, candesartan 8 mg od, and amlodipine 10 mg od. She had a history of hypertension and transient ischaemic attacks. Examination was unremarkable.

```
Investigations:
  Hb                              80 g/L
  Hct                             0.27
  MCV                             110 fl
  Platelets                       171 × 10⁹/L
  WCC                             4.2 × 10⁹/L
  CRP                             3 mg/L
  Reticulocyte                    0.2%
  INR                             1.0
  B12                             896 ng/L
  Folate                          8.4 µg/L
  Ferritin                        213 µg/L
  Janus kinase 2 (JAK2)           negative
  Bone marrow aspirate/trephine   hypercellular marrow with
                                  hyposegmented granulocytes
                                  and megakaryocytes,
                                  6% blasts
```

Which of the following is true?

A. A prior history of chemotherapy with alkylating agents would adversely affect prognosis

B. G-CSF (granulocyte-colony stimulating factor) treatment will improve survival

C. Her best chance of long-term survival is with an autologous stem cell transplant

D. She has transformed to acute myeloid leukaemia (AML)

E. The JAK2 result rules out myelodysplasia

98. A) Stage IIIA Hodgkin's lymphoma

The above biopsy shows Reed-Sternberg cells which are pathognomonic for Hodgkin's lymphoma. These large cells have a bilobed nucleus and prominent nucleoli, forming the characteristic appearance of 'owl eyes'.

Staging of Hodgkin's lymphoma is based on the Cotswolds modified Ann Arbor Staging system which is shown in Table 5.1.

Table 5.1 Ann Arbor staging system for Hodgkin's lymphoma

Stage	Definition
I	Involvement of a single lymph node region or lymphoid structure
II	Involvement of ≥2 lymph node regions on the same side of the diaphragm
III	Involvement of lymph node regions or lymphoid structures on both sides of the diaphragm
IV	Involvement of extranodal site/s other than those designated as 'E'; more than one extranodal deposit at any location; or any involvement of liver or bone marrow
A/B	Absence/presence of B-symptoms: weight loss >10%, fever, drenching night sweats
E	Extranodal extension or single, isolated site of extranodal disease
X	Bulk >10 cm

Extracted from Lister T, Crowther D, Sutcliffe S, et al. (1989). Report of a committee convened to discuss the evaluation and staging of patients with Hodgkin's disease: Cotswolds meeting. *Journal of Clinical Oncology* 7(11): 1630–1636.

However, as the spleen is counted as a lymphoid structure, not an extranodal site, this patient has stage III disease.

The patient does not have any of the so-called B-cell symptoms, which are:

a) Unexplained weight loss of >10% of the body weight during the six months prior to staging investigations.

b) Unexplained, persistent or recurrent fever with temperatures >38°C during the previous month.

c) Recurrent drenching night sweats during the previous month.

Alcohol-induced pain is *not* a B-symptom, and is relatively rare. It can be present at diagnosis, and also at relapse.

Tutorial

Hodgkin's disease is one of the most common malignancies in young adults aged 16–35, with a second peak over the age of 50. Increased rates have been noted amongst siblings

(2–5 fold) and in those of Jewish ancestry. The most common presentation is with non-tender lymphadenopathy, generally in the cervical, supraclavicular, or axillary regions. One third of patients will have B symptoms at diagnosis, although they can also present with more unusual symptoms including severe pruritis, alcohol-induced pain, paraneoplastic syndromes, and erythema nodosum.

Diagnosis is generally made on a core biopsy, as an FNA often does not give sufficient structural information to confirm the type of lymphoma. Hodgkin's disease can be subtyped as nodular sclerosing (the majority), mixed cellularity, lymphocyte predominant, or lymphocyte depleted. Staging investigations include LDH, ESR, FBC, biochemistry profile, CT neck/chest/abdo/pelvis, and a bone marrow biopsy. PET scans are often used, and can be helpful in clarifying the correct stage by differentiating between reactive and involved nodes. They are also commonly used at completion of treatment to determine biochemical remission. It is common practice in the UK to undertake an interim PET after two cycles for advanced stage Hodgkin's and to adjust future treatment plans on this—so-called response adapted therapy (from the RATHL study). Poor prognostic indicators include: age (>60 years); male gender; elevated LDH and/or ESR; anaemia; stage III or IV disease; and presence of systemic (B) symptoms.

Treatment is dependent on stage at diagnosis, age, and co-morbidities. Those with stage III or IV disease require chemotherapy: the commonly used regimens are ABVD and BEACOPP. Consolidation radiation treatment may be required for those with bulky disease (>7 cm diameter) following chemotherapy. Those with stage II disease may be treated with 2–3 cycles of chemotherapy followed by involved field radiation; while stage I disease may be treated the same way, or with radiation alone in those wishing to avoid chemotherapy, or those with good prognosis disease.

Most patients with Hodgkin's disease have an excellent prognosis, with long-term survival of 50–90% depending on stage and treatment. Those with relapsed disease may still be salvaged with further chemotherapy and autologous stem cell treatment. Long-term complications of treatment for survivors include: increased risk of second malignancy (especially non-Hodgkin's lymphoma/haematological malignancy); subfertility; lung damage; increased risk of cardiac disease; and radiation-induced malignancy in radiation field. This risk is particularly significant for smokers who have received mediastinal radiation (lung cancer) and females who previously received mantle irradiation (breast cancer). Hodgkin's patients also require irradiated cellular blood components for life.

Further Reading

Barrington S, Kirkwood A, Franceschetto A, et al. (2016). PET-CT for staging and early response: results from the Response-Adapted Therapy in Advanced Hodgkin Lymphoma study. *Blood* 127(12): 1531–1538.

Lister T, Crowther D, Sutcliffe S, et al. (1989). Report of a committee convened to discuss the evaluation and staging of patients with Hodgkin's disease: Cotswolds meeting. *Journal of Clinical Oncology* 1989 7(11): 1630–1636.

99. A) ANA (antinuclear antibody)

This patient has presented with a significant thrombosis whilst on therapeutic warfarin, and has episodic severe abdominal pain associated with a decrease in haemoglobin. Haptoglobin levels decrease during episodes of intravascular haemolysis as the haptoglobin binds to free haemoglobin. A normal level of haptoglobin can occur with extravascular haemolysis. If elevated, serum bilirubin will also suggest haemolysis as the cause of anaemia.

The abdominal ultrasound should be performed with Dopplers to investigate the abdominal vasculature, as thrombosis of the mesenteric or hepatic vessels may be the cause of the severe abdominal pain in someone with known multiple thrombotic events. It would also investigate other causes for intermittent abdominal pain, including ovarian cysts or underlying malignancy.

Haemoglobinuria may be spasmodic or absent in intravascular haemolysis disorders such as paroxysmal nocturnal haemoglobinuria, which is the diagnosis in this patient.

There is no role for ANA testing in this patient, as this diagnosis is not associated with autoimmune disorders. If lupus is suspected, lupus anticoagulant testing (performed as part of the thrombophilia screen) and dsDNA testing are more appropriate.

Tutorial

Paroxysmal nocturnal haemoglobinuria (PNH) is a rare acquired haemolytic disorder caused by complement-mediated intravascular destruction of red blood cells. It results from an inactivating somatic mutation in a gene found on the X chromosome, known as PIG-A (phosphatidylinositol glycan A). This is required for the synthesis of the glycosyl phosphatidylinositol anchor (GPI) which attaches proteins to the cell surface. It is the absence of two of these proteins (CD55 and CD59)—both complement defence proteins—which results in the sensitivity to lysis and the abnormal initiation of clotting. If this mutation is expressed in a haematopoietic stem cell then all of its lineage will share the defect.

The three common signs are venous thrombosis, haemolytic anaemia and deficient haematopoiesis. The characteristic sign of haemoglobinuria ('Coca-Cola urine') is generally intermittent and often missed. Some patients will never have this. It most commonly occurs when complement is activated, such as during an infection.

Venous thrombosis is more common in those of European origin (up to 40–50% of patients), although less common in other ethnic groups. The most common vessels involved are intra-abdominal, such as mesenteric, hepatic, and portal veins. It can also cause Budd-Chiari syndrome, congestive splenomegaly, and severe abdominal pain. It can affect the usual venous targets (DVT and PE), and the cerebral venous sinuses. Thrombosis is one of the most common causes of death in PNH.

The diagnosis of PNH was previously made using the Ham test (acidified serum lysis test) but more recently, monoclonal antibodies against the GPI-anchored proteins have been used (usually CD55, CD59), together with flow cytometry.

The only curative treatment is allogeneic stem cell transplant, for those with a matched donor, although spontaneous remission may occur. There is a significant crossover with aplastic anaemia, and patients may progress from one condition to another. A monoclonal antibody directed against C5, eculizumab, was approved for treatment in 2007. It has been shown to reduce thrombotic events, episodes of haemolysis, and decrease red cell transfusion requirements; but increases the risk of infection with encapsulated bacteria, particularly *Neisseria meningitides,* hence vaccination for *Neisseria* prior to starting eculizumab is recommended. Treatment with eculizumab is controversial as it costs $440,000 per year (USD). Prior to this, treatment was supportive, including steroids during episodes of haemolysis, anticoagulation for those with a history of thrombosis (although this does not always prevent further episodes), and transfusion.

Further Reading

Brodsky R (2008). Advances in the diagnosis and therapy of paroxysmal nocturnal haemoglobinuria. *Blood Reviews* 22: 65–74.

Hillmen P, Young N, Schubert J, et al. (2006). The complement inhibitor eculizumab in paroxysmal nocturnal hemoglobinuria. *New England Journal of Medicine.* 355: 1233–1243.

100. B) Hepatitis A

This woman is at risk of having contracted HIV and hepatitis C as a result of her previous lifestyle, and both can cause thrombocytopaenia, both as autoimmune manifestations and as late changes.

Lupus is a common cause of thrombocytopaenia, although usually to a milder level, and hence testing for lupus with dsDNA is reasonable. Quinine antibodies are useful in eliminating this as a cause of severe thrombocytopaenia, as she has been drinking spirits, which may include mixers such as tonic (some forms of which include quinine). Hepatitis A, however, is not associated with ITP, although chronic hepatitis can cause low platelet levels for other reasons. There are rare reports of ITP secondary to hepatitis B.

Tutorial

This patient has ITP (idiopathic thrombocytopaenia purpura) caused by platelet antibodies which accelerate platelet destruction and inhibit platelet production. The most common manifestation is bleeding and excessive bruising. The majority of cases are primary, while others may be secondary to co-existing conditions. These are highlighted in Table 5.2.

Table 5.2 Common secondary causes of ITP

Cytomegalovirus	Acute secondary ITP is more common in children but is associated with ~1/30 of adults with ITP. The thrombocytopaenia generally recovers after the acute viral infection resolves.
Hepatitis C	This accounts for 20% of patients presenting with ITP. The pathophysiology is not well known. Anti-platelet antibodies are common, as is reduced production of thrombopoietin. Megakaryocytes may also be infected with Hep C, leading to further reduction in platelet production. The degree of thrombocytopaenia is less severe than in primary ITP. Steroids should be avoided as they may increase the viral load and transaminases.
HIV	HIV-related ITP was common prior to HAART (highly active antiretroviral therapy), but is now much less common (~4% patients). Rates are doubled in patients with AIDS. The mechanism is related to cross-reactivity of viral antibodies and GPIIIa. Patients may develop isolated thrombocytopaenia years before developing AIDS. Short-term treatment with prednisone, or splenectomy, is appropriate, although response rates are lower amongst IV drug users.
Haematological	CLL, Hodgkin's lymphoma, large granular T-lymphocyte leukaemia, and common variable immune deficiency are all rare causes of secondary ITP.
SLE	Some degree of thrombocytopaenia develops in up to one third of patients with SLE, with the most common causes antibodies to platelet glycoproteins and immune complexes. Severe thrombocytopaenia may develop during episodes of vasculitis. Antiphospholipid syndrome may also cause secondary thrombocytopaenia.

Reprinted from *The Lancet Oncology*, 15, 12, SV Rajkumar et al. (2014). International Myeloma Working Group updated criteria for the diagnosis of multiple myeloma, e538–e548, Copyright 2014, with permission from Elsevier.

The clinical course of ITP varies hugely: some require a single course of steroids to achieve remission, whilst others will require splenectomy, and may still go on to have further relapses even when asplenic. The latter group of patients is more likely to have inhibition of megakaryocytes and enhanced clearance of platelets.

The bleeding manifestations of this disorder also vary from patient to patient. Some will have frequent bleeding with platelet counts of ≥20, whilst others do not have bleeding with counts of 5. Thrombocytopaenia may also increase the risk of thrombosis in some patients, although whether this may be due to the co-existence of an anti-phospholipid disorder is not clear.

Further Reading

Cines D, Bussel J, Liebman H, Luning Prak E (2009). The ITP syndrome: pathogenic and clinical diversity. *Blood* 113: 6511–6521.

101. D) HbH disease

The results show a microcytic, hypochromic anaemia, with normal ferritin, folate, and B$_{12}$ levels. The level of ferritin rules out iron-deficiency anaemia; with a normal CRP, it is unlikely to be elevated as an acute phase reactant. The reticulocyte percentage is normal. That leaves the thalassaemia options. Of the alpha-thalassaemias, only HbH is associated with a significant microcytic anaemia (the other two generally have normal haemoglobin levels). Beta-thalassaemia trait is associated with microcytosis and hypochromia, but not with significant anaemia.

Tutorial

Thalassaemia is due to reduced production of the α or β-globin chains, resulting in abnormal haemoglobin molecules with reduced oxygen transport capacity and anaemia; and an inability to produce normal foetal haemoglobin (made up of 2α and 2γ chains) or adult haemoglobin (made of 2α and 2β chains). The condition may be asymptomatic or severe, depending on the number of genes affected, and the number of copies of the chains able to be synthesized.

Alpha-thalassaemia is caused by mutations or deletions affecting one or more of the α-globin genes, leading to decreased or absent α-globin production from the affected gene. Normally, each person has two alpha-globin genes on each copy of chromosome 16 (four genes per person in total). Those with inactivation or deletion of one gene cause few problems (alpha-thalassaemia carrier: -α/αα); those with two gene deletions/inactivations (alpha-thalassaemia trait: --/αα or -α/-α) have microcytic, hypochromic cells but levels of red cells are generally at the lower limit of normal. Those lacking three genes (HbH disease: --/-α) have moderate anaemia, marked microcytosis, and hypochromia, along with an excess of β-globin chains that form β4 tetramers (HbH). In alpha-thalassaemia major, those lacking all α-globin genes (also known as Hb Barts) die *in utero* or shortly after birth (hydrops foetalis) as they are unable to make normal foetal or adult haemoglobin.

HbH is an unstable tetramer and forms intracellular precipitates when oxidized, which can cause intramedullary erythroid cell death and ineffective production of erythrocytes. Precipitates that form in circulating red cells cause membrane dysfunction and decreased red cell survival. However, the main cause of anaemia in HbH is haemolysis. Episodes of haemolysis may be precipitated by fever/infections, parvovirus B19 infection, hypersplenism, and pregnancy. Haemolysis causes severe anaemia and requires transfusion.

HbH is also associated with iron overload, which is independent of previous transfusions or iron supplementation. This is most likely due to increased iron absorption, with overload particularly problematic in heavy alcohol drinkers. This can progress to diabetes, cardiac iron overload, and cirrhotic liver disease.

The beta-thalassaemias occur when there is reduced or absent synthesis of the beta-globin genes. Over 200 gene mutations of the β-globin genes have been identified, with the highest incidence generally found in those of Cypriot, Greek, Asian, Chinese, and Afro-Caribbean descent. There is generally consistent synthesis of the gamma-globin genes, which results in higher levels of foetal haemoglobin (also known as HbF, α2γ2). The severity of the condition depends on the number and type of abnormal genes involved, and can be divided into three main categories: thalassaemia major, thalassaemia intermedia, and thalassaemia minor.

Beta-thalassaemia major occurs when two separate mutations of the β-globin genes are inherited, resulting in either β0 where the β-globin chains are absent, or β + thalassaemia where there are partial β-chains. Both are associated with severe anaemia, hypertrophy of the bone marrow with secondary skeletal changes, and marked hepatosplenomegaly. Anaemia generally presents after three months of age, when children would generally switch from producing γ chains (HbF) to β-chains. Those with partial chains may not present until they are aged 3–4 years. Children generally present with failure to thrive, symptomatic anaemia, and hepatosplenomegaly. Extra-medullary haematopoiesis occurs as a response to the anaemia, and can result in 'thalassaemia facies' with facial bossing and an enlarged maxilla. The characteristic change noted on X-rays is referred to as 'hair on end'.

Blood transfusions are usually required every 6–8 weeks to maintain haemoglobin levels, and patients require iron chelation therapy to prevent iron overload syndrome. Children (and surviving adults) are generally functionally asplenic, and at risk of infection from encapsulated bacteria such as *Pneumococcus, Meningococcus,* and *Haemophilus.*

Thalassaemia intermedia is a clinical diagnosis, usually caused by mild defects in the β-globin chain synthesis that may still allow for some normal chain production. The anaemia is generally milder, and the need for blood transfusion is much less.

Thalassaemia minor (also known as thalassaemia trait) includes those heterozygous for β-thalassaemia and carriers. They are generally asymptomatic, with very mild anaemia, as the remaining normal gene synthesises adequate amounts of β-globin chains. Populations with high carrier rates of thalassaemia are advised to undergo screening.

Further Reading

Chui D, Fucharoen S, Chan V (2003). Haemoglobin H disease: not necessarily a benign disorder. *Blood* 101: 791–800.

102. B) Bone marrow biopsy

This patient presented with a combination of anaemia, impaired renal function, hypercalcaemia, and lytic bone lesions with a normal bone scan. This should indicate multiple myeloma, despite the normal serum electrophoresis, as light chain myeloma will show a normal electrophoresis pattern. This can be confirmed by bone marrow biopsy, where clonal plasma cell infiltration will be observed. Some of these factors (impaired renal function, hypercalcaemia) may occur in renal cell cancer, but this is seldom associated with anaemia unless due to large amounts of haematuria. Urine cytology is a helpful screen for bladder cancer but not renal cancer.

Parathyroid-related peptide levels are non-diagnostic and will only demonstrate that the hypercalcemia is from some form of malignancy. Finally, biopsy of a lytic lesion will show high levels of bone turnover, but is unlikely to yield enough cells to be diagnostic.

Tutorial

Multiple myeloma makes up 13% of haematological malignancies. It is characterized by a clonal proliferation of malignant plasma cells in the bone marrow, monoclonal protein in the urine or blood, and secondary organ impairment, such as renal failure. It most commonly produces IgG paraprotein (70%); 20% produce IgA, 5–10% will have light chain myeloma, and 1% of patients have IgM myeloma, IgD, IgE, or non-secretory myeloma.

Myeloma may be asymptomatic or symptomatic, based on whether or not there is organ dysfunction such as hypercalcaemia, anaemia, renal impairment, or bone involvement. The most common manifestations at diagnosis are anaemia (~75%, usually secondary to renal impairment or marrow infiltration), bone disease (~80%), and renal impairment (20–40%, caused by direct tubular toxicity from high protein loads, dehydration, hypercalcaemia, and nephrotoxic medication).

The recommended workup for myeloma includes routine blood and urine tests, bone marrow sampling and imaging:

- FBC with differential and blood film.
- Biochemistry including renal function and bone profile.
- Serum protein electrophoresis with immunofixation.

- Immunoglobulins.
- Routine urinalysis and 24-hour urine collection for proteinuria, electrophoresis, and immunofixation.
- Quantification of urine M-component level and albuminuria.

Bone marrow aspirate and trephine should be sent with testing for cytogenetics, FISH, and immunophenotyping. Imaging should include a bone survey; low-dose whole-body CT or MRI, and PET-CT.

It is possible to have a normal serum protein electrophoresis result in light chain myeloma, but patients will have elevated levels of either kappa or lambda light chains. The rare subtype of non-secretory myeloma will have both normal levels of serum free light chains and normal serum electrophoresis, but will show myeloma clones on bone marrow sampling.

The International Myeloma Working Group (IMWG) published the following revised criteria for diagnosis of myeloma to include three 'myeloma defining events'. If at least one of these events is present, then that is sufficient for the diagnosis of multiple myeloma regardless of the absence of symptoms or end-organ dysfunction: these events have been shown to be associated with at least an 80% risk of developing myeloma-related organ damage within two years. The new definition of multiple myeloma is:

≥10% clonal bone marrow plasma cells OR biopsy-proven bony or extramedullary plasmacytoma *and* any one of more of the following 'CRAB' features or myeloma-defining events:

- ◆ 'CRAB' features: evidence of myeloma-related organ dysfunction:
- ◆ Hyper**C**alcaemia (serum Ca >2.75 mmol/L)
- ◆ **R**enal impairment (creatinine >177 μmol/L)
- ◆ **A**naemia (haemoglobin <100 g/L)
- ◆ **B**one disease (one or more lytic lesion on X-ray/CT or PET-CT)

Reprinted from *The Lancet Oncology*, 15, 12, SV Rajkumar et al., International Myeloma Working Group updated criteria for the diagnosis of multiple myeloma, e538-e548, Copyright 2014, with permission from Elsevier

- Myeloma-defining events: biomarkers of malignancy:
  - ◆ Sixty per cent or greater clonal plasma cells on bone marrow biopsy.
  - ◆ Serum involved/uninvolved free light chain ration of 100 or greater, provided the absolute level of the involved light chain is at least 100 mg/L.
  - ◆ More than one focal lesion on MRI that is at least 5 mm or greater in size.

Patients with <10% clonal bone marrow plasma cells, serum monoclonal protein <30 g/L, and no evidence of organ dysfunction are classified as having MGUS (monoclonal gammopathy of uncertain significance), which may progress to myeloma and therefore should be followed up regularly.

There are a number of variables important to prognosis for myeloma, including tumour-specific features such as IgA myeloma (versus other subtypes); levels of β-2 microglobulin; immunoglobulins and LDH; the percentage of bone marrow plasmacytosis; the presence of renal failure and significant hypercalcaemia. Patient factors such as age, albumin level, performance status, and co-morbidities are also important, particularly in determining treatment options.

There is no advantage to early treatment and therefore asymptomatic patients may be observed until symptoms develop. Conversely, the treatment of symptomatic myeloma should begin immediately and should be tailored to the age and general fitness of the patient. Aggressive treatment for young patients generally involves induction chemotherapy followed by stem cell transplant. Those aged over 65 generally receive chemotherapy alone, with induction chemotherapy followed by maintenance treatment. The use of drugs such as thalidomide/lenalidomide and bortezomib have greatly increased life expectancy; but even with the most aggressive treatment, complete response rates are low and relapses are common.

Symptomatic treatment is an important aspect of the management of myeloma. Anaemia can be treated with drugs such as erythropoietin and blood transfusions. Bisphosphonates are useful for those with bony disease or hypercalcaemia, and have been shown to reduce the rate of pathological fractures as well as new bone disease. They require dose adjustment in patients with significant renal impairment, and all patients should have a baseline dental assessment due to the risk of osteonecrosis of the jaw. Finally, radiation treatment can be useful for those with painful bony metastases or those with spinal cord compression.

Further Reading

Palumbo A, Anderson K (2011). Multiple myeloma. *New England Journal of Medicine* 364: 1046–1060.

Rajkumar S, Dimopoulos M, Palumbo A, et al. (2014). International Myeloma Working Group updated criteria for the diagnosis of multiple myeloma. *Lancet Oncology* 15(12): e538–548.

103. A) Autoimmune haemolytic anaemia

This patient has autoimmune haemolytic anaemia secondary to chronic lymphocytic leukaemia. This affects up to 5% of patients with CLL at some point in their illness. Red cell aplasia is another manifestation of anaemia related to CLL, but this presents with normal haptoglobin levels and low levels of reticulocytes; however, this patient has low haptoglobins and elevated reticulocytes in keeping with haemolysis. The normal urea and lack of melaena or haematemesis make GI losses less likely; and this patient does not clinically describe aortic stenosis, which is associated with gastrointestinal vascular malformations. Myelofibrosis would not give an elevated lymphocyte count or lymphadenopathy, and is not associated with transformation to CLL.

Tutorial

Between 10–20% of patients with chronic lymphocytic leukaemia (CLL) will develop autoimmune cytopaenias, of which autoimmune haemolytic anaemia (AIHA) is the most common at 7%, although immune thrombocytopaenia (2–5%), pure red cell aplasia (<1%), or autoimmune granulocytopaenia (<1%) can also occur. Autoimmune haemolytic anaemia may occur before patients require treatment for their CLL, although the risk is highest in advanced disease. A similar picture can occur with bone marrow infiltration, and occasionally with cold-agglutinin disease.

AIHA is also reported in other haematological malignancies such as non-Hodgkin's lymphoma. Conversely, patients with AIHA are at an increased risk of developing non-Hodgkin's lymphoma, multiple myeloma, CLL, or other myeloid malignancies.

The classical presentation of AIHA related to CLL is symptomatic anaemia with the associated features from increased red cell breakdown: an isolated fall in haemoglobin accompanied by a positive direct antiglobulin test (DAT) with a reticulocytosis, raised bilirubin, elevated LDH and decreased haptoglobins. A positive DAT without haemolysis is more frequent than AIHA in CLL and myelodysplastic syndrome (MDS). The diagnosis should be confirmed with flow cell cytometry with a bone marrow aspirate/trephine reserved for cases of greater diagnostic uncertainty. Similar findings can occur with other causes of anaemia, such as red cell aplasia. It is also possible that other factors such as recent chemotherapy (particularly fludarabine) and bone marrow infiltration may impact on aspects of the typical presentation such as reticulocytosis. CMV and parvovirus B19 infection should also be excluded.

ITP has no precise diagnostic test but a fall in platelet count with no other cause for thrombocytopaenia is suggestive; it may occur in conjunction with AIHA as Evans syndrome. Pure red cell aplasia is a less common cause of anaemia in CLL, and typically presents with a normochromic, normocytic anaemia with low reticulocytes and a negative DAT. Pure red cell aplasia may be precipitated by infection with Epstein-Barr virus, cytomegalovirus, and parvovirus B19. A bone marrow aspirate and biopsy will generally show arrest of erythroblast maturation.

There are no controlled trials or studies on the management of AIHA in CLL, but a trial of steroids is the usual first line. If this fails, other agents such as ciclosporin or rituximab can be trialled, or combination chemo-immunotherapy for the CLL itself. In severe cases, splenectomy can be considered.

Further Reading

British Society for Haematology (2017). *British Society for Haematology Guidelines: Management of Drug-Induced Immune and Secondary Autoimmune Haemolytic Anaemia April 2017*. British Society for Haematology, London.

Hodgson K, Ferrer G, Pereira A, Moreno C, Montserrat E (2011). Autoimmune cytopaenia in chronic lymphocytic leukaemia: diagnosis and treatment. *British Journal of Haematology* 154: 14–22.

Mauro F, Foa R, Cerretti R, et al. (2000). Autoimmune haemolytic anaemia in chronic lymphocytic leukaemia: clinical, therapeutic, and prognostic features. *Blood* 95: 2786–2792.

104. A) She does not require any anticoagulation treatment

This screen was prompted by thrombotic events in her mother, which occurred following provocation (pelvic surgery), which carries a relatively high risk of thrombosis. There is no suggestion that her mother had clots in pregnancy which is a relatively high-risk situation. This woman does not have any personal history of clots and therefore there is no current indication to commence anticoagulation with these results.

Anti-phospholipid syndrome is a common cause of recurrent miscarriage, but she tests negative for this and has no personal history of miscarriage. Her risk of miscarrying with Factor V Leiden deficiency is not particularly high. If patients are commenced on treatment dose LMWH in pregnancy, they should have regular anti-Xa level monitoring.

Tutorial

Thrombophilia, or a predisposition to thrombotic events, may be inherited or acquired. Each has different underlying mechanisms and associated risks of thrombosis. In addition to the acquired syndromes, there are also temporary conditions which increase the risk of a thrombotic event such as pregnancy, oral contraceptive use, surgery (particularly pelvic or orthopaedic), or prolonged immobility.

A deficiency in the anticoagulant proteins antithrombin, Protein C, and Protein S, can all result in thrombosis. Heterozygotes (with 50–60% deficiency) in each condition have a ten-fold increased risk of venous thromboembolism (VTE) compared to the general population. Homozygosity for antithrombin is incompatible with life; whilst homozygotes for Protein C or Protein S generally present with purpura fulminans soon after birth, with major thromboembolic complications. Each of these can be tested for using functional or immunological assays, to assess the amount and activity of each protein present.

In contrast, increased levels of pro-coagulant proteins (generally through gain-of-function mutations) can also cause thrombophilia. Of these, the most common is heterozygosity for a Factor V Leiden mutation (also known as activated protein C (APC) resistance), which is present in 3–5% of the European population. This is the most common cause of unprovoked deep vein thromboses and pulmonary emboli in Caucasian populations, although the overall risk in heterozygotes is only increased by 2.5-fold. Those who are homozygous for Factor V Leiden have an 80-fold increased risk.

The other common pro-coagulant mutation is the prothrombin G20210A gene mutation. This mutation causes a substitution from guanine (G) to adenine (A) at position 20210 on the gene, resulting in increased circulating levels of prothrombin. Heterozygotes have a 2–3-fold risk of VTE compared to the general population.

Antiphospholipid syndrome is an acquired autoimmune disorder, defined as the persistence of one or more antiphospholipid antibodies measured at least 12 weeks apart (anti-cardiolipin antibody or lupus anticoagulant or anti-β2-glycoprotein I antibody), together with either morbidity in pregnancy or ≥1 episode of arterial, venous, or small vessel thrombosis. Pregnancy complications include: three or more unexplained consecutive spontaneous miscarriages before ten weeks of pregnancy; one or more otherwise unexplained intrauterine deaths at or beyond ten weeks (i.e. normal foetus with normal placenta); or one or more premature births before 34 weeks as a result of pre-eclampsia, eclampsia, or recognized features of placental insufficiency. Anti-phospholipid syndrome may be primary or secondary to other conditions (most often systemic lupus erythematosus). It is important to note that antiphospholipid antibodies can occur transiently due to infections such as HIV, hepatitis C, and malaria; lymphoproliferative conditions such as lymphoma; and some drugs, such as anticonvulsants. Therefore, in order to diagnose antiphospholipid syndrome, the patient must have two positive tests for an antiphospholipid antibody at least 12 weeks apart.

Although the relative risk of VTE is increased by 4–6-fold in pregnancy and post-partum, the absolute risk is low with an overall incidence of 1–2 per 1000 pregnancies: up to half of these occur in women with an underlying procoagulant condition. The most common of these is Factor V Leiden heterozygosity, although this is one of the lower risk thrombophilias. Inherited thrombophilias may also be associated with other adverse events in pregnancy such as early pregnancy loss, late pregnancy loss (beyond first trimester), pre-eclampsia, placental abruption, and intrauterine growth retardation.

Thrombophilias in pregnancy can be risk-stratified in order to guide thrombo-prophylactic management, and risk stratification as well as treatment advice can be found in guidelines by the Royal College of Obstetrics and Gynaecology on *Thrombosis and Embolism during Pregnancy and the Puerperium*. Where anticoagulation is advised, low molecular weight heparin is the anticoagulant agent of choice for antenatal and postnatal thromboprophylaxis and is safe in breastfeeding.

New oral anticoagulants (NOACs) should be avoided in pregnancy and are not currently recommended in women who are breastfeeding. Warfarin is only used in patients in whom LMWH is deemed unsuitable: for example women with mechanical heart valves as warfarin crosses the placenta and is associated with an increased risk of congenital abnormalities

Further Reading

Keeling D, Mackie I, Moore G, Greer I, Greaves M (2012). Guidelines on the investigation and management of antiphospholipid syndrome. *British Journal of Haematology* 157: 47–58.

Lim W, Eikelboom J, Ginsberg J (2007). Inherited thrombophilia and pregnancy associated venous thromboembolism. *British Medical Journal* 334: 1318–1321.

Royal College of Obstetrics and Gynaecologists (2015). *Thrombosis and Embolism during Pregnancy and the Puerperium, Reducing the Risk* (Green-top Guideline No. 37a). Royal College of Obstetrics and Gynaecologists, London.

105. C) Febrile non-haemolytic transfusion reaction

Inclusion of donor leucocytes in red blood cell units is the most common cause of febrile non-haemolytic transfusion reactions (FNHTR). Delayed haemolytic transfusion reactions and transfusion-related acute lung injury are also immune responses, but leucodepletion does not reduce the risk of either of these. The risk of graft-versus-host disease is reduced but not removed by leucodepletion. ABO incompatibility reactions are not related to the presence of white cells in the blood.

Tutorial

The transfusion of blood products saves many lives per year and modern transfusions are much safer than those of years ago. There have been many advances in the preparation of red blood cells, designed to minimize complications and reactions, but some reactions remain a life-threatening risk.

Leucodepletion (removal of white cells) of red blood cell units reduces the most common reaction: FNHTR. It also reduces transmission of cytomegalovirus (CMV) and HLA alloimmunization. Prior to leucodepletion, the fever/chill reaction was estimated to occur in 20–25% of transfusions, but is now reported in 1:300 transfusions. The fever was caused by the immune response of the transfusion recipient directed against the white cells from the donor.

Transfusion-associated graft-versus-host disease is a rare but very serious complication of transfusion in immunosuppressed patients, which can result in multi-organ failure. It generally presents 4–30 days after the transfusion, with fever, rash, diarrhoea, hepatitis, lymphadenopathy, and pancytopaenia. Those most at risk are: those on immunosuppressive agents such as fludarabine; recipients of allogeneic stem cell transplants; those with congenital immunodeficiencies; and those receiving *in utero* transfusions. The risk can be reduced significantly by irradiating the red blood cells to prevent the proliferation of donor lymphocytes within the immunocompromised recipient, but those who develop the syndrome have a mortality rate of ~90%.

ABO incompatibility resulting in anaphylaxis is now a very rare complication, and generally occurs with accidental mis-labelling of blood. Improvements in techniques mean this is now very rare, and is estimated to occur in less than 1:38000 transfusions.

Haemolytic reactions are also due to immune-mediated reactions: they can range from immediate, fulminant haemolysis to mild, delayed (>24 hours post-transfusion) haemolytic reactions which result in mild jaundice and a drop in haemoglobin over the following week. The degree and rapidity of reaction is dependent on the amount of complement and cytokines released. Most are due to non-ABO antibodies: serious reactions occur in 1:76000 transfusions, although this figure is improving with increasing recognition and matching for antibodies.

TRALI (transfusion-related acute lung injury) is the most frequent cause of transfusion-related mortality reported to the FDA (Food and Drug Administration). It is currently estimated to occur in 1:5000 reactions and can occur with most plasma-containing blood components. It is caused by host antibodies directed against a variety of antigens, and presents within 1–2 hours of transfusion with chills, fever, non-productive cough, dyspnoea, cyanosis, and hypotension or hypertension. X-ray findings most typically show bilateral infiltrates without cardiomegaly, leading to its previous name of non-cardiogenic pulmonary oedema.

For all transfusion reactions, the blood transfusion should be stopped and 0.9% NaCl delivered via a different giving set. The patient ID, blood label, and blood bank number should be re-checked and vital signs monitored. Further investigation and monitoring should be tailored to the patient's status and the nature of their reaction; however, in all cases, blood bank should be notified and a transfusion reaction sample sent to the lab (EDTA sample and red top) with sufficient clinical information to guide appropriate type and speed of investigations.

Further Reading

Clarke G (2017). Investigation and management of non-infectious transfusion reactions. *Vox Sanguinis* 12: 80–86.

Tinegate H, Birchall J, Gray A, et al. (2012). Guideline on the investigation and management of acute transfusion reactions prepared by the BCSH Blood Transfusion Task Force. *British Journal of Haematology* 159: 143–153.

106. A) Acquired factor VIII inhibitor

Spontaneous bleeding into the muscle or joints is generally a sign of haemophilia. However, in this patient, there was no history of bleeding until three months previously. This suggests an acquired deficiency, especially given the previous uncomplicated surgery. The initial APTT correction might suggest that there is indeed a factor deficiency, but this reverses at two hours. This suggests that there is an inhibitor which often takes time to inhibit the respective clotting factors. Von Willebrand disease does not generally result in spontaneous muscle bleeding. Anti-thrombin III deficiency causes a thrombophilic state, not spontaneous bleeding, hence this is not the correct answer. There are normal levels of platelets, ruling out ITP.

Tutorial

Circulating inhibitors are generally IgG antibodies that deplete or inhibit coagulation factors, the most common of which are factor VIII and von Willebrand factor. Inhibitors against other coagulation factors are only occasionally reported. Anti-factor VIII antibodies can occur as a secondary phenomenon in patients who are post-partum, have autoimmune conditions or AIDS, but 50% of patients will have no other underlying conditions. These are listed in Table 5.3. The incidence follows a double peak, with an initial peak between the ages of 20 and 40, but most commonly presents during the second peak around 75–80 years old. The incidence is around 1.5 per million per year.

Table 5.3 Common causes of acquired haemophilias

Cause	Examples
Idiopathic (approx. 50%)	
Autoimmune disease	Rheumatoid arthritis, polymyalgia rheumatica, systemic lupus erythematous, Graves' disease
Malignancy	CLL, non-Hodgkin's lymphoma, breast cancer, colorectal cancer
Drugs	Penicillin, sulphonamides, clopidogrel
Infection	Acute hepatitis B and C, *Mycoplasma pneumonia*, HIV
Skin conditions	Pemphigoid
Pregnancy	

Acquired factor VIII inhibition, or acquired haemophilia A (AHA), differs from congenital haemophilia A in the pattern of bleeding. More than 80% of those with acquired factor VIII inhibitors have haemorrhages into the muscle, skin, soft tissue, or mucosal membranes; however, the trademark haemarthroses of congenital haemophilia are very rare. The critical test is the failure of normal plasma to correct the prolonged APTT, as the patient's plasma will progressively inactivate the coagulation protein. The diagnostic dilemma in a patient with suspected AHA is generally between an isolated factor deficiency, lupus anticoagulant, and AHA. In patients in whom classical haemophilia has been excluded (generally on the basis of medical history and presentation), then a screening test of PT, APTT, and mixing studies should be performed to confirm the cause. Mixing studies are performed by mixing normal plasma with patient plasma and incubating for one or two hours because factor VIII inhibitory antibodies are often time-dependent; they are also temperature-dependent. The presence of lupus anticoagulant can mimic factor VIII inhibitors, and therefore the guidelines recommend its exclusion in the diagnostic tree (Figure 5.1). ELISA-based assays have been reported for factor VIII inhibitor detection which may avoid interference by lupus anticoagulant.

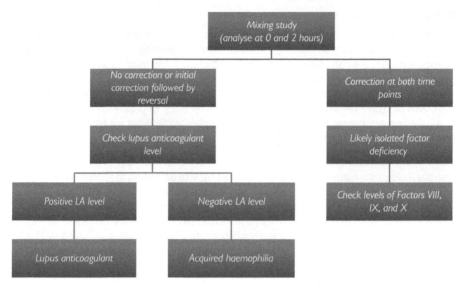

Figure 5.1 Diagnosis tree to investigate a prolonged APTT. LA: lupus anticoagulant.

Many patients with AHA will require only observation due to the relatively quick spontaneous remission most patients have. Those who do require treatment during an acute bleed should be discussed with a haematologist to achieve prompt haemostatic control whilst avoiding the increased risk of thrombosis associated with treatment by bypassing agents. The most popular bypassing agents used are recombinant factor VIIa (rFVIIa; NovoSeven) and the activated prothrombin complex concentrate (aPCC) factor VIII inhibitor bypassing activity (FEIBA).). A period of treatment at reduced dose and frequency after initial control has been achieved is often needed to prevent recurrence and should be assessed on a case-by-case basis.

Treatment with human FVIII concentrates is less effective unless combined with immunoadsorption or plasmapheresis. Desmopressin has also been used in patients with low titres of inhibitor; however, clinical response is unpredictable and not as good as that seen with bypassing agents. Adjunct therapies such as tranexamic acid and IV Ig have also been used.

Immunosuppression to eradicate the inhibitor should be started as soon as the diagnosis has been made to reduce the time the patient is at risk of bleeding. First-line treatment is with prednisolone 1 mg/kg/day either alone or combined with cyclophosphamide 1–2 mg/day: the latter probably results in a higher complete remission but long-term outcome in terms of disease-free and overall survival is unaffected. If there is poor response in the first month, second-line therapies such as rituximab combined with calcineurin inhibitors can be trialled. IV Ig is not recommended as a treatment for inhibitor eradication. Patients should be followed up at least monthly for the first six months because relapse is common.

Further Reading

Collins W, Chalmers E, Hart D, et al. (2013). A United Kingdom Haemophilia Centre Doctors' Organization (UKHCDO) guideline approved by the British Committee for Standards in Haematology; Diagnosis and management of acquired coagulation inhibitors: a guideline from UKHCDO. *British Journal of Haematology* 162: 758–773.

Franchini M, Targher G, Montagnana M, Lippi G (2008). Laboratory, clinical and therapeutic aspects of acquired haemophilia A. *Clinica Chimica Acta* 395: 14–18.

107. A) A prior history of chemotherapy with alkylating agents would adversely affect prognosis

This patient has myelodysplasia, as evidenced by the dysplastic marrow and macrocytic anaemia with normal B$_{12}$, folate, and ferritin and reticulocytopaenia suggesting a primary marrow problem. The blast cell count is below the 20% required to diagnose transformation to acute myeloid leukaemia. JAK2 is much more commonly abnormal in myelofibrosis and other myeloproliferative disorders; it is only positive in 5% of myelodysplasia, and therefore a normal result would not rule out the diagnosis. The treatment for myelodysplasia includes observation and supportive treatment with red blood cell transfusion and G-CSF when required. However, G-CSF treatment (useful for neutropaenia, especially if the patient has recurrent infections) has not been shown to improve overall survival. Up to a third of patients will die of other causes. At 81 years old, with ischaemic co-morbidities, this patient is likely to have a significant risk of morbidity and mortality with autologous stem cell transplant, thus excluding this treatment option for her, although it can be useful for younger patients without significant co-morbidities. A prior history of chemotherapy with alkylating agents would indicate that the myelodysplasia is secondary to the previous chemotherapy, and patients with secondary myeloid neoplasms have a shorter median survival than those who have *de novo* myelodysplastic syndrome. Therefore, the prognosis is much poorer in those with previous chemotherapy.

Tutorial

The myelodysplastic disorders are a heterogeneous group of disorders, all of which involve ineffective blood cell production from a cellular bone marrow, producing dysplastic changes in one or more cell lineages, cytopaenias, and a variable predilection to progress to AML. It most commonly presents in patients over 65. The incidence is approximately 4 in 100,000 per year but in over-70 population it increases to >30 in 100,000 per year. It is usually an incidental finding on routine blood tests. A non-age related secondary MDS can occur secondary to previous treatment, usually alkylating chemotherapy given for previous malignancy (haematological or solid tumours). Treatment-associated MDS is associated with a more rapid transformation to an acute leukaemia and is much more resistant to treatment.

The presentation of symptomatic patients is usually with gradual onset of fatigue, pallor, and dyspnoea, but only 50% are symptomatic with diagnosis. Examination is usually unremarkable other than signs of anaemia, although ~20% will have splenomegaly. Occasionally skin conditions such as Sweets syndrome can occur.

A bone marrow is required for diagnosis and differentiation from leukaemia. The marrow is generally hypercellular or normocellular, with specific changes related to the specific myelodysplastic syndrome (such as ringed sideroblasts). However, common changes include hyposegmented, hypogranulated granulocytes, nuclear abnormalities in erythroblasts, and megaloblastic cells. The presence of 20% of blasts in marrow is generally considered the defining feature of acute leukaemia, rather than MDS.

The underlying problem in MDS is a clonal haemapoietic stem cell population with cytogenetic abnormalities present in about 50% of patients. These can be important for prognosis with some, such as del(5q), associated with a much better prognosis, while others (any chromosome 7 mutation) have a much shorter prognosis. These genetic alterations lead to the increased apoptosis of marrow cells, disordered iron metabolism, and ineffective erythropoiesis. Cytogenetic analysis should be performed on all patients diagnosed with MDS.

The prognosis of patients varies from months to many years. A scoring and prognostic system, revised by the 2012 International Prognostic Scoring System (IPSS-R), can help guide treatment. In general more severe cytopaenias, higher the bone marrow blast percentage, and certain cytogenetic mutations all confer a worse prognosis.

Treatment of MDS varies based on age and co-morbidity. Younger patients should be considered for stem cell transplant, which is the only curative option, but this comes with significant morbidity and mortality. Supportive treatment with antibiotics, transfusion, G-CSF, and erythropoietin have been shown to improve symptoms in those with neutropaenia or anaemia, but have not been shown to improve overall survival. Many patients will require frequent transfusions and are at risk of iron overload and secondary haemochromatosis. Chemotherapy is not particularly successful in elderly patients, but agents like melphalan or cytarabine are occasionally used.

Further Reading

Greenberg P, Tuechler H, Schanz J, et al. (2012). Revised international prognostic scoring system for myelodysplastic syndromes. *Blood* 120(12): 2454–2465.

Killi, S, Carter C, Culligan D, et al. (2014). British Committee for Standards in Haematology: guidelines for the diagnosis and management of adult myelodysplastic syndromes. *British Journal of Haematology* 164: 503–525.

Vardiman J (2010). The World Health Organization (WHO) classification of tumours of the haematopoietic and lymphoid tissues: an overview with emphasis on myeloid neoplasms; *Chemical Biological Interactions* 184: 16–20.

108. **A 17-year-old boy was visiting the UK on a school trip from Brazil. He presented with a five-day history of fever, sore throat, and lethargy. On examination, there was pronounced tender cervical lymphadenopathy and a greyish membrane overlying his tonsils. His temperature was 37.5°C, pulse rate was 70 beats per minute, and respiratory rate was 16 breaths per minute.**

What is the most likely diagnosis?

A. Diphtheria
B. Hodgkin's lymphoma
C. Infectious mononucleosis (EBV)
D. Oral candidiasis
E. Streptococcal pharyngitis

109. **A 45-year-old Caucasian man presented with a five-month history of lethargy, non-bloody diarrhoea, and weight loss. He had noticed his stool was difficult to flush. He also complained of joint aches and pains in his knees. His wife had noticed that he had become increasingly depressed over the last few months and had no interest in doing things. He had lost 10 kg of weight over a three-month period. He had a 20-pack year history of smoking and drank 30 units of alcohol a week. He had no significant past medical history.**

   Examination revealed a temperature of 37.3°C, a pulse rate of 80 beats per minute, and a BP of 145/92 mmHg. There was no lymphadenopathy. The abdomen was soft and non-tender with bowel sounds present. There were no masses felt. Neurological examination was normal.

   ```
   Investigations:
     Hb                        91 g/L
     MCV                       89 fL
     Eosinophils               0.2 × 10⁹/L
     Platelets                 550 × 10⁹/L
     WCC                       7.6 × 10⁹/L
     Albumin                   32 g/L
     CRP                       47 mg/L
     Na                        128 mmol/L
     K                         3.4 mmol/L
     Amylase                   70 iU/L
   Abdominal X-ray: normal bowel gas distribution
   Endoscopic duodenal biopsy: infiltration of macrophages
     within the lamina propria staining positive for PAS
     (periodic acid Schiff) positive material.
   ```

   Given the likely diagnosis, what is the most appropriate treatment course?

   A. Gluten-free diet

   B. Intravenous ceftriaxone (two weeks) then oral co-trimoxazole (one year)

   C. Ivermectin

   D. Oral metronidazole course

   E. Oral prednisolone and mesalazine

110. **A 34-year-old farmer presented to the emergency department with a frontal headache, muscle pains, and fever. He had not had any diarrhoea or vomiting, and he had not travelled abroad for over two years. Examination revealed a temperature of 38.3°C and there was conjunctival suffusion in both eyes. There was mild jaundice in the sclera. There was no rash or photophobia. Heart sounds were normal and breath sounds were vesicular. The abdomen was soft with no organomegaly.**

```
Investigations:
   Hb                    123 g/L
   Platelets             300 × 10⁹/L
   WCC                   10 × 10⁹/L
   Na                    143 mmol/L
   K                     3.6 mmol/L
   Urea                  7.3 mmol/L
   Creatinine            100 µmol/L
   Bilirubin             50 µmol/L
   ALT                   70 IU/L
   ALP                   350 IU/L
   Urine dipstick        blood +
```

What is the most likely diagnosis?

A. Brucellosis

B. Dengue fever

C. Enteric fever

D. Leptospirosis

E. Lyme disease

111. **A 65-year-old gentleman presented with a two-week history of malaise, weakness, and fevers. Sudden onset intermittent severe right hypochondrial pain prompted his presentation. He had a past medical history of type II diabetes and diverticular disease. There was no history of recent travel, he had never used intravenous drugs, and was with a long-term partner. Examination revealed a temperature of 38.3°C and marked tenderness over the right upper quadrant. There was no rebound tenderness. There was 2 cm hepatomegaly. Cardiac, respiratory, and neurological examinations were normal. There was no focal neurology.**

```
Investigations:
  Hb                      122 g/L
  WCC                     14.2 × 10⁹/L
  ALT                     120 IU/L
  ALP                     350 IU/L
  Bilirubin               23 µmol/L
  Albumin                 30 g/L
  Urea                    6 mmol/L
  Creatinine              89 µmol/L
  Na                      136 mmol/L
  K                       3.4 mmol/L
  CRP                     249 mg/L
  Chest X-ray             raised right hemi-diaphragm. Lung
                          fields had no focal consolidation.
  CT Abdomen:             Figure 6.1
```

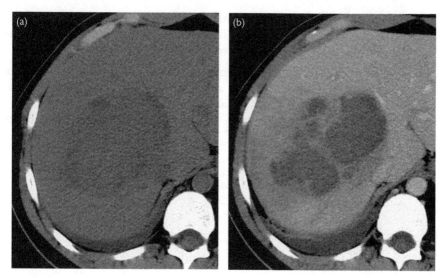

Figure 6.1 CT abdomen.

What is the most likely diagnosis?

A. Amoebic liver abscess

B. Hepatocellular carcinoma

C. Hydatid cyst

D. Pyogenic liver abscess

E. Simple liver cysts

112. **A 54-year-old Mediterranean gentleman with known HIV infection presented with a three-week history of increasing fever, dyspnoea, and cough. He was poorly compliant with anti-viral medication.**

    Examination revealed a temperature of 38.3°C, pulse rate of 100 beats per minute, BP of 110/80 mmHg, and respiratory rate of 24 per minute. Oxygen saturations were 90% on air. Heart sounds were normal with no murmurs. Breath sounds were vesicular; diffuse crackles were heard across both lung bases.

    ```
    Investigations:
      Hb                      122 g/L
      WCC                     5.1 × 10⁹/L
      Neutrophils             4.2 × 10⁹/L
      Urea                    8 mmol/L
      Creatinine              140 µmol/L
      CRP                     41 mg/L
      CD4 Count               150 cells/µL (500–1500)
      HIV RNA                 230,000 copies/mL
      ABG on room air:
        pH                    7.31
        pO2                   8.2 kPa
        pCO2                  3.8 kPa
        HCO3                  18 mmol/L
        BE                    −3 mmol/L
        Lactate              1 mmol/L
        Glucose              10.2 mmol/L
      Chest X-ray:            bilateral infiltrates
      Subsequent HRCT: bilateral ground glass shadowing.
    ```

    What is the most appropriate next management step?

    A. Clindamycin IV + oral primaquine

    B. No need to check G6PD, immediate IV co-trimoxazole + steroids

    C. Pentamidine IV + IV steroids

    D. Send G6PD levels, await result before starting IV co-trimoxazole + steroids

    E. Send G6PD levels, start IV co-trimoxazole + steroids without waiting for levels

113. **A 45-year-old man presented with fever, headache, and rash. His temperatures had started three days before when he awoke with an itchy maculopapular rash over his forearms and legs, sparing his palms and soles. He developed a severe headache with retro-orbital pain. He had no past medical history. He took no regular medication. He had a regular female partner with whom he had recently travelled to Thailand.**

Examination revealed a temperature of 38.8°C, with a confluent rash overlying the arms with sparing of small islands of normal skin. Pulse rate was 110 beats per minute and BP was 150/80 mmHg. There was no photophobia or neck stiffness.

```
Investigations:
   Hb                    135 g/L
   WCC                   3.1 × 10⁹/L
   Platelets             30 × 10⁹/L
   ALT                   110 IU/L
   ALP                   100 IU/L
   Albumin               28 g/L
   Urea                  6.8 mmol/L
   Creatinine            69 μmol/L
   Na                    140 mmol/L
   K                     4.2 mmol/L
   Urine dipstick        protein ++
   During phlebotomy, the patient developed minor bleeding
      and a haematoma around the venipuncture site. A clinical
      diagnosis of Dengue fever was made.
```

Which of the following is not a 'warning sign' for progression to severe dengue infection?

A. Clinical fluid accumulation (e.g. ascites)

B. Decrease in haematocrit

C. Liver enlargement >2 cm

D. Mucosal bleeding

E. Persistent vomiting

114. **A 35-year-old male presented with a rash a few days after visiting the New Forest. He developed a flu-like illness during the last few days of his holiday which he put down to swimming in the lake in the evening. He was otherwise well and had no other past medical history. Examination revealed a pulse of 60 beats per minute, BP of 115/ 85 mmHg and temperature of 36.8°C. There were no abnormalities found on examination of the cardiovascular, abdominal, or neurological systems.**

```
Investigations:
  Hb                   142 g/L
  Platelets            401 × 10⁹/L
  WCC                  9.2 × 10⁹/L
  CRP                  <0.6 mg/L
  ALT                  27 IU/L
  Bilirubin            5 µmol/L
  ALP                  88 IU/L
  Image:               Figure 6.2.
```

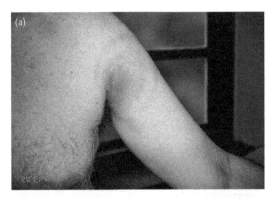

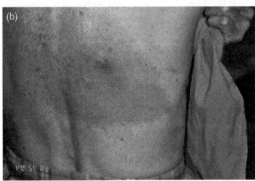

Figure 6.2 Patient's rash.

Reproduced with permission from *Oxford Textbook of Medicine*, Fifth Edition. Edited by David A Warrell, Timothy M Cox, and John D Firth, Fig. 7.6.32.2, p. 862. Oxford University Press, Oxford, UK, Copyright © 2010.

What is the most likely diagnosis?

A. Cat scratch fever
B. Cellulitis
C. Cutaneous anthrax
D. Lyme disease
E. Rocky mountain spotted fever

115. **A registrar sustained a needlestick injury whilst inserting a central line on the intensive care unit. The patient was an intubated and ventilated 45-year-old Chinese gentleman who was admitted three days previously with severe chest sepsis.**

The doctor was wearing gloves at the time and was pierced with a hollow-bore needle which was exposed to the patient's blood. She immediately washed her hands with soap and water and went to occupational health. She had been vaccinated against hepatitis B virus (HBV) infection five years previously and was told that she was a 'responder' to the vaccine.

Blood tests from the patient were taken to screen for blood-borne viruses.

```
HIV                        negative
HCV Ab                     negative
HBV surface antigen        negative
HBV surface antibody       positive
HBe antigen                negative
HBe antibody               positive
HBV core antibody IgG      positive
```

What is the most appropriate next action?

A. Booster vaccine

B. Booster vaccine and hepatitis B immunoglobulin (HBIG)

C. Hepatitis B immunoglobulin

D. No further action required

E. Start tenofovir

116. **A 23-year-old woman presented with fever, abdominal pain, and vaginal discharge. The pain was sharp and pleuritic in nature in the right upper quadrant of her abdomen and radiated to the right shoulder. Her periods were usually regular but she reported inter-menstrual bleeding and she also reported pain on intercourse.**

Examination reveals a pulse of 90 beats per minute, respiratory rate of 18 breaths per minute, BP of 125/87 mmHg, and her temperature was 37.8°C. There was tenderness over the lower abdomen and over the right upper quadrant with guarding. Bowel sounds were present. Bimanual pelvic examination revealed adnexal tenderness.

```
Investigations:
  Hb                      128 g/L
  WCC                     14.2 × 10⁹/L
  CRP                     155 mg/L
  Creatinine              57 µmol/L
  Urea                    4.2 mmol/L
  Bilirubin               13 µmol/L
  ALT                     57 IU/L
  ALP                     134 IU/L
  Na                      136 mmol/L
  K                       3.9 mmol/L
  Urine                   β-HCG negative
  Urine dipstick          Leukocytes +
  Chest X-ray             No consolidation, no free air under
                          the diaphragm
```

What is the most likely diagnosis?

A. Bacterial vaginosis

B. Cholecystitis

C. Fitz-Hugh Curtis syndrome

D. Pyelonephritis

E. Tubulo-ovarian abscess

117. **A 24-year-old pregnant teacher attended the emergency department after suspected exposure to chickenpox. A pupil she was tutoring the day before had called in sick with fever, an itchy rash, and spots which were coming up in crops. She was at 20 weeks gestation and did not recall having chickenpox as a child. She was brought up in Malaysia and was unsure of her vaccination history.**

What is the next most appropriate management step?

A. Acyclovir
B. Check varicella antibodies
C. Reassurance
D. Varicella immunization
E. VZIG (varicella immunoglobulin)

118. **A 30-year-old Somalian man presented to the sexual health clinic with a genital ulcer. He had no other symptoms. He had a background of HIV infection and was adherent to medication. His baseline CD4 count was 350 cells/μL and HIV RNA was undetectable. He had last had unprotected sexual intercourse one week previously with a new female partner. He complained that the ulcer was very painful to touch and bled easily on contact.**

Examination revealed a deep ulcer overlying the coronal sulcus of the penis. There was painful lymphadenopathy over the left inguinal lymph nodes. He was otherwise afebrile with a pulse rate of 67 beats per minute and BP of 115/82 mmHg.

What is the most likely diagnosis?

A. Chancroid
B. Genital herpes
C. Granuloma inguinale (donovanosis)
D. Lymphogranuloma venereum
E. Syphilis

119. **A 25-year-old male presented with fever and sore throat, which had been ongoing for six days. A trial of amoxicillin prescribed by his GP had had no effect on symptoms. He subsequently developed a new rash across his upper chest, neck, and face which was mildly itchy. He had no significant travel history. He had no significant previous medical problem, regular medication, or history of drug allergies. Sexual history revealed he had had two casual male partners over the preceding three months. However, his most recent sexual health screen two weeks previously was negative for any blood-borne viruses.**

Examination revealed a temperature of 38.9°C and palpable axillary lymphadenopathy. There was a generalized maculopapular rash across his face and upper trunk with well circumscribed oval pink macules. Examination of the mouth revealed pharyngeal oedema and hyperaemia but no tonsillar enlargement or exudate.

```
Investigations:
   WCC                      3.1 × 10⁹/L
   Platelets                75 × 10⁹/L
   Na                       140 mmol/L
   K                        4.4 mmol/L
   Urea                     3 mmol/L
   Creatinine               63 µmol/L
   CRP                      7 mg/L
   Bilirubin                13 µmol/L
   ALT                      68 IU/L
   ALP                      84 IU/L
```

What is the most likely diagnosis?

A. EBV mononucleosis

B. Hepatitis C

C. HIV seroconversion illness

D. Pityriasis rosea

E. Syphilis

120. **A 45-year-old male with advanced HIV disease (baseline CD4 count 35 cells/µL, HIV RNA 600,000 copies/ml) presented 20 days post initiation of HAART (highly active anti-retroviral therapy) with fever and breathlessness. Diagnosis had been made recently when he was investigated for a prolonged productive cough, weight loss, and pulmonary infiltrates on chest X-ray. He was found subsequently to have tuberculosis and had been on anti-TB therapy for nearly six weeks. Examination revealed cervical lymph nodes which the patient reported as having increased in size. Chest X-ray demonstrated more extensive pulmonary infiltrates than those seen six weeks previously.**

```
Investigations:
  Hb                      123 g/L for men
  WCC                     6 × 10⁹/L
  Urea                    5 mmol/L
  Creatinine              65 µmol/L
  Na                      133 mmol/L
  K                       3.5 mmol/L
  CRP                     45 mg/L
  Bilirubin               16 µmol/L
  ALT                     44 IU/L
  ALP                     76 IU/L
  HIV RNA                 20,000 copies/ml
  CD4 count               135 cells/µL)
```

What is the most likely diagnosis?

A. Drug hypersensitivity reaction

B. Failure of TB therapy

C. Immune reconstitution inflammatory syndrome (IRIS)

D. Interaction between HAART and anti-TB drugs

E. Poor compliance with anti-retroviral therapy

121. **A 36-year-old homeless man was admitted to hospital after being found collapsed. He was known to have a past medical history of substance abuse, including use of intravenous drugs. On examination he was afebrile with a pulse of 95 beats per minute, BP of 98/50 mmHg, a respiratory rate of 12 per minute, and oxygen saturations were 94% on room air. There was evidence of skin-popping on his arms. Cranial nerve examination revealed bilateral ptosis with a pupil size of 4 mm bilaterally with sluggish responsiveness to light. There was a reduced range of eye movement and diplopia in all directions with bilateral nystagmus. There was also global facial weakness with slurred speech. Peripheral neurological examination revealed predominantly upper limb weakness in the proximal muscles. Reflexes were depressed bilaterally and plantars were down going.**

```
Investigations:
    Hb                      122 g/L
    WCC                     11.1 × 10⁹/L
    Neutrophils             9.1 × 10⁹/L
    Urea                    7 mmol/L
    Creatinine              80 µmol/L
    Albumin                 35 g/L
    CRP                     95 mg/L
    Chest X-ray             normal lung fields
    CT head                 no space occupying lesions, haemorrhage
                            or infarction
    Lumbar puncture:
    Normal opening pressure
    No organisms
    No white cells
    Normal glucose
    Protein                 0.5 g/l (0.2-0.4 g/l)
```

What is the most likely diagnosis?

A. Botulism

B. Lambert Eaton syndrome (LEMS)

C. Miller-Fisher syndrome

D. Myasthenia gravis (MG)

E. Stroke

122. **A 56-year-old Nigerian woman was admitted to hospital with a one-month history of fever and generalized joint pains. Examination revealed a temperature of 38°C and arthritis of the left knee, both ankles, and second metacarpophalangeal joint of the left hand. There was erythema nodosum on her lower legs. There was no history of mouth ulcers or recent sexual contacts. There was no cough, haemoptysis, or shortness of breath. She had a background of diabetes controlled with metformin and had tuberculosis as a child. She took no regular medications.**

```
Investigations:
  Hb                        101 g/L
  WCC                       13.1 × 10⁹/L
  Platelets                 180 × 10⁹/L
  Urea                      5.2 mmol/L
  Creatinine                93 µmol/L
  ALT                       18 IU/L
  ALP                       105 IU/L
  Corrected calcium         2.55 mmol/L
  ESR                       80 mm/hr
  Anti-CCP                  positive
  Rheumatoid factor         positive
  HBV/HCV/HIV               negative
  Synovial fluid left knee:
    WCC                     8 × 10⁹/L
    No crystals
    No organisms (Gram and Ziehl-Neelsen stain)
    Left knee X-ray:        normal
    Chest X-ray:            normal
```

What is the most likely diagnosis?

A. Lofgren's syndrome
B. Poncet's disease
C. Rheumatoid arthritis
D. Still's disease
E. Syphilis

123. **A 42-year-old Indian man visiting the UK on a business trip presented with a six-day history of arthralgia, fevers, and rigors. His only medical history included hypertension for which he was taking lisinopril. On examination, he had a temperature of 39.1°C, a heart rate of 120 beats per minute and a BP of 126/85 mmHg. He had no meningism or localizing signs of infection.**

```
Investigations:
  Hb                      138 g/L
  WCC                     8.8 × 10⁹/L
  Platelets               84 × 10⁹/L
  Creatinine              120 µmol/L
  ALP                     75 U/L
  ALT                     47 U/L
  Bili                    26 µmol/L
  CRP                     48 mg/L
```
Thick and thin blood smears stained with Giemsa showed *Plasmodium vivax* parasites at 0.7% parasitaemia in multiples stages of development (ring forms with Shüffner's dots and gametocytes).

What is the recommended treatment?

A. Artemether-lumefantrine (Riamet®)

B. Artesunate followed by doxycycline

C. Atovaquone-proguanil (Malarone®)

D. Chloroquine followed by primaquine

E. Quinine and doxycycline

124. A 36-year-old Caucasian man presented to the emergency department with a tonic-clonic seizure following a two-week history of headache and vomiting and one day of intermittent drowsiness. He had been diagnosed with HIV infection four years previously but proved non-compliant with treatment and was lost to follow-up. His last CD4 count, one year previously, was 95 cells/μl.

On examination, he appeared emaciated. His temperature was 38.2°C, and he scored 12/15 on the Glasgow Coma Scale. Cardiovascular examination was unremarkable. Neurological examination revealed no focal deficit or nuchal rigidity.

```
Investigations:
  WCC                      5.2 × 10⁹/L
  Neutrophils              4.1 × 10⁹/L
  Lymphocytes              0.51 × 10⁹/L
  Platelets                106 × 10⁹/L
  CRP                      1 mg/L
  Chest X-ray:             normal
  T1 weighted MRI head:    Figure 6.3
```

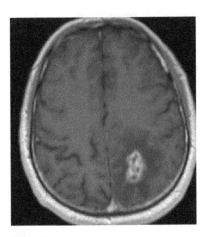

Figure 6.3 One weighted MRI head.

Reproduced with permission from *The Neurosurgeon's Handbook*. Edited by George Samandouras, Fig. 7.6.2, p. 337. Oxford University Press, Oxford, UK, Copyright © 2010.

What is your treatment of choice?

A. Amphotericin B and flucytosine

B. Ceftriaxone and metronidazole

C. Clindamycin and primaquine

D. Pyrimethamine and sulfadiazine

E. Rifampicin, isoniazid, pyrazinamide, and ethambutol

125. **A 42-year-old Nigerian man living in the UK was admitted to hospital with a gradual deterioration over four weeks. His speech had become incomprehensible and he had been noted to walk into door frames and walls.**

On examination, his temperature was 37.3°C, and his vital signs were within normal limits. He had oral thrush. His pupils were equal and reactive to light. However, he was unable to count fingers with either eye. He had an expressive dysphasia but no other focal neurology.

```
Investigations:
   WCC                      3.6 10⁹/L
   Neutrophils              2.2 × 10⁹/L
   Lymphocytes              0.71 × 10⁹/L
   Platelets                136 × 10⁹/L
   CRP                      3 mg/L
   HIV-1 serology           positive

Cerebrospinal fluid analysis:
   Microscopy
   White cells              2 × 10⁶/L (<5)
   Red cells                2 × 10⁶/L (<10)
   Gram stain               no organisms seen
   CSF protein              0.35 g/L (0.15-0.45)
   CSF glucose              4.4 mmol/L
   Serum glucose            6.2 mmol/L
   CT head:                 Unremarkable
```

Which of the following tests on the cerebrospinal fluid is most likely to reveal the underlying diagnosis?

A. Cryptococcal antigen

B. Herpes simplex virus (HSV) polymerase chain reaction (PCR)

C. JC virus PCR

D. *Mycobacterium tuberculosis* (TB) PCR

E. Toxoplasma PCR

126. A 35-year-old Estonian man presented with a four-week history of productive cough, fever, night sweats, and weight loss. He had been in the UK for 18 months working in the construction industry. He had no past medical history of note and took no regular medications. He smoked 15 cigarettes per day. He had spent time incarcerated in prison in Estonia before emigrating to the UK. Examination revealed a thin man with a temperature of 37.7°C and normal vital signs. No abnormal findings were present on cardiovascular and respiratory examination. There was no lymphadenopathy or organomegaly.

Investigations:

WCC	6.8×10^9/L
Neutrophils	3.8×10^9/L
Lymphocytes	1.9×10^9/L
ESR	45 mm/h
CRP	19 mg/L
Sputum auramine stain	positive for acid-fast bacilli
HIV test	negative
Chest X-ray:	B/L upper lobe changes

What is your next investigation?

A. Bronchoscopy
B. Early morning urines cultures for acid-fast bacilli
C. High-resolution CT scan of the chest
D. Interferon-gamma release assay (IGRA)
E. Sputum PCR for TB and *rpoB* gene mutations

127. A 17-year-old student presented with a three-week history of painful red lumps on her right arm and armpit and intermittent fevers, sweats, and shivers. Her GP had prescribed a one-week course of flucloxacillin with no effect. She noticed a small papule on her right index finger, which predated the lumps by two weeks. Her only animal contact was with her three cats. She was fully immunized and had no other medical history of note.

Examination revealed very tender right axillary and epitrochlear lymphadenopathy and a faint maculopapular rash over the shoulders and torso. The remainder of her examination was unremarkable.

Investigations:

WCC	8.6×10^9/L
Neutrophils	6.7×10^9/L
Lymphocytes	1.4×10^9/L
ESR	45 mm/h
CRP	15 mg/L

What is the most likely diagnosis?

A. *Bartonella henselae*
B. *Bordetella pertussis*
C. *Borrelia burgdorferi*
D. *Brucella melitensis*
E. *Coxiella burnetii*

128. **A 43-year-old sheep abattoir worker presented with a three-week history of malaise, weight loss, intermittent fevers, and progressive shortness of breath. His past medical history was significant for a patent foramen ovale which had not been repaired. He had no history of foreign travel.**

On examination, he had a temperature of 38.3°C and but was not haemodynamically compromised. An early diastolic murmur was audible in his left sternal edge and bibasal crepitations were present in his chest.

```
Investigations:
  Hb                        138 g/L
  WCC                       5.3 × 10⁹/L
  ESR                       45 mm/h
  CRP                       79 mg/L
  ALT                       79 U/L
  Blood cultures            ×3 negative
Transthoracic echocardiogram:
  Moderate aortic regurgitation and vegetation seen on aortic
    valve
```

What is the most likely diagnosis?

A. *Bartonella quintana*
B. *Brucella melitensis*
C. *Chlamydia psittaci*
D. *Coxiella burnetii*
E. *Tropheryma whipplei*

129. **A 62-year-old woman of Jamaican origin presented to A&E with fever, abdominal pain, haematemesis, and worsening shortness of breath two weeks after her first cycle of chemotherapy with cyclophosphamide, dexamethasone, and thalidomide for multiple myeloma. She had lived in the UK for 20 years and had no recent travel history.**

    On examination she had a distended and diffusely tender abdomen. She was in type I respiratory failure due to acute respiratory distress syndrome (ARDS) and required intubation and mechanical ventilation.

    ```
    Investigations:
      Hb                       110 g/L
      WCC                      8.9 × 10⁹/L
      Neutrophils             6.8 × 10⁹/L
      Lymphocytes             0.7 × 10⁹/L
      eosinophils             0.3 × 10⁹/L
      CRP                      58 mg/L
      Chest X-ray:            bilateral infiltrates
      Endotracheal aspirate:  larva of parasite
    ```

    What is the diagnosis?

    A. Giardiasis

    B. Schistosomiasis

    C. Strongyloidiasis

    D. Toxoplasmosis

    E. Tropical pulmonary eosinophilia

130. An 80-year-old man developed severe diarrhoea (Bristol type 7 stool, up to six times a day) during a prolonged hospital admission for pneumonia and poorly controlled type II diabetes. His stool sample was found to be *Clostridium difficile* toxin positive, although his abdomen was soft and he remained afebrile. He was commenced on oral vancomycin. Unfortunately, his pneumonia failed to improve and he was also diagnosed with a Gram-negative bacteraemia likely due to urinary tract infection, thus intravenous piperacillin-tazobactam was also commenced. His blood tests at initiation of vancomycin and piperacillin-tazobactam (day 1), and after one week of treatment (day 7), are shown below. The diarrhoea was persistent, but there were no new clinical symptoms or signs.

	Day 1	Day 7
Hb (g/L)	107	102
WCC (× 109/L)	15.3	16.1
Plt (× 109/L)	330	418
Urea (mmol/L)	8.2	13.5
Creatinine (umol/L)	74	129
C-reactive protein (mg/L)	124	261

What is the most appropriate next step in management?

A. Abdominal X-ray

B. Convert oral vancomycin to intravenous vancomycin

C. CT abdomen

D. Stop piperacillin-tazobactam

E. Stop vancomycin and commence fidaxomicin

131. **A 23-year-old student from Korea presented with a one-week history of increasing headache and lethargy. Over the previous three weeks she had developed a non-productive cough and fever. There was no history of coryza or sore throat and no contact with other sick people. She had no past medical history of note and took no regular medications. She had no pets at home and her last travel was to the east coast of the USA four months previously.**

On admission her Glasgow Coma Scale was 14/15, and her temperature was 38.7°C with stable haemodynamic parameters. Her chest auscultation revealed bilateral scattered crepitations. Her cardiovascular and abdominal examinations were unremarkable. Neurological assessment revealed no focal deficit. However, there was definite nuchal rigidity.

```
Investigations:
  CSF microscopy
  Polymorphs              5 × 10⁶/L (<5)
  Lymphocytes             83 × 10⁶/L (<5)
  Red cells               10 × 10⁶/L (<10)
  Gram stain              no organisms seen
  Auramine stain          no acid fast bacilli seen
  CSF protein             >2 g/L (0.15-0.45)
  CSF glucose             1.8 mmol/L
  Serum glucose           5.3 mmol/L
  CT head:                hydrocephalus, no focal brain
                          lesions
```

What is the likely diagnosis?

A. Herpes simplex virus meningo-encephalitis

B. Japanese encephalitis virus meningo-encephalitis

C. Pneumococcal meningitis

D. Tuberculous meningitis

E. West Nile virus meningitis

108. A) Diphtheria

Diphtheria is caused by toxin producing Gram positive bacillus, *Corynebacterium diphtheria* or *Corynebacterium ulcerans*. It is spread through droplets and contaminated objects from an infectious person. Although uncommon in the UK due to the immunization programme, it remains endemic in parts of the world, including India, Southeast Asia, Brazil, and Russia. Patients often present with fever and lymphadenopathy; a firmly adherent diphtheritic 'pseudo-membrane' over the tonsils and pharynx is a classical feature.

Streptococcal pharyngitis may also present with sore throat and reactive cervical lymphadenopathy. However, a membranous pharyngitis is not present. Oral lesions of candidiasis form white plaques which can be easily removed; treatment is initially with nystatin liquid or pastilles. Infectious mononucleosis has a longer incubation period of usually 4–6 weeks, and usually presents with significant cervical lymphadenopathy and splenomegaly. Hodgkin's disease presents with enlarged, rubbery, non-tender lymph nodes and constitutional symptoms may be observed in up to 25% of patients. It is a tissue diagnosis requiring lymph node biopsy; the Reed-Steenberg cell is characteristic.

Tutorial

Diphtheria comes from the Greek word for leather, due to the characteristic appearance of an adherent greyish pseudo-membrane which forms within the upper respiratory tract. The standard incubation period is 2–5 days. Untreated, individuals may be infectious for up to a month. Asymptomatic carriers have the potential to transmit infection for longer.

Although a common disease in the 1940s, the national vaccination programme has vastly reduced the number of cases within the UK. However, cases are still widely reported in India, Africa, Southeast Asia, and South America. Release of diphtheria exotoxin causes local tissue necrosis and membranous pharyngitis which can be accompanied by fever, cervical lymphadenopathy, and oedema of soft tissue, producing a 'bull neck' appearance. Cutaneous diphtheria is also seen. Systemic effects of the exotoxin include cardiotoxicity with myocarditis, segmental demyelinative neuropathy, and paralysis of the palate, pharyngeal, respiratory, and limb muscles. Diagnosis is dependent on bacterial culture from throat and nasal swabs. The toxin-producing gene can be identified by PCR.

Diphtheria is a notifiable disease in the UK. Contacts should be investigated and prophylactically treated with a course of erythromycin or penicillin and vaccinated.

Suspected cases are given diphtheria antitoxin (without waiting for bacterial confirmation). The anti-toxin is derived from horse serum, therefore clinicians should be aware of a risk of hypersensitivity reaction. Antibiotic treatment with a macrolide is additionally required for clearance of bacteria. In addition, immunization status should be confirmed; immunized individuals should receive a single reinforcing dose of a diphtheria containing vaccine. Unimmunized patients should complete immunization as per the UK schedule. As the pseudo-membrane provides a risk of oropharyngeal obstruction, if the airway is compromised then referral to intensive care specialists for intubation should be considered early.

Further Reading

Public Health in England (2013). Chapter 15: Diphtheria. The Green Book. pp. 109–225. Available at: https://www.gov.uk/government/publications/diphtheria-the-green-book-chapter-15

109. B) Intravenous ceftriaxone (two weeks) then oral co-trimoxazole (one year)

The most likely diagnosis is Whipple's disease. The causative organism is *Tropheryma whipplei*. Clinical presentation is often with diarrhoea, abdominal pain, and weight loss secondary to malabsorption (*Tropheryma* was named from the Greek: *trophe* (nourishment) and *eryma* (barrier)). Diagnosis is by biopsy of small bowel tissue demonstrating presence of inclusion bodies within macrophages which stain positive for PAS positive material. PAS staining is negative for the other malabsorptive syndromes. Coeliac disease is one of the commonest causes of malabsorption. Proteins in dietary rye, barley, and wheat induce T cell responses which drive intestinal inflammation and villous atrophy, resulting in chronic diarrhoea, steatorrhea, weight loss, and fatigue. Treatment is strict avoidance of gluten in the diet. Ivermectin is the treatment of choice for strongyloidiasis; this is more common in people who have lived in the tropics or subtropics. Chronic asymptomatic infection is common. Patients often have an eosinophilia. Infection with the flagellate protozoan, *Giardia intestinalis* can cause watery diarrhoea, weight loss, and malabsorption. However, this is acquired by drinking water containing cysts and is often associated with traveller's diarrhoea. Treatment is with metronidazole. Oral prednisolone and mesalazine could be used if Crohn's disease was suspected.

Tutorial

Whipple's disease, a rare-multisystem disorder, is caused by the Gram-positive intracellular bacterium *Tropheryma whipplei*. Patients present with arthralgia, abdominal pain, diarrhoea, and weight loss. Up to 60% of cases may have neurological or psychiatric involvement, including cognitive change, supranuclear ophthalmoplegia, or upper motor neuron signs. Other presentations may include culture-negative endocarditis, isolated arthritis, or uveitis. Classically, the patient is a middle-aged Caucasian male. Diagnosis is based on histological features, including infiltration of macrophages into the lamina propria of the small intestine, staining brilliant magenta with PAS reagent. Diagnosis is confirmed by identification of *Tropheryma whipplei* DNA by polymerase chain reaction (as the inclusion bodies of *Mycobacterium avium-intracellulare* may also stain positive for PAS). Treatment is with a bactericidal agent with CSF penetration; an initial course of ceftriaxone or meropenem is followed by prolonged co-trimoxazole. Unrecognized disease can eventually be fatal.

Further Reading

Fenollar F, Puéchal X, Raoult D (2007). Whipple's disease. *New England Journal of Medicine* 356: 55–66.

110. D) Leptospirosis

Brucellosis, leptospirosis, and Q fever are infections of livestock and can be transferred as a zoonosis to individuals such as farmers who are in close contact. Conjunctival suffusion is a typical feature of leptospirosis but not universally present. Brucellosis has been virtually eradicated from the UK through vaccinations of animals. Lyme disease is transferred through tick bites in forested areas of Europe and the USA. The first indication is usually a characteristic rash, erythema migrans, in addition to a flu-like illness. Untreated disease may lead to neurological, cardiac, and joint involvement. A lack of travel history makes dengue and typhoid fever unlikely. The former is caused by inoculation of dengue virus from mosquitos, which can result in sudden onset of febrile illness with headache, retro-orbital pain, myalgia, and arthralgia. In a small proportion of cases this progresses to severe dengue with evidence of systemic capillary leakage and fluid accumulation, haemorrhage, and shock. Enteric fever is caused by *Salmonella typhi* or *paratyphi*; it is spread by the faeco-oral route in developing countries. Presentation is with abdominal pains and fever, but dysentery is present in only 20–40% of patients. Signs include rose spots on the trunk and a relative bradycardia—but these are rare.

Tutorial

Leptospirosis is a zoonosis caused by transfer of spirochaete bacteria, *leptospirae* from animals (the maintenance hosts) to humans (accidental hosts). It is a biphasic illness. After an incubation period of typically 7–21 days, the initial bacteraemic phase is characterized by a flu-like illness with abrupt onset of headache, fever, muscle aches, and vomiting; some patients develop meningitis. Conjunctival suffusion is often a telltale sign. In some cases this may be followed by an immune phase. Severe leptospirosis is commonly known as Weil's disease, and features: jaundice, renal failure, haemorrhage, and myocarditis with arrhythmias. Leptospirosis induced pulmonary haemorrhage with respiratory failure has a mortality rate of greater than 50%. The vast majority of cases, however, are sub-clinical.

Leptospirosis is primarily a disease of tropical and subtropical areas. The commonest animal reservoirs include rodents and cattle; infected animals carry bacteria in their kidneys and excrete *Leptospira* in their urine. Infection can be acquired by contact with infected animal urine or tissue secretions (often in contaminated water or moist soil) through abrasions in the skin or mucous membranes. There are 50–60 cases of leptospirosis per year in the UK; risk groups include farmers and those who have contact with water, for example divers and canoeists.

Diagnosis is often clinical; however, this can be aided by serological detection of leptospiral IgM antibodies (positive from five days of symptom onset), microscopic agglutination test (MAT; positive from tenth day of illness), or PCR. Treatment is with antibiotics; high dose intravenous penicillins are preferable for severe illness and oral doxycycline can be given for milder disease. Jarisch-Herxheimer reactions may occur after penicillin treatment. Prompt treatment can result in complete recovery.

Further Reading

Haake D, Levett P (2015). Leptospirosis in humans. *Current Topics in Microbiology and Immunology* 387: 65–97.

111. D) Pyogenic liver abscess

Simple liver cysts are not usually associated with constitutional symptoms or abdominal pain. Unilocular fluid-filled lesions are seen on ultrasound scan and well-circumscribed lesions that do not enhance with contrast are seen on CT scan. Hydatid disease is caused by ingestion of the eggs of the dog tapeworm, *Echinococcus granulosus*. The ingested eggs hatch into larvae that penetrate through the gut wall into the portal system and are carried to the liver (cysts can also disseminate to the lungs, bone, and brain). It is more commonly acquired in areas such as the Middle East, North and South America, and Australasia; the course of disease is insidious and patients are often asymptomatic (unless cysts rupture). Enlarging hepatic cysts may result in progressing right upper quadrant swelling and jaundice due to obstruction of bile canaliculi. Fever is usually absent with hepatocellular carcinoma. Histology would confirm the diagnosis. Differentiating an amoebic abscess from a pyogenic liver abscess (PLA) can be difficult; however, it is important as the management is different.

Amoebic abscesses are commonly solitary and occur in younger males. There may be a preceding or associated bloody diarrhoea, and patients are usually very unwell. Aspiration may yield an 'anchovy paste' sterile aspirate, whereas in a PLA, often mixed organisms will be cultured. Treatment of an amoebic abscess is with metronidazole and aspiration of abscess contents, and a luminal agent may be needed to clear cysts from the gut. The correct answer here is PLA. Amongst the predominant organisms are commensals from the gastrointestinal tract including *E.coli*, *Enterococcus faecalis*, and anaerobes. A history of diverticular disease may provide an initial source for dissemination of bacteria.

Tutorial

PLAs account for over 80% of liver abscesses. Microbes are introduced by either:

1. Direct spread from contiguous infection (biliary tract disease is the commonest cause of PLA).
2. Septic emboli from the gastrointestinal tract arriving through the hepatic portal vein (diverticulitis, inflammatory bowel disease, appendicitis).
3. Haematogenous spread in a septic patient (e.g. from endocarditis).

Patients may present with fevers, rigors, and right upper quadrant pain, or even non-specifically with anorexia and weight loss. Hiccups due to diaphragmatic irritation have also been reported. Investigations invariably reveal a raised ALP. Around half of patients will also develop derangement in AST, ALT, and bilirubin. Other features include leukocytosis and a normochromic anaemia (anaemia of 'chronic disease').

Blood cultures are positive in less than 50% of cases and so diagnosis is often from culture of aspiration fluid. Radiological imaging is also important in establishing diagnosis, not least because it allows for targeted aspiration of the abscess. Ultrasound demonstrates a variably echoic lesion, whilst contrast enhanced CT abdomen will usually show hypodense liver lesions. It is worth noting that PLAs are often multiple.

If amoebic abscess is suspected, a serum antibody test for *Entamoeba histolytica* or antigen testing/PCR of aspirated abscess fluid can confirm the diagnosis. In the event of concurrent bloody diarrhoea, a 'hot' stool, in which *Entamoeba histolytica* trophozoites engorged with blood are seen on microscopy, is diagnostic. Whilst this test is specific, it often lack sensitivity and thus many laboratories can also test for the organism by running a multiplex PCR on the stool sample looking for evidence of amoebic DNA.

The mainstay of treatment for liver abscesses is percutaneous drainage and prolonged antibiotic course. Surgical drainage or resection is associated with improved outcome for large multi-loculated abscesses >5 cm in diameter. If the history, exposure, or imaging is consistent with a diagnosis of hydatid, special care and specialist intervention may be needed to avoid the potential complication of hydatid rupture which is associated with anaphylaxis.

Further Reading

British Medical Journal (2016). Best Practice. Liver abscess. Available at: http://bestpractice.bmj.com/best-practice/monograph/640.html

112. E) Send G6PD levels, start IV co-trimoxazole + steroids without waiting for levels

Treatment for pneumocystis is based on severity of disease. Disease is classified as mild if *all* of the below criteria are met:

1. Dyspnoea on exertion
2. Oxygen saturations over 96% on air
3. PaO_2 >11 kPa on air
4. Normal or minor peri-hilar shadowing on CXR

Treatment for mild disease is oral trimethoprim and sulphamethoxazole (co-trimoxazole). Individuals with a PaO_2 less than 9.3 kPa or oxygen saturations <92% on room air should additionally be treated with oral steroids (or intravenous if oral not tolerated). Alternatives for mild-moderate disease in the case of intolerance include trimethoprim and dapsone, clindamycin and primaquine, or atovaquone (in mild disease).

Patients with more severe disease are treated first line with intravenous trimethoprim-sulphamethoxazole. Up to one third of patients may fail to respond to treatment and require salvage treatment. Second-line options include intravenous/oral trimethoprim and dapsone, clindamycin and primaquine, or intravenous pentamidine.

Glucose-6-phosphate dehydrogenase (G6PD) is an enzyme required in red blood cell metabolism. It is required for production of reduced glutathione which mops up excess free radicals and prevents red cell haemolysis during oxidative stress; infection or medications including sulphonamides, dapsone, primaquine, and pentamidine can induce oxidative stress. Therefore, individuals should be screened for G6PD deficiency (more prominent in Mediterranean populations) to reduce the risk of red cell haemolysis after treatment with the above medications. Treatment should not be delayed for the results, however, and can be discontinued or altered later in the event of a positive result or development of haemolysis.

Tutorial

Fungal infection with *Pneumocystis jirovecii* is an AIDS defining illness most commonly occurring in patients with a CD4 count less than 200 cells/μL. It can also occur in the absence of AIDS in patients who are receiving chronic immunosuppressive agents, for example.

The clinical course in HIV is often protracted over weeks, with development of malaise, dry cough, progressive dyspnoea, and low-grade fever. On examination, there may be tachycardia and tachypnoea with typically normal findings on lung auscultation. End-inspiratory crackles and wheeze are less commonly heard. Desaturation upon exercise is highly suggestive of pneumocystis pneumonia. In terms of imaging, it is worth noting that around 40% of patients have a normal chest X-ray. Other radiological abnormalities include perihilar haze, 'interstitial infiltrates', and pneumothoraces. There is relative sparing of the apices. In the presence of a normal X-ray, high resolution CT of the chest may show ground glass shadowing.

Desaturation upon exercise is often quoted as a giveaway sign for PCP, but it is not specific for this condition as it occurs in many other parenchymal lung diseases as well (any condition which impairs diffusion of oxygen from the alveoli into the capillaries). Microbiological investigations historically relied on visualization of the organism via histochemical 'silver stain' or immunofluorescent stains, as pneumocystis cannot be cultured *in vitro*, However, PCR is now the usual diagnostic test and will still be positive a few days after treatment has started as DNA from dead organisms is still relatively stable. Expectorated sputum does not provide an adequate alveolar sample. Induced sputum can be obtained initially or alternatively, samples from broncho-alveolar lavage. Tissue diagnosis with open lung biopsy is used only for patients with negative tests by other methods who are clinically not improving on empirical therapy.

Treatment of PCP, depending on severity, is discussed above. However, all HIV-positive patients with a CD4 T cell count less than 200 cells/μL should receive prophylaxis with co-trimoxazole. Failing that, second-line treatment is pentamidine nebulizers. Many specialties involved with organ transplantation (e.g. kidneys) will also routinely prescribe prophylactic co-trimoxazole to their patients as induction immune-suppression will render them at risk of PCP as well.

Further Reading

Nelson M, Dockrell D, Edwards S (2011). British HIV Association and British Infection Association Guidelines for the Treatment of Opportunistic Infection in HIV-seropositive Individuals. *HIV Medicine* 12(2): 1–5.

Thomas C, Limper A (2004). Pneumocystis pneumonia. *New England Journal of Medicine* 350: 2487–2498.

113. B) Decrease in haematocrit

Appropriate triage of a patient with dengue is required to assess their risk of developing potentially life-threatening severe dengue and dengue shock syndrome. A presumptive diagnosis can be made on the clinical history and laboratory tests which commonly reveal a mild to moderate thrombocytopenia and usually also a leukopaenia. The tourniquet test can be helpful in diagnosis (see below for explanation). In a small proportion of patients, the initial febrile phase may be followed by a 'systemic vascular leak syndrome' associated with haemo-concentration (therefore a rising haematocrit), hypoproteinaemia, and subsequent pleural effusions and ascites. The rising haematocrit is concurrent with a rapid decrease in platelets. A narrowing of pulse pressure by 20 mmHg or less and signs of peripheral vascular collapse may then suggest impending dengue shock syndrome.

Because of this, patients who have any of the following warning signs should be referred for in-hospital care and closely monitored:

- Abdominal pain/tenderness
- Persistent vomiting
- Clinical fluid accumulation
- Mucosal bleeding
- Lethargy, restlessness
- Liver enlargement >2 cm
- Laboratory: increase in haematocrit concurrent with rapid decrease in platelets

Tutorial

Dengue is a *Flavivirus*, a single stranded RNA virus of the Flavivirus genus which has four serotypes (DEN-1, DEN-2, DEN-3, and DEN-4). Recovery from infection by one provides lifelong immunity against that particular serotype only. Subsequent infections by other serotypes are thought to increase the risk of developing severe dengue. This is because cross-immunity to the other serotypes post-recovery is only partial, thus eliciting a severe but not completely effective immune response. The virus is spread between humans by the *aedes* mosquito which is a daytime feeder. It is endemic in most tropical and subtropical regions. The incubation period is 5–8 days, and presentation is with sudden onset of fever, arthralgia, myalgia (often involving the back, hence the term 'breakbone fever'), headache, and a maculopapular rash.

Patients may have signs of haemorrhage including petechiae, purpura, menorrhagia, or gastrointestinal bleeding. Application of a tourniquet, followed by deflation may result in formation of petechiae due to capillary fragility; the test is positive if >20 petechiae are found in an area of 2.5 cm squared.

The febrile phase is followed by a critical phase around the time of defervescence and then a spontaneous recovery phase. The recent WHO classification now differentiates patients into three groups: dengue without warning signs, dengue with warning signs, and severe dengue. Severe dengue is associated with complications including shock, accumulation of serosal fluid, severe bleeding, or severe organ impairment.

Detection of virus nucleic acid by RT-PCR or NS-1 protein performed by ELISA, from serum samples, is diagnostic. Serological tests may also be used; serum IgM to dengue virus antigens may be detected by four days after fever onset. A single raised IgM level provides a presumptive diagnosis (alongside the clinical picture). IgG seroconversion between paired samples is confirmatory.

Management is supportive, with principles focusing on fluid resuscitation. In severe cases patients may require intensive monitoring and even cardiovascular support. Avoidance of mosquito bites is the mainstay of prophylaxis. A vaccine is available but not routinely available.

Further Reading

Simmons C, Farrar J, van Vinh Chau N, Wills B (2012). Dengue. *New England Journal of Medicine* 366(5): 1423–1432.

World Health Organization and the Special Programme for Research and Training in Tropical Diseases (TDR) (2009). *Dengue Guidelines, for Diagnosis, Treatment, Prevention and Control*. World Health Organization, Geneva.

114. D) Lyme disease

This rash is erythema migrans and develops 7–10 days after a bite from a tick carrying *Borrelia burgdorferi*. It is associated with Lyme disease (named after a cluster of cases developed in Old Lyme, Connecticut). The lesions of cutaneous anthrax are painless and may result in papular, vesicular, and ulcerated stages before progression to a black eschar with surrounding extensive oedema. This is now very rare, but is more common in individuals working with animal hides, post-office staff who sort mail, or intravenous drug users.

Cat scratch disease (CSD) is caused by *Bartonella henselae*; the history involves contact with cats and a papular rash develops at the site of inoculation; patients develop regional lymphadenopathy. Rocky mountain spotted fever is another tick-borne infection, caused by *Rickettsia rickettsii*, an intracellular bacterium. Typical features include a blanching maculopapular rash, headache, and fever, and neurological sequelae are not uncommon.

Tutorial

Lyme disease is caused by the tickborne spirochaete *Borrelia burgdorferi*. Transfer of these intracellular bacterium via *ixodic* (hard) ticks often occurs in forested areas. The most common sign of early infections is erythema migrans at the site of the tick bite. This is a slowly expanding skin lesion with a central densely red macule (site of bite), a surrounding clear centre and an erythematous periphery, often said to look like a 'target lesion'. It is important to note, however, that central clearing may not be present and that the rash may have a homogenous appearance. Early infection is often accompanied with flu-like symptoms. After several weeks, if untreated, neurological involvement may also occur; lymphocytic meningitis, cerebellar ataxia, unilateral or bilateral facial palsies, or motor or sensory radiculoneuritis can manifest. Months after the initial inoculation, a second phase of joint swelling and pain can manifest in up to 60% of untreated patients. Lyme arthritis is more common in patients who acquired the infection in the USA compared to Europe.

Diagnosis is based on clinical findings, for example erythema migrans and history of tick bites. The most common investigation is serology for antibodies to *Borrelia burgdorferi*. However, antibody titres take several weeks to reach a detectable level so may be negative during the early stages, and may also be falsely negative if patients have been treated early, which may result in a lack of seroconversion. Serology is thus not required for diagnosis with a classical rash and exposure history. Samples which give an equivocal result for presence of antibodies are subjected to a second stage test by western blotting.

Treatment is with doxycycline 100 mg twice a day or amoxicillin 500 mg three times a day for two weeks for erythema migrans. A prolonged course is used for Lyme arthritis, and ceftriaxone may be used for cardiac or neurological involvement.

Further Reading

Steere A (2001). Lyme disease. *New England Journal of Medicine* 345(2): 115–125.

115. A) Booster vaccine

This patient has resolved HBV infection evidenced by the lack of HBsAg and the development of anti-HBs and anti-core IgG antibodies, suggesting prior exposure. Accidental exposure in a vaccinated individual warrants a booster vaccine unless given within the last year. HBIG, which provides additional temporary passive immunity, is not given unless the patient is known to be HBsAg positive (i.e. has current acute or chronic HBV infection), or the subject who has received the injury is a non-responder to the vaccine (i.e. anti-HBs <10 IU). A significant exposure with confirmed HBsAg positive blood in a vaccinated but non-responder health worker is best managed with both a booster vaccine and HBIG together.

Relative risk of exposure following percutaneous injury is often quoted as one in three for hepatitis B (but depending on e antigen status can be as high as 60%), 1 in 30 for hepatitis C, and 1 in 300 for HIV. The use of a hollow-bore needle, visible blood on the device, a deep injury, and terminal HIV-related illness carry a higher risk of exposure.

Tutorial

Hepatitis B virus is a DNA which has infected over two billion people worldwide. Over 250 million individuals have developed chronic infection, which confers a huge global disease burden as patients prematurely develop liver cirrhosis and hepatocellular carcinoma (an estimated 600,000 deaths annually are attributed to HBV related liver disease). The end point of anti-viral therapy is to improve quality of life and survival and to delay development of end-stage liver disease and death. Therapy is lifelong, non-curative, and often costly. Resistance may develop although is rarer with tenofovir.

Development of chronic infection is much more likely if infection is transferred vertically from mother to newborn. Adults, with developed immune systems, who acquire infection through sexual contact or through exposure to needles clear the infection spontaneously in 95% of cases. In these individuals, the clinical course may be asymptomatic, or patients may develop a flu-like illness and jaundice around 12 weeks after exposure. Only 1% of individuals develop fulminant hepatitis.

Acute infection is therefore not routinely treated. Therapy is generally commenced for patients with chronic infection if their HBV DNA levels are greater than 2000 IU/ml, ALT levels are above the upper limit of normal, and there is evidence of moderate to severe active necro-inflammation, for example on liver biopsy or transient elastography (FibroScan). Treatment strategies include first-line treatment with either pegylated interferon with ribavarin or a nucleoside analogue with good resistance profile (e.g. tenofovir).

A suggested algorithm for interpreting HBV serology is shown in Figure 6.4.

Further Reading

European Association for the Study of the Liver (EASL) (2017). Clinical practice guidelines on the management of hepatitis B virus infection. *Journal of Hepatology* 67(2): 1370–1398.

116. C) Fitz-Hugh Curtis syndrome

This is a case of peri-hepatitis associated with pelvic inflammatory disease (PID): Fitz-Hugh Curtis syndrome. The incidence ranges from 4% to 14% in women with PID. In this case, the presentation of a young woman with abdominal pain and vaginal discharge raises the possibility of PID. Peri-hepatitis is thought to be due to peritoneal and lymphatic spread of pelvic chlamydial/gonococcal infection to the hepatic capsule. Notably, the liver parenchyma is not affected, and patients therefore have normal or mildly raised liver function tests only. Bacterial vaginosis is asymptomatic in 50% of individuals; vaginal discharge is characteristically grey-white with a fishy smell. Patients are systemically well. The history is not in keeping with cholecystitis and one may expect a higher ALP with this diagnosis. Pyelonephritis often presents with a triad of fever, vomiting and loin to groin or back pain, along with a recent history of lower urinary tract symptoms such as dysuria. In this case, a urine dipstick showing only 1+ leukocytes goes against this diagnosis. Tubulo-ovarian abscess may also present in a similar manner with fever, abdominal pain, dyspareunia, and vaginal discharge, and

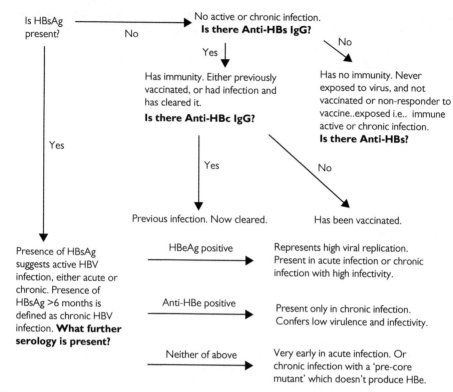

Is HBsAg present? — No → No active or chronic infection. **Is there Anti-HBs IgG?**

Yes ↓

Has immunity. Either previously vaccinated, or had infection and has cleared it. **Is there Anti-HBc IgG?**

No ↘

Has no immunity. Never exposed to virus, and not vaccinated or non-responder to vaccine..exposed i.e.. immune active or chronic infection. **Is there Anti-HBs?**

Yes ↓ → Previous infection. Now cleared.

No ↘ → Has been vaccinated.

Yes ↓

Presence of HBsAg suggests active HBV infection, either acute or chronic. Presence of HBsAg >6 months is defined as chronic HBV infection. **What further serology is present?**

HBeAg positive → Represents high viral replication. Present in acute infection or chronic infection with high infectivity.

Anti-HBe positive → Present only in chronic infection. Confers low virulence and infectivity.

Neither of above → Very early in acute infection. Or chronic infection with a 'pre-core mutant' which doesn't produce HBe.

Figure 6.4 Interpreting hepatitis B serology algorithm.

remains an important differential to consider but would not account for the right upper quadrant pain and guarding. The next investigation would be a pelvic and abdominal ultrasound which would help guide diagnosis.

Tutorial

Fitz-Hugh Curtis syndrome is associated with pelvic inflammatory disease in which there is direct spread of infection from the fallopian tube to the liver capsule (Gleeson's capsule) and peritoneum causing a peri-hepatitis. This causes acute onset of right upper quadrant pain which is sharp in nature and may radiate to the back and shoulder tip. Pain is exacerbated by deep inspiration and movement. Around 50% of patients are pyrexic. Symptoms can include bilateral lower abdominal pain, dyspareunia, vaginal bleeding (post-coital, menorrhagia, inter-menstrual), and purulent discharge. Examination findings on bimanual pelvic exam include adnexal tenderness and cervical motion tenderness. Pyrexia is a common feature. Diagnosis is usually clinical, but can be confirmed by swabs positive for *N. gonorrhoeae* and/or *C. trachomatis*. It is also important to ensure that an ectopic pregnancy has been excluded as it may present in a similar manner.

Management of the case requires analgesia and prompt antibiotics initially. This is likely to be IV ceftriaxone 2 g od in the first instance with PO doxycycline 100 mg bd, with conversion to oral therapy (ceftriaxone being substituted for PO metronidazole) when clinically indicated (falling inflammatory markers, usually 48–72 hours into treatment). Patients are advised to avoid sexual intercourse until completion of treatment and follow-up. Contact screening as well as testing for other sexually transmitted infections is also important. Whilst there is no other specific treatment for Fitz-Hugh-Curtis syndrome, severe pain main require laparoscopy for division of hepatic lesions.

Pelvic inflammatory disease is most often caused by sexually transmitted infection with chlamydia (50–65% of cases) and gonorrhea (18% of cases). Rarer causes include introduction of bacteria after IUD insertion, post-partum, or during abortion or miscarriage. Infection ascends from the endocervix causing endometritis, salpingitis, oophoritis, tubulo-ovarian abscess, and pelvic peritonitis.

Further Reading

Ross J, McCarthy J (2011). UK National Guideline for the Management of Pelvic Inflammatory Disease 2011. Clinical Effectiveness Group. British Association for Sexual Health and HIV. Available at: https://www.bashh.org/documents/3572.pdf

117. B) Check varicella antibodies

In the first instance, serum should be tested for varicella zoster virus (VZV) IgG. Serum will also have been saved from her booking bloods which can also be tested. Women from tropical and subtropical areas are more likely to be seronegative and are more susceptible to development of chickenpox. Around 80–90% of women tested will have varicella antibodies and can be reassured. If the pregnant woman is not immune and there was a significant exposure (face-to-face contact, contact in the same room for 15 minutes or more, or on a ward setting) then VZIG should be given as soon as possible; this is effective if given up to ten days after contact. Of note, chickenpox is infectious 48 hours before the rash appears and until the vesicles crust over.

Pregnant women who have been exposed to chickenpox or shingles who go on to develop a rash should notify their doctor. Oral acyclovir should be prescribed for pregnant women with chickenpox if they present within 24 hours of onset of rash and if they are more than 20 weeks gestation. VZIG has no therapeutic benefit once chickenpox has developed. The varicella vaccine is an option to prevent future chickenpox for women found seronegative for VZV IgG before pregnancy or during the post-partum period, but this is not current practice in the UK.

Tutorial

Varicella zoster virus is a herpes virus transmitted in respiratory droplets and by personal contact through vesicle fluid. The incubation period is 1–3 weeks and it is characterized by fever, malaise, and a pruritic rash that develops into crops of vesicles. The patient is no longer infectious once all the vesicles have crusted over.

Maternal risk

Varicella infection in adults has increased morbidity associated with development of pneumonia, hepatitis, and encephalitis. Women who are immunosuppressed, or develop chest/neurological symptoms or a haemorrhagic rash and bleeding should be referred to hospital and nursed in isolation from babies, susceptible pregnant women, or non-immune staff. Delivery during the viraemic phase confers a higher risk of bleeding/thrombocytopenia, DIC, and hepatitis; supportive treatment and intravenous acyclovir can be given.

Foetal risk

Varicella infection during the first 28 weeks of pregnancy confers a small risk of foetal varicella syndrome, characterized by eye defects, limb hypoplasia, skin scarring, and neurological abnormalities including microcephaly. Infection at term confers a significant risk of neonatal varicella infection. Elective delivery should be avoided until 5–7 days after onset of maternal rash to allow transfer of antibodies from mother to child. VZIG should be given to the neonate.

Further Reading

Royal College of Obstetricians and Gynaecologists (2015). Green Top Guidelines No. 13. Available at: https://www.rcog.org.uk/en/guidelines-research-services/guidelines/gtg13

118. A) Chancroid

Options A and B are associated with painful genital ulcers, whereas C, D, and E usually present with painless ulcers. Until the early 1990s, chancroid, caused by *Haemophilus ducreyi*, used to be the most common cause of genital ulceration worldwide. It presents with a deep necrotic ulcer with tender regional lymphadenopathy in 50% of cases. Prodromal symptoms are uncommon.

Donovanosis is mostly found in the tropics, and is caused by *Klebsiella granulomatis*. Patients may initially present with a firm papule/nodule which then ulcerates. Ulcers are usually painless and may be single or multiple. There is usually no regional lymphadenopathy. The incubation period is estimated to be 3–40 days and treatment is with either azithromycin or ciprofloxacin until lesions have healed.

Genital herpes, acquired through contact with infected genitalia (HSV-2) or transmitted by contact with infected oro-labial mucosa (HSV-1), is becoming increasingly common. Two thirds of patients acquire the virus from someone who is asymptomatic. Constitutional symptoms can occur within the first week, including fever, headache, and myalgia. Ano-genital lesions appear as vesicles which may become pustular, degrading to form tender ulcers with localized oedema. Complications in males include phimosis and in females cervicitis. Recurrence within the first year is common. Viral culture or real time polymerase chain reaction of vesicle fluid obtained from a swab is diagnostic. Initial infection can be managed with saline lavage and analgesia. Anti-virals given within five days of onset (e.g. acyclovir 200 mg ×5/day for five days) reduced duration of symptoms by 50% and viral shedding.

Lymphogranuloma venereum is caused by serotypes L1–L3 of *Chlamydia trachomatis*. It presents with painless, small ulcers and tender lymph nodes which discharge.

Primary syphilis may present as a hard, ulcerated, painless chancre; secondary syphilis is associated with a flu-like illness and 'snail track' ulcers in the oropharynx and on genitalia. Diagnosis is by dark ground microscopy for treponemes or serological testing. Of note, non-sexually transmitted disorders which result in genital ulceration include Behçets disease, leishmaniasis, and schistosomiasis.

Tutorial

Chancroid is caused by *H. ducreyi*, a Gram-negative coccobacillus. It is common in tropical and subtropical areas including Africa, South West Asia, the Caribbean, and South America. The incubation period is 4–10 days. Males present with single or multiple deep, necrotic ulcers and painful regional lymphadenitis. Lesions in females often occur at the entrance of the vagina. Diagnosis can be made by microscopy (62% sensitive) or culture (75% sensitive), although PCR is more sensitive (95%) and is being done by in-house assays in specialist research laboratories. Typical appearances on microscopy are of small Gram-negative coccobacilli forming chains or 'shoals of fish'. However, this test has low sensitivity and is not recommended for diagnosis. Treatment is either with single dose therapy with azithromycin or ciprofloxacin; WHO recommends a seven-day course of high-dose erythromycin as first-line therapy. Of note, chancroid is an important risk factor for bi-directional spread of HIV infection; ulcers may also take longer to heal in the setting of HIV-related immune suppression. As with all sexually transmitted infections, patients should be screened for other potentially transmittable diseases, and partners who have had sexual contact within ten days should be treated *for H. ducreyi* even if asymptomatic.

Further Reading

O'Farrell N, Lazaro N (2014). UK National Guideline for the management of chancroid 2014. BASHH National guidelines. Available at: https://www.bashh.org/guidelines.

119. C) HIV seroconversion illness

This case is a presentation of acute HIV seroconversion illness. By contrast, pityriasis rosea is an acute, self-limiting skin disease (unknown aetiology, potential viral trigger) which presents with a characteristic 'herald patch' lesion followed by an eruption of salmon-coloured oval lesions which distribute in a 'Christmas tree' pattern over the trunk and proximal limbs. Prodromal constitutional symptoms occur only in a minority of individuals and laboratory findings are usually normal. Acute hepatitis C virus infection is often asymptomatic; 25% of patients may develop jaundice. The rash described above would be uncommon, and liver function tests may show a transaminitis (commonly 6–12 weeks after exposure). If acute hepatitis C virus infection is suspected, patients should be tested for HCV RNA in the serum which is detectable by PCR within days after exposure. Rash is uncommon with EBV, although ampicillin/amoxicillin can induce a non-allergic rash in almost all patients with EBV mononucleosis. Tonsillar hypertrophy and exudate are common in EBV, whereas non-exudative pharyngitis predominates during acute HIV infection. Laboratory findings demonstrate a lymphocytosis rather than lymphopenia and elevated transaminases. Secondary syphilis can also present with a maculopapular rash and mucocutaneous ulcers. However, the patient usually develops red-brown macules over the palms and soles. Currently, sensitive fourth-line assays which test for both HIV antibodies and p24 antigen simultaneously can detect HIV infection at around four weeks (though in some cases it can even be detected as early as 15 days post-infection). Hence, newly acquired infection less than a month before testing does not mean HIV infection is excluded.

Tutorial

Epidemiology

Over 33 million individuals are living with HIV infection worldwide; 2.6 million people are newly infected every year. One third of HIV infection in UK adults remains undiagnosed. At diagnosis, 25% of individuals are 'late presenters' with a CD4 count already less than 200 cells/µL; these individuals suffer increased morbidity and may demonstrate an impaired response to HAART therapy. Diagnosis may initially be missed by healthcare professionals due to the non-specific syndrome associated with acute disease.

Pathology

Around 80% of HIV-1 is acquired through mucosal surfaces: genital tract or rectal mucosa. The HIV virion binds via a surface protein (gp120) to immune cells bearing the CD4 molecule; this includes CD4 T-cells, macrophages, and dendritic cells. HIV virions have different tropisms. Virions that preferentially enter macrophages also bind to the CCR5 co-receptor. Virions that bind to CXCR4 preferentially enter CD4 T cells. There is an initial eclipse phase of 7–21 days when the virus is replicating in the mucosa and sub-mucosa virions are undetectable in the plasma. The intestinal mucosa is also a target for initial viral replication. Depletion of CD4 T-cells results in a rapid increase in viraemia, which then precipitously drops after development of an acquired CD8 T cell immune response.

Testing

Serological testing is with fourth-generation assays which simultaneously test for HIV antibody and p24 antigen. This assay has the advantage of a reduced time between infection and testing positive to one month, but can be positive in a significant number of people even earlier if performed during symptomatic seroconversion. Point-of-care tests also exist and can give results from fingerpricks or mouth swabs in just a few minutes. They have a low specificity, however, which often results in false positives and thus all positive results must be confirmed by serological tests.

Treatment

Previously treatment was recommended to start only if a patient had any of the following: neurological involvement, an AIDS-defining illness, or a CD4 count <350 cells/µL. However, numerous trials have shown that starting medication early not only improves long-term recovery of CD4 counts, but by suppressing viral load helps prevent spread of the infection. As such, it is now recommended that patients are started on ART as soon as possible. Post-exposure prophylaxis (PEP) is also readily available at sexual clinics for members of the public who may have been exposed to the virus. PEP consists of triple ART therapy—usually emtricitabine, tenofovir, and raltegravir. It is most effective if taken within 72 hours of exposure and must be taken for a month in total. Recent studies have also shown that pre-exposure prophylaxis, that is, taking the medication before engaging in behaviour associated with infection, also helps reduce risk of transmission. However, whether these drugs will be funded on the NHS is at present unclear.

Treatment options often need to be tailored to the individual according to co-morbidities, side effects, drug interactions with other medications, the patient's compliance with medication, and viral resistances. However, the principal is to use triple therapy. This usually consists of two nucleotide reverse transcriptase inhibitors and a third agent of another class. A common regimen might be tenofovir and emtricitabine (usually as a combined tablet—Truvada) and then either a protease inhibitor (e.g. atazanavir), an integrase inhibitor (e.g. raltegravir), or a non-nucleoside reverse transcriptase inhibitor (e.g. efavirenz)). In addition, the clinician should discuss secondary prevention, including partner notification. HIV is now a treatable chronic condition; patients compliant with therapy can expect a normal life expectancy.

Further Reading

British Medical Journal (2016). Best Practice. HIV infection. Available at: http://bestpractice.bmj.com/best-practice/monograph/555.html

120. C) Immune reconstitution inflammatory syndrome (IRIS)

IRIS is a diagnosis of exclusion and most commonly occurs during advanced HIV infection when the CD4 count is less than 200 cells/uL. After initiation of HAART there is significant reduction in HIV viraemia, with recovery of CD4 T cell counts. However, the reconstituted immune system then reacts to infectious and non-infectious antigens that have been thus far ignored and mounts an inflammatory response. Patient non-compliance, adverse drug reactions and allergy, drug-resistant infection, and bacterial super-infection must be excluded prior to making the diagnosis. Mycobacterium tuberculosis is most often associated with IRIS in HIV-infected individuals. The risk of IRIS is greater when HAART is started within the first two months of TB therapy and in patients with CD4 counts <100 cells/uL as in this case.

In this scenario, poor compliance with anti-retroviral therapy would not result in a reduction in HIV viraemia and reconstitution of CD4 T cell count as observed. The clinical syndrome is not typical of a hypersensitivity reaction. Rifampicin, part of the initial therapy regimen during the first two months of TB treatment, is a CYP3A enzyme inducer and may result in increased metabolism and suboptimal levels of anti-viral drugs. However, this would not explain the worsening of clinical features and chest X-ray findings which are more consistent with paradoxical reaction to mycobacterial antigens. Multi-drug resistant TB (resistance to both isoniazid and rifampicin) is a rising global health threat; risk factors include previous TB treatment failure, HIV, male gender, and birth in a foreign country with a high incidence of MDR-TB (e.g. former Soviet Republics). The clinical history is similar to that of normal TB infection. The temporal association between initiation of HAART and clinical symptoms makes drug resistance less likely to cause the clinical scenario described.

Tutorial

IRIS is defined as a paradoxical deterioration of clinical status secondary to recovery of the immune system during HAART therapy. It is more common in patients with HIV infection, particularly those who have advanced disease with a low baseline CD4 count. The immune-pathogenesis of IRIS is only partially understood. It is thought that a rapid recovery of CD4 T cells is associated with a pathological host immune response to antigenic stimuli, resulting in tissue-destructive immunity and symptoms consistent with infection or an inflammatory condition. Often the immune response is targeted against opportunistic pathogens which have at one time infected the host and have remained latent; most commonly mycobacteria (tuberculosis and MAC), herpes zoster, CMV, varicella zoster, hepatitis B and C, and *Pneumocystis jirovecii* and *Cryptococcus neoformans*. Clinical manifestations are therefore diverse. *Mycobacterium tuberculosis* is most frequently associated with IRIS. Clinical presentation might include fever, worsening respiratory symptoms, or new or increased lymphadenopathy. Reactions occur at a median of 15 days, and most cases within two months of HAART. Inflammation of skin over nodes can be a feature, and nodes may spontaneously rupture. Chest radiography may reveal worsening parenchymal infiltrates or new pleural effusions. Paradoxical reactions can occur following HAART (or anti-TB therapy) in patients with known TB, or can also unmask previously undiagnosed TB. A rapid recovery of CD4 count is often seen on blood tests.

Diagnosis is one of exclusion. Differentials include drug hypersensitivity reactions and exacerbation of TB infection due to treatment failure. Moderate or high dose corticosteroids may be used for symptom control. However, the risk of developing serious infection such as CMV retinitis is increased with such treatment. Reactions are self-limiting and if not severe, should be managed with non-steroidal agents without a change in HAART therapy. Recurrent needle aspiration of abscesses or nodes if tense/inflamed can prevent spontaneous rupture and decrease the chance of scarring and sinus formation.

Further Reading

Barber D, Andrade B, Sereti I, Sher A (2012). Immune reconstitution inflammatory syndrome: the trouble with immunity when you had none. *Nature Reviews Microbiology* 10(2): 150–156.

121. A) Botulism

Given the history of neuromuscular weakness affecting both cranial nerves and peripheral nerves, along with a history of intravenous drug use with evidence of skin-popping, botulism is the most likely explanation here. The neurotoxin produced by *C. botulinum* impairs acetylcholine release at pre-synaptic nerve terminals affecting both the peripheral nervous system and autonomic nervous system. This causes widespread neuromuscular weakness and also autonomic dysfunction, though this often manifests later on.

Guillain-Barré syndrome (GBS), or acute inflammatory demyelinating polyradiculopathy (ADIP) as it is also known, is a post-infectious syndrome which classically presents with an ascending paralysis and can have a sensory component. Miller-Fisher syndrome is a rare variant of GBS that actually presents with a descending paralysis but is usually only limited to eye muscle weakness. Whilst there is often ataxia and areflexia, limb weakness is uncommon. Autonomic dysfunction would also be absent.

In LEMS, antibodies against pre-synaptic voltage-gated calcium channels impair pre-synaptic acetylcholine release also. The syndrome presents with proximal muscle weakness and autonomic symptoms including dry mouth, impotence, and postural hypotension. It is more insidious in its presentation than botulism and is strongly associated with small-cell lung cancer.

Myasthenia gravis remains an important differential diagnosis in this case. Whilst there is evidence of autonomic symptoms in this case—low BP, one could argue that the patient may also have an infection (as suggested by the raised CRP) and may also be dehydrated—having been found on the floor. Various investigations can distinguish botulism from GBS and MG, including antibody tests (C. botulinum antibodies vs AchR antibodies in MG), CSF protein (mildly raised in botulism, increased in GBS), and perhaps most discriminatory—neurophysiological studies.

A cerebrovascular accident would commonly cause unilateral weakness and upper motor neuron findings, rather than a flaccid paralysis.

Tutorial

Clostridium botulinum bacteria produce a neurotoxin which can result in a potentially life-threatening syndrome characterized by an afebrile, descending flaccid paralysis. The toxin binds to a receptor synaptotagmin II, which impairs acetylcholine release from the pre-synaptic nerve terminal at ganglia and neuro-muscular junctions. The toxin does not cross the blood brain barrier, hence causes diseases in the peripheral cholinergic nervous system. There are three main forms: food-borne, wound botulism, and intestinal colonization botulism, which occurs mainly in infants.

Patients may present with blurred or double vision (fixed pupillary dilatation, III, IV, VI cranial nerve palsies), slurred speech, facial weakness, and difficulty swallowing. Untreated, paralysis can progress to arms, legs, trunk, and respiratory muscles. Due to interruption of acetylcholine release, patients may also suffer autonomic dysfunction, manifest as dry mouth, dilated pupils, urinary retention, and constipation. Recovery can take up to six months as return of synaptic function requires generation of a new pre-synaptic terminal.

Diagnosis is by detection of botulinum toxin in serum, or isolation of *C. botulinum* from wound swabs or pus, biopsy tissue after surgical debridement or from post-mortem specimens. Botulinum anti-toxin is effective at reducing disease severity if given early. This should not be delayed for laboratory testing if the clinical suspicion is high. Antibiotics to treat this Gram-positive, spore-forming obligate anaerobe include benzylpenicillin and metronidazole.

Wound botulism is more common in injecting drug users with heroin contaminated with spores of *C. botulinum* (especially if injecting into muscle or under the skin where anaerobic conditions are favourable). These heat resistant spores germinate with subsequent production of neurotoxin.

Further Reading

Cherington M (2004). Botulism: update and review. *Seminars in Neurology* 24(2): 155–163.

122. B) Poncet's disease

Poncet's disease is an aseptic, reactive arthritis seen in patients with active TB. Lofgren's syndrome is an acute form of sarcoidosis characterized by a triad of erythema nodosum, hilar lymphadenopathy, and arthritis; it is less likely in this case in view of the normal chest X-ray findings. Rheumatoid arthritis is a symmetrical inflammatory polyarthritis; false positive anti-CCP results can occur during tuberculosis infection. Still's disease is a diagnosis of exclusion and is usually seen in children. Adult-onset Still's disease is characterized by ongoing fevers and may present with a transient salmon-coloured, flitting rash. Diagnosis is by clinical clues on laboratory testing including a leukocytosis and a very high serum ferritin. Anti-nuclear antibody and rheumatoid factor are negative. Syphilis has a wide spectrum of clinical presentations, including infective arthritis.

Tutorial

Musculoskeletal TB accounts for 5–10% of extrapulmonary TB cases. The majority of cases are due to tuberculous spondylitis (Pott's disease) affecting lower cervical and upper thoracic vertebrae. Other syndromes include tuberculous monoarthritis of joints or more rarely as in this case, a reactive sterile arthritis with no objective evidence of active TB infection (Poncet's disease). Unlike the monoarthritis, this results in an acute, symmetrical polyarthritis of large and small joints; there is often a good response to anti-TB treatment with no residual joint destruction. Interestingly, patients who receive intravesical BCG for bladder cancer can also develop Poncet's syndrome after therapy, usually after 2–3 weeks. Symptoms usually abate with steroids, but stronger immunosuppression is sometimes needed.

In terms of erythema nodosum, around 30–50% of cases are idiopathic. Of the remainder, the causes include:

- Infection: TB, streptococcal pharyngitis, enterovirus, EBV, mycoplasma pneumonia
- Systemic disease: sarcoidosis, inflammatory bowel disease, Behçet's disease
- Drugs: sulphonamides, penicillin, oral contraceptive pill

Further Reading

Dall L, Long L, Stanford J (1989). Poncet's disease: tuberculous rheumatism. *Reviews of Infectious Diseases* 11(10): 105–107.

123. D) Chloroquine followed by primaquine

This is the correct answer as it is the only option that will ensure eradication of both the erythrocyte and hypnozoite forms of *P. vivax*.

Chloroquine remains a recommended first-line treatment for the erythrocytic forms of all non-falciparum malaria species (*P. vivax*, *P. ovale*, *P. malariae*). It is no longer recommended for the treatment of *P. falciparum* due to widespread resistance. Chloroquine-resistant *P. vivax* is uncommon but its prevalence is increasing particularly in Papua New Guinea and Indonesia. Primaquine should follow chloroquine therapy in *P. vivax* and *P. ovale* to eradicate the hypnozoite (liver) stage and prevent relapse. *P. falciparum* and *P. malariae* have no hypnozoite stage. G6PD activity must be measured prior to starting primaquine due to the risk of precipitating haemolysis and methaemoglobinaemia in individuals with deficiency in this enzyme. Primaquine is contraindicated in pregnancy and its use should be delayed until after delivery.

The remaining agents (A–C, E) are all recommended therapies for *P. falciparum*. Artemether-lumefantrine (preferred option), atovaquone-proguanil, and quinine with doxycycline, are all recommended in non-severe, uncomplicated *P. falciparum* infections. Artemether-lumefantrine is also recommended for the treatment of the acute stage of non-falciparum malaria, and should be considered particularly when chloroquine resistance is suspected. It lacks activity against hypnozoites so requires follow-on therapy with primaquine. In clinical trials, intravenous artesunate has been shown to improve survival and rates of parasite clearance in severe *P. falciparum* infection compared to intravenous quinine (SEAQUAMAT study, Dondorp et al., 2005). It is the drug of choice for all cases of severe *P. falciparum* but remains unlicensed in the UK and many hospitals may not keep a supply. Intravenous quinine administration should not be delayed whilst waiting for artesunate in cases of severe falciparum malaria.

Tutorial

Malaria is a disease caused by parasitic protozoans of the *Plasmodium* type. It is transmitted by the bite of infected female Anopheles mosquitos and is one of the most important travel-related infections with 1300–1800 cases diagnosed in the UK annually. An estimated 75–80% of cases are caused by *P. falciparum* most of which are acquired in sub-Saharan Africa, and 10–15% by *P. vivax* acquired mainly in South Asia. Most cases occur in individuals of African or Asian descent who visit friends and family in their country of origin and have not taken malaria prophylaxis. Less than ten fatalities due to malaria were recorded in the UK last year, almost exclusively in *P. falciparum*, although deaths due to *P. vivax* have been reported. All travellers returning from the tropics with a fever, or a history of fever should have an urgent blood film for malaria. Patients with falciparum malaria generally present within a month of returning from the tropics but 10% of cases present up to three months after travel. Patients with vivax or ovale malaria can present many months later, sometimes years.

Patients with falciparum malaria can deteriorate rapidly, even with the correct treatment and generally all patients with falciparum malaria should be admitted. It is important that you are aware of how to identify severe infection. Features of complicated or severe infection include, but are not limited to, parasitaemia of >10%, cerebral involvement, anaemia, acidosis, renal impairment, pulmonary oedema, hypoglycaemia, shock, spontaneous bleeding, and haemoglobinuria. Parasitaemia >2%, or <2% with schizonts on the blood film indicate an increased risk of developing severe infection. Generally speaking, patients with non-falciparum malaria can be managed as outpatients unless features of severity are present or they are unable to tolerate oral treatment.

The gold standard for diagnosis remains thick and thin blood films read by an experienced microscopist; typically three negative films over three days are required to exclude the diagnosis. Increasingly, rapid diagnostic antigen tests are being used as an adjunct to blood films. However, they do not provide an indication of burden of infection/parasitaemia. PCR is the most sensitive test but it is not used routinely in clinical practice.

A number of interventions can reduce the risk of acquiring malaria when travelling to endemic areas, including chemoprophylaxis, use of mosquito-repellent spray, sleeping under mosquito nets, and wearing long sleeves and trousers after dusk.

Further Reading

Dondorp A, Nosten F, Stepniewska K, Day N, White N, and South East Asian Quinine Artesunate Malaria Trial (SEAQUAMAT) group (2005). Artesunate versus quinine for treatment of severe falciparum malaria: a randomised trial. *Lancet* 366: 717–725. Available at: https://pubmed.ncbi.nlm.nih.gov/16125588/

Lalloo D, Shingadia D, Bell D, Beeching N, Whitty C, Chiodini P, and PHE Advisory Committee on Malaria Prevention in UK Travellers (2016). UK malaria treatment guidelines 2016. *Journal of Infection* 72(6): 635–649.

124. D) Pyrimethamine and sulfadiazine

Pyrimethamine and sulfadiazine are the drugs of choice for toxoplasmosis. The history, which is consistent with a space-occupying lesion and the radiological appearances of ring-enhancing lesion with surrounding oedema and mass effect, in the context of advanced HIV, point to the likely diagnosis of cerebral toxoplasmosis. Pyrimethamine and sulfadiazine should be administered with folinic acid to prevent bone marrow suppression caused by the antifolate effect of pyrimethamine.

Amphotericin B and flucytosine would cover fungal infections such as *Cryptococcus neoformans*, a common cause of meningitis in advanced HIV. Cryptococcal meningitis usually presents with fever and headache and can be complicated by hydrocephalus and raised intracranial pressure resulting in confusion and reduced GCS. It is rare for cryptococcal meningitis to produce space-occupying lesions in the brain (cryptococcomas), and when seen these are smaller than those we see on this imaging. Ceftriaxone and metronidazole would be the treatment of choice for bacterial brain abscesses. These would present similarly to this case both clinically and radiologically. However, in the context of advanced HIV, toxoplasmosis is a more likely diagnosis. Primaquine and clindamycin are second-line agents for the treatment of *Pneumocystis jirovecii* infection. This does not usually cause intracranial involvement. Rifampicin, isoniazid, pyrazinamide, and ethambutol are first-line agents for the treatment of tuberculosis. Tuberculosis of the central nervous system could present in a similar fashion but is a less likely diagnosis in this epidemiological context.

Tutorial

Cerebral toxoplasmosis is the most common cause of a space-occupying lesion in patients with advanced HIV. Following the introduction of antiretroviral therapy (ART) the incidence of this condition has greatly decreased. *Toxoplasma gondii* is a protozoan parasite with a complex life cycle. Cats are the definite hosts, with humans and other mammals being intermediate hosts. Humans are infected through ingesting food or water contaminated by oocysts from cat faeces, or through eating undercooked meat containing cysts. Toxoplasmosis is also an important cause of severe congenital infections. Primary infection in immunocompetent patients is usually asymptomatic or can resemble a self-limiting infectious mononucleosis-like illness. Latent cysts can reactivate in immunosuppressed individuals, classically causing cerebral abscesses in patients with HIV and a CD4 count <200 cells/μl. The clinical presentation is subacute, with focal neurology, seizures, or signs of raised intracranial pressure. It can also cause chorioretinitis and pneumonia.

The diagnosis is based on the demonstration of usually multiple ring-enhancing lesions on CT or MRI brain. If lumbar puncture is not contraindicated, *Toxoplasma* PCR on CSF can be helpful in confirming the diagnosis, but the sensitivity is only 50%. *Toxoplasma* serology is less helpful in the acute setting, as a positive IgG merely confirms previous acquisition of infection. IgG titres can rise as a result of reactivation. First-line treatment is with pyrimethamine and sulfadiazine (folinic acid is also given to prevent bone marrow suppression caused by pyrimethamine). The main differential is primary central nervous system lymphoma (PCNSL). In practice, patients are started on toxoplasmosis treatment as 90% with the correct diagnosis should improve within two weeks. Single-photon emission CT (SPECT), positron emission tomography (PET), and lumbar puncture can assist in differentiating PCNSL from an abscess. In the absence of improvement, histological/ microbiological diagnosis should be sought.

Prophylaxis against cerebral toxoplasmosis is recommended in all HIV patients with CD4 count <200 cells/μl and a positive *Toxoplasma* serology, in the form of co-trimoxazole (which is also indicated for *Pneumocystis* prophylaxis).

For a comprehensive discussion of CNS manifestations of HIV, please see the tutorial to question 148.

Further Reading

British HIV Association (2011). Treatment of opportunistic infection in HIV-seropositive individuals 2011. *HIV Medicine* 12(2): 1–140. Available at: http://www.bhiva.org/OI-guidelines

125. C) JC virus PCR

This is a classic presentation of progressive multifocal leukoencephalopathy (PML) demonstrating gradual onset of worsening neurological deficits (usually motor, speech, and visual deficits), in the absence of fever or headache. As well as through confirmation of the presence of JC viral DNA in the CSF, radiological appearances are also characteristic, with subcortical white matter changes best visualized on MRI.

Toxoplasmosis is the commonest cause of space-occupying lesion in AIDS but patients typically present more acutely with fever, reduced conscious level, and focal neurological deficits including seizures. MRI classically shows ring-enhancing lesions with associated mass effect. HSV encephalitis usually has an acute onset and is characterized by fever, headache, confusion, and behavioural change. The CSF is lymphocytic with a raised protein. Radiological changes in HSV encephalitis are most commonly seen in the temporal lobes. Central nervous system tuberculosis would fit with an insidious onset and should always be considered in a patient from sub-Saharan Africa. Patients often have fever and reduced conscious level, especially in the context of TB meningitis (TBM). The CSF would classically have an elevated lymphocyte count with a markedly raised protein and a low glucose (<50% of serum value). An MRI may show meningeal enhancement and/or tuberculomas.

Cryptococcal meningitis is the commonest CNS AIDS defining illness. Patients have fever and nuchal rigidity but parenchymal brain changes are not common.

Of note, in advanced HIV multiple opportunistic infections can co-exist and may appear occasionally atypically; all of the above tests would be useful in practice.

Tutorial

PML is caused by a polyomavirus named JC after the initials of the first patient in whom it was identified. It is an opportunistic infection in the context of advanced HIV infection, haematological malignancy, or organ transplantation. Rare cases have also been reported as a complication of natalizumab treatment (antibody against alpha-4 integrins) in multiple sclerosis.

Initial infection is thought to occur asymptomatically via the respiratory route at a young age, with up to 70% seropositivity in adults. JC virus establishes latency in the kidneys and in B lymphocytes. In advanced immunosuppression (in HIV, CD4 counts tend to be less than 200), infection can spread to oligodendrocytes in the brain leading to irreversible demyelination of white matter. The presentation is insidious, with focal neurological deficits, which can include cortical blindness and occasionally seizures.

The gold standard for diagnosis has been brain biopsy, but nowadays, characteristic MRI appearances coupled with a positive JC virus PCR on CSF are considered diagnostic. MRI changes consist of asymmetrical, bilateral white matter changes, which are hyperintense on T2-weighted and hypointense on T1-weighted images, in the absence of mass effect or enhancement. The sensitivity of JC virus PCR on CSF is approximately 70–90% in the absence of ART.

Prognosis is poor, especially in patients with brainstem involvement, those with high CSF JC viral load, or CD4 count <100 cells/μl. The mainstay of treatment is introduction of ART, with a one-year survival rate up to 50% compared to 10% in the absence of treatment. Cidofovir and cytarabine have been trialled but have shown no benefit when used with ART.

Further Reading

Tan C, Koralnik I (2010). Progressive multifocal leukoencephalopathy and other disorders caused by JC virus: clinical features and pathogenesis. *Lancet Neurology* 9(4): 425–437.

126. E) Sputum PCR for TB and *rpoB* gene mutations

The diagnosis of tuberculosis is strongly suggested by the characteristic presentation, chest X-ray changes, and the presence of acid-fast bacilli in sputum. This patient has recognized risk factors for multi-drug resistant (MDR) tuberculosis as listed by the National Institute for Health and Clinical Excellence (NICE) guidance for TB (2016): birth in a foreign country with high-incidence for MDR TB (>5% of new diagnoses) and possible contact with known cases of drug-resistant TB given his previous incarceration in prison in Estonia. A further risk factor (not known to apply to this patient) is a history of previous TB treatment (suspected failure, in particular in the context of poor adherence to therapy).

As culture results and phenotypic susceptibility testing take several weeks, rapid diagnostic tests such as PCR can influence treatment in a timely fashion. PCR probes can confirm presence of *Mycobacterium tuberculosis* DNA and additionally can detect the common mutations in the *rpoB* (RNA polymerase B subunit) gene that confers resistance to rifampicin.

Bronchoscopy is not indicated for diagnostic purposes as sputum is already positive for AFB and it may actually put the operators at risk of exposure to drug-resistant TB. A CT chest may give useful information about the extent of disease but will not influence therapeutic options at this stage. An IGRA is useful in screening for latent TB but its role in diagnosing active TB is less clear; it is not indicated here given the positive microbiology. Similarly, early morning urine specimens for AFB can detect systemic/miliary dissemination but are less useful in this context.

Tutorial

Early ascertainment of the risk for drug-resistant TB is not only important for establishing the patient on appropriate therapy, but also for infection control and public health reasons. Drug-resistance is most commonly to isoniazid with a rate of ~7% in the UK. MDR TB is defined as resistance to both isoniazid and rifampicin, the two most potent bactericidal agents that form the backbone of TB therapy, and accounts for slightly over 1% of all TB cases in the UK. Much higher rates of MDR TB are found in the former Soviet Republics, including the Baltic states. Rapid molecular amplification tests directly from clinical specimens can detect the commonest *rpoB* gene mutations which confer rifampicin resistance. This is important because 80% of these strains will also prove to be resistant to isoniazid and therefore be MDR. Molecular tests for *rpoB* gene mutations are now recommended by the NICE guidelines for all patients with smear positive samples or positive cultures and suspected MDR TB.

The treatment of MDR TB is challenging, as available agents are less effective and more toxic compared to first-line drugs, resulting in lower success rates. Treatment duration is longer and more costly. Patients with suspected or confirmed infectious MDR TB should be nursed in a negative-pressure side-room. Public Health and the local TB services should be involved for screening close contacts and for determining when the patient is safe for discharge from a public health perspective.

Further Reading

Nathanson E, Nunn P, Uplekar M, et al. (2010). MDR tuberculosis—critical steps for prevention and control. *New England Journal of Medicine* 363(11): 1050–1058.

National Institute for Clinical Excellence (2019). Tuberculosis [NG23]. January 2016, updated September 2019. Available at: https://www.nice.org.uk/guidance/ng33

127. A) *Bartonella henselae*

The presentation is characteristic for CSD caused by *Bartonella henselae*. This is a common cause of lymphadenopathy in children and young adolescents. The papule likely represents the initial inoculation injury, followed by the lymphadenopathy, fever, and rash.

Bordetella pertussis causes whooping cough, which is still a significant cause of childhood morbidity and mortality in the developing world. Immunization in childhood should confer protective immunity, although this wanes with age and outbreaks in adolescents and adults are well described.

Borrelia burgdorferi is the causative agent of Lyme disease, a tick-borne infection that manifests typically with rash known as erythema migrans and can be complicated by arthritis, neurological or cardiac conduction defects.

Brucellosis is a zoonotic infection caused by consumption of unpasteurized dairy products or direct contact with animal tissues and fluids, hence it is often associated with occupational exposure. It is particularly prevalent in the Mediterranean basin and the Middle East, the Indian subcontinent, Africa, and Central and South America but has been eradicated in the UK. Brucellosis has a broad clinical spectrum including acute febrile illness with or without localizing signs of infection, the most common being osteoarticular involvement. Lymphadenopathy is present in 10–20% of cases.

Coxiella burnetii, the cause of Q fever, is a zoonotic infection that is prevalent worldwide with only a few exceptions. It is associated with occupational exposure (e.g. in veterinarians and farm workers) to farm animal products, birth products posing the greatest risk. It can cause a self-limiting febrile illness, or organ-specific syndromes including pneumonia, endocarditis, hepatitis, and meningoencephalitis.

Tutorial

CSD is a zoonotic infection caused by *Bartonella henselae*. It is thought to be transmitted to humans by cat bites and scratches or by flea bites. Transmission between cats is by fleas, causing an asymptomatic bacteraemia which can last for up to a year. It usually affects immunocompetent children and young adults and infrequently causes severe illness, although patients with disseminated disease (liver, spleen, eye, central nervous system) can have life-threatening complications.

Around 85–90% of patients with CSD present with a self-limiting localized cutaneous and lymph node disorder up to seven weeks after the inoculation injury. The inoculation site is a small papule which develops 3–10 days after initial scratch or bite, often going unnoticed. Fever and generalized malaise are present in about half of the cases, and a transient rash may be present in some. Other rare forms of the disease include Parinaud's oculoglandular syndrome (consisting of granulomatous conjunctivitis and ipsilateral preauricular lymphadenopathy), hepatosplenomegaly, retinitis, endocarditis, or encephalitis. In immunocompromised patients the infection can lead to a severe life-threatening condition called bacillary angiomatosis.

The diagnosis should be suspected based on the history, clinical findings, and absence of an alternative diagnosis (including other infections and haematological malignancy). It can be supported by laboratory tests including serology. However, some experts suggest that serology is limited by poor specificity, significant cross-reactivity, and the fact that rates of seroprevalence in the community can lead to false positives and this test is no longer provided by Public Health England. There is limited use for blood and tissue culture as the organism is fastidious and slow growing. Warthin-Starry staining of tissue from lymph nodes and the primary inoculation site may demonstrate *B. henselae* bacilli, although is not definitive. PCR can be used but sensitivity has been reported in the range of 43–76%.

Antibiotics, including rifampicin, azithromycin, and doxycycline, are recommended in disseminated disease and, whilst appropriate antibiotics (usually macrolides) can reduce the period of lymphadenopathy, some experts do not recommend treatment in mild cases.

Further Reading

Margileth A (2000). Recent advances in diagnosis and treatment of cat scratch disease. *Current Infectious Disease Reports* 2(2): 141–146.

Rolain J, Brouqui P, Koehler J, Maguina C, Dolan M, Raoult D (2004). Recommendations for treatment of human infections caused by Bartonella species. *Antimicrobial Agents Chemotherapy* 48(6): 1921–1933.

128. D) *Coxiella burnetii*

This is a case of blood culture-negative endocarditis (BCNE) in a patient with a congenital heart anomaly (which is not considered high risk for endocarditis). Whilst all the suggested organisms are potential causes of BCNE, the epidemiological exposure to potentially contaminated meat puts this patient at risk of occupational acquisition of *Coxiella burnetii*, the aetiologic agent of Q fever, which is a zoonotic infection that is prevalent worldwide including the UK (especially in the south west and Wales). It is associated with occupational exposure (e.g. in veterinarians and farm workers) to farm animal products, birth products posing the greatest risk. It can cause a self-limiting febrile illness, or organ-specific syndromes including pneumonia, endocarditis, hepatitis, and meningoencephalitis.

Bartonella quintana causes trench fever. It is a re-emerging infection with cases in the UK associated with patients of Eastern European origin and poor socioeconomic status including homelessness and alcoholism. It is transmitted by louse vectors.

Brucella melitensis is the cause of brucellosis, a common zoonotic disease worldwide which can also cause endocarditis. It is transmitted by ingestion of unpasteurized dairy products or direct contact with animal tissues and fluids and is an occupational hazard. However, it has been eradicated in the UK and most cases diagnosed in the UK would have acquired the infection in a Mediterranean or Middle Eastern country. *Chlamydia sp.* including *C. pneumoniae* and *C. psittaci* were previously thought to be a significant yet rare cause of BCNE, but recent large series have failed to identify any cases. *C. psittaci* is associated with bird contact.

Tropheryma whipplei causes Whipple's disease, a rare multisystem chronic infection affecting middle-aged men and characterized by arthralgia, weight loss, and gastrointestinal symptoms. It can, however, also present as isolated endocarditis.

Tutorial

The incidence of BCNE varies according to studies and is influenced by local epidemiological factors, host susceptibility, and prior use of antibiotics that can suppress growth of the common causative pathogens such as streptococci. In a recent large multicentre survey of 2781 adults with endocarditis, 10% were culture-negative. In the largest case series of BCNE performed in France, 759 patients underwent an extensive panel of serological and molecular amplification testing in blood to determine the aetiology. They also performed 16S rDNA PCR and sequencing (a broad-range PCR to specifically detect ribosomal bacterial DNA) on explanted heart valves. An infective cause was identified in 62.7% of cases, and a non-infectious cause in 2.5%. The commonest pathogens were *Coxiella burnetii* (agent of Q fever) in 37% and *Bartonella spp.* in 12.4%, with *Tropheryma whipplei* accounting for 2.6% of cases. Fungi should also be considered, especially in immunocompromised patients or those with prosthetic devices. Non-infective causes, including lupus and marantic endocarditis (associated with underlying malignancy), were important differentials. The authors suggested testing all patients with BCNE using Coxiella and Bartonella serology or PCR and ANA in the first instance (of note, Bartonella serology is no longer offered in the UK). Second- and third-line testing would include Whipple's PCR, panfungal PCR, and Brucella, Mycoplasma and Legionella serology. Most of these recommendations have been endorsed by the British Society for Antimicrobial Chemotherapy and the European Society of Cardiology endocarditis guidelines.

Of note, HACEK organisms (*Haemophilus spp.*, *Aggregatibacter actinomycetemcomitans* (formerly *Actinobacillus*), *Cardiobacterium hominis*, *Eikenella spp.* and *Kingella spp.*) should grow with the use of modern blood culture systems and are not considered causes of BCNE in the absence of prior suppressive antibiotic use.

Further Reading

Fournier P, Thuny F, Richet H, et al. (2010). Comprehensive diagnostic strategy for blood culture-negative endocarditis: a prospective study of 819 new cases. *Clinical Infectious Diseases* 51(2): 131–140.

Murdoch D, Corey G, Hoen B, et al. (2009). Clinical presentation, etiology, and outcome of infective endocarditis in the 21st century: The International Collaboration on Endocarditis—prospective cohort study. *Archives in Internal Medicine* 169(5): 463–473.

129. C) Strongyloidiasis

This dramatic presentation is typical for *Strongyloides stercoralis* hyperinfection (or hyperinfestation) syndrome. *S. stercoralis* is endemic in the tropics and subtropics and can establish a chronic intestinal infection, which is often asymptomatic but usually accompanied by eosinophilia. The infection can persist for decades through cycles of autoinfection but has the potential to flare up in the context of immunosuppression, in particular corticosteroids which suppress blood and tissue eosinophilia, and cause life-threatening, disseminated infection. In hyperinfection, the eosinophilia typically disappears as the immune system fails to control the parasite.

Giardiasis is a parasitic gastrointestinal infection often encountered in returning travellers, causing chronic diarrhoea and malabsorption. It is diagnosed by stool microscopy or duodenal biopsy. It does not cause invasive disease and is not associated with eosinophilia. Schistosomiasis, also known as bilharzia, is acquired by contact with freshwater containing the infectious cercariae. It can lead to chronic infection causing hepatosplenomegaly or urinary tract disease depending on the infective species, and is associated with bladder cancer.

Toxoplasmosis usually establishes asymptomatic infection with chronic carriage. Reactivation can occur in immunosuppressed individuals causing retinitis or encephalitis. It is not associated with eosinophilia.

Tropical pulmonary eosinophilia is a rare hypersensitivity reaction to the lymphatic filariae *Wuchereria bancrofti* or *Brugia malayi*, leading to fever, dry cough, pulmonary infiltrates, and marked eosinophilia.

Tutorial

Strongyloides stercoralis is a nematode endemic in tropical and subtropical areas and certain warm temperate regions. It is commonly acquired through bare feet, for example from walking on soil or haematogenously to the lungs, ascending the bronchial tree until it is swallowed and reaching the small intestine where they mature to the adult form which produces eggs. Unlike other parasites, the eggs hatch in the intestine forming non-infectious rhabditiform larvae which are then excreted in the stool. Once outside the body they can complete a sexual life cycle and infect new hosts. Alternatively, and unlike other helminthic parasites, *S. stercoralis* can complete its life cycle in the human host through autoinfection: the rhabditiform larvae mature to the infective filariform larval stage in the gastrointestinal tract and reinfect the original host by penetrating the intestinal mucosa or perianal skin. This can lead to persistence of the infection for decades.

The infection is commonly asymptomatic and may be accompanied by eosinophilia. The most common symptoms include gastrointestinal disturbance, dry cough or irritation, and a pruritic erythematous rash that migrates (larva currens). The rare, life-threatening hyperinfection syndrome occurs in patients immunosuppressed with steroids or chemotherapy, and in those coinfected with human T-lymphotropic virus type 1 (HTLV-1). The clinical manifestations include paralytic ileus, Gram-negative bacterial sepsis from intestinal translocation (which can also present as meningitis), and ARDS. Eosinophilia is usually absent in this context.

The diagnosis is established by stool microscopy for detection of the larvae or by serology. Patients with hyperinfection should be screened for HTLV-1 infection.

The treatment of choice is ivermectin. It is important to screen all migrants from endemic countries using *Strongyloides* serology and treating those infected prior to commencing any immunosuppressive therapy in order to prevent development of the hyperinfection syndrome.

Further Reading

Checkley A, Chiodini P, Dockrell D, et al. (2010). British Infection Society and Hospital for Tropical Diseases. Eosinophilia in returning travellers and migrants from the tropics: UK recommendations for investigation and initial management. *Journal of Infection* 60(1): 1–20. Available at: http://www.cdc.gov/parasites/strongyloides/

130. E) Stop vancomycin and commence fidaxomicin

This question tests the candidate's knowledge of the management of *Clostridium difficile* infection (CDI). The management of CDI includes immediate enteric isolation, discontinuation of non-CDI antibiotics if clinically appropriate, and commencement of oral metronidazole for non-severe CDI, or oral vancomycin for those with signs and symptoms of severe CDI. The features of severe CDI are any of: white cell count >15, acutely rising creatinine (i.e. >50% increase over baseline), temperature >38.5, or evidence of colitis (abdominal signs or radiologically). In this case, the white cell count of 15.3 meant that vancomycin was started as first line, rather than metronidazole.

The patient developed no new features suggestive of an acute colitis, and thus abdominal imaging (X-ray or CT) was not routinely indicated, but should be performed if there are any localizing abdominal signs or concern about megacolon. Stopping the piperacillin-tazobactam, or narrowing the antibiotic spectrum, would be preferable. However, the typical duration of treatment for a Gram-negative bacteraemia, such as urinary tract sepsis in a male, is 10–14 days, and an alternative antibiotic is not offered, hence stopping the piperacillin-tazobactam is not appropriate at day 7. Converting the oral vancomycin to intravenous does not add to efficacy in CDI. For patients unable to take tablets, the intravenous vials can be administered through nasogastric tubes. According to Public Health England guidance, fidaxomicin may be considered for severe CDI cases not responding to oral vancomycin, following consultation with microbiologists. Therefore, in this instance the most appropriate next step is to switch to fidaxomicin.

Tutorial

Clostridium difficile is a Gram-positive, anaerobic, spore-forming bacillus that is responsible for the development of antibiotic-associated diarrhoea and colitis. Approximately 20% of individuals who are hospitalized become colonized with *C. difficile*, and more than 30% of these patients develop diarrhoea. Thus, *C. difficile* colitis is currently one of the most common hospital-acquired infections. Once infected with *C. difficile*, the rate of disease recurrence is 20–40%, especially when first-line agents such as metronidazole and vancomycin are not successful.

Testing for *C. difficile* toxin should only be performed on diarrhoeal stool, unless there is suspicion of ileus due to CDI. Testing in asymptomatic individuals is not recommended due to the difficulty in distinguishing asymptomatic carriage from infection. For similar reasons, repeat testing for 'cure' of CDI is also not recommended. Stool cultures are the most sensitive tests for detecting *C. difficile*, but due to the longer turnaround time, immunoassays for *C. difficile* toxins A and B are typically used (sensitivity 80%). The immunoassay for *C. difficile* glutamate dehydrogenase (GDH) is sometimes used as a screening test, as the sensitivity is higher (85–100%), although the specificity is slightly lower than the toxin assays, thus treatment is not usually commenced unless the patient is toxin positive.

Until recently there were only two main alternatives (metronidazole or vancomycin) for the treatment of CDI. However, two recent, multicentre randomized, double-blind trials compared oral fidaxomicin (200 mg bd for 10–14 days) with oral vancomycin (125 mg qds for 10–14 days), both demonstrating non-inferiority of fidaxomicin in the initial clinical cure of CDI, and superiority in reducing recurrence. Other potential options include the addition of oral rifampicin (rifaximin), intravenous immunoglobulin, or faecal transplantation.

Further Reading

Public Health England (2013). Updated guidance on the management and treatment of *Clostridium difficile* infection. Available at: http://www.gov.uk/phe

131. D) Tuberculous meningitis

There are many features in this presentation that point to the diagnosis of tuberculosis (TB). There is a subacute presentation with a respiratory illness that failed to respond to conventional antibiotic therapy. There is basal meningitis leading to hydrocephalus (none of the other choices would usually be associated with hydrocephalus). The CSF is lymphocytic with a very high protein and low glucose, very suggestive of TB. The AFB stain is negative but sensitivity of this test is poor compared to cultures and a negative stain does not exclude the diagnosis.

Streptococcus pneumoniae would fit with a respiratory illness associated with meningitis. However, the CSF in *S. pneumoniae* would show predominantly polymorphs and the presentation would be more acute. HSV encephalitis also presents acutely. The CSF is predominantly lymphocytic but the glucose ratio compared to serum is >40%. Japanese encephalitis and West Nile virus are not endemic in the UK. A travel history to the USA is relevant (West Nile virus) as is the Korean origin (Japanese encephalitis virus). However, the incubation period is up to two weeks in immunocompetent individuals. The patient's presentation is also highly suggestive of meningeal involvement (nuchal rigidity with hydrocephalus due to obstruction of the arachnoid villi resulting from the meningeal inflammation), which goes against the latter two choices.

Tutorial

TBM complicates approximately 1% of active TB infections. Following establishment of primary lung infection or during late reactivation, TB can disseminate haematogenously and form subpial and subependymal foci. TBM results from rupture of these foci into the subarachnoid space. In the UK, it is mostly seen in young adults, mainly immigrants from high prevalence countries. The risk of TBM is increased in patients with HIV.

The presentation of TBM is insidious and characterized by headache, fever, vomiting, and weight loss, which progress to neck stiffness, focal neurological deficits, lethargy, and coma. It is an important cause of basal meningitis, which can be complicated by cranial nerve palsies and hydrocephalus. CSF examination is crucial for establishing the diagnosis: it is characterized by lymphocytosis, elevated protein, and <0.5 CSF/serum glucose ratio. In some series, smear for acid fast bacilli has been reported positive in up to 80% of cases, but high yields are dependent on examination of high volumes of CSF and multiple samples. TB PCR can give a rapid result but sensitivity is in the range of 50%, hence a negative result does not exclude the diagnosis. Culture remains the gold standard for diagnosis but can take weeks for a positive result. Miliary dissemination is present in up to a third of cases so imaging to detect other foci and fundoscopy can aid in the diagnosis. CT or MRI of the brain can reveal basal meningeal enhancement, hydrocephalus, vasculitic infarcts, and tuberculomas.

The duration of treatment for TBM is twice that for pulmonary TB. For susceptible organisms, it consists of standard quadruple therapy for the first two months (rifampicin, isoniazid, pyrazinamide, and ethambutol), followed by ten months of rifampicin and isoniazid. Adjunctive dexamethasone has been shown to improve short-term mortality, but this effect wanes with time.

Further Reading

National Institute for Clinical Excellence (2019). Tuberculosis [NG23]. January 2016, updated September 2019. Available at: https://www.nice.org.uk/guidance/ng33

Thwaites G, Fisher M, Hemingway C, Scott G, Solomon T, Innes J (2009). British Infection Society guidelines for the diagnosis and treatment of tuberculosis of the central nervous system in adults and children. *Journal of Infection* 59(3): 167–187.

INDEX

Notes: Page numbers in *q* refer to Question and *a* refer to Answer.